IMMUNOLOGY OF OCULAR TUMORS

Immunology

of

Ocular Tumors

——

MANFRED ZIERHUT
Department of Ophthalmology, University of Tübingen, Germany

MARTINE J. JAGER
Department of Ophthalmology, Leiden University Medical Center, Leiden,
The Netherlands

BRUCE R. KSANDER
Schepens Eye Research Institute, Harvard Medical School, Boston, USA

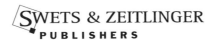
SWETS & ZEITLINGER
PUBLISHERS

LISSE   ABINGDON   EXTON (PA)   TOKYO

Library of Congress Cataloging-in-Publication Data

Applied for

Cover design: Studio Jan De Boer, Amsterdam

Typesetting: CharonTec, India

Printed in the Netherlands by Krips The Print Force, Meppel

Copyright © 2002 Swets & Zeitlinger B.V., Lisse, The Netherlands

Published by: Swets & Zeitlinger Publishers

www.szp.swets.nl

ISBN 90 265 1931 1

Contents

Foreword

————

The eye and the ocular adnexa may give rise to over 300 histologically different tumors. This is by far the largest tumor variety of the human body. While histological features of these tumors have long been recognized, the immunological behaviour of ocular tumors has been explored only in some cases.

The eye is an immune privileged site in which cells that express forcign antigens escape immune mediated elimination. If a tumor forms within this privileged environment, it is not required to develop mechanisms that allow them to escape immune surveillance; the surrounding ocular environment already provides this protection. This is not the case for tumors that develop outside the eye, or eye tumors that metastasize. These tumors must establish their own "privileged" environment. In this regard, there are many similarities between how the eye establishes immune privilege and how tumors that form at non-ocular sites establish their own privileged environment. Therefore, understanding ocular immune privilege has important implications for understanding how tumors, in general, evade the immune system. This will help us understand how, on the one hand, tumor cells express a variety of tumor and differentiation antigens that can be recognized by cytotoxic T lymphocytes and, on the other hand, these antigens fail to elicit protective anti-tumor immunity in patients with progressively growing tumors.

This book will highlight aspects of ocular and general tumor immunology. Mayor chapters summarize the role of the immune system and how tumor tissue can influence various parameters (T-cells, NK-cells, HLA-expression, apoptosis), leading to escape mechanisms used by the tumor. Beside this, the immunological behaviour of skin melanoma will be compared to choroidal melanoma, and basal cell carcinoma of the ocular lid will be compared to those of the skin. Ocular lymphoma, developing on the conjunctiva and the retina, also became a main point of interest in the last years. Intraocular lymphoma represents the ocular malignancy with the lowest 5-year-survival-rate. In recent years, paraneoplastic syndromes became much better understood.

Finally, new therapeutic regimens, urgently wanted by our patients, are summarized, which hopefully help in the fight against ocular malignancies.

We hope that this book can stimulate research in the field of ocular tumor and help to initiate new ideas.

MANFRED ZIERHUT
MARTINE JAGER
BRUCE KSANDER

Clinical remarks on intra- and periocular tumors

Abstract

Histologically, more than 300 different tumors of the eye and its adnexa can be differentiated. Pathogenic mechanisms for intra- and periocular tumor formation include 1. irreversible, autonomous cell proliferation, 2. hamartomas and choristomas, 3. inflammatory infiltration, 4. cyst formation, 5. deposits and exudation, and finally 6. spread of tissue. Most eye tumors can be classified on clinical grounds. Histology is the diagnostic method of choice, but it is often difficult to perform in intraocular neoplasms. Rapid growth is an indicator but not a proof of malignity as some malignant tumors may grow slowly while some benign lesions may develop quickly. Ocular tumors may "hide" behind an inflammation, a hemorrhage, a retinal detachment, a cataract or a secondary glaucoma, thus causing a "masquerade-syndrome."

Keywords: Ocular tumors, pathogenesis, diagnosis, growth characteristics, masquerade syndromes

Tumor definition and general considerations

There is some disagreement between "general clinicians (ophthalmologists)" on the one hand and pathologists (and oncologists) on the other concerning the *definition of a "tumor"*. For the latter, a "real tumor" is an irreversible, autonomous growth excess [1]. In benign tumors this growth excess is limited while in malignant tumors it is unlimited. However, although neuroblastoma, retinoblastoma, or cutaneous and uveal melanoma are clearly malignant tumors their growth may in single cases be limited, and even regression may occur.

"General clinicians" define a tumor as a "circumscribed swelling of tissue which is normally absent". But even this wide tumor definition is not

University Eye Clinic Dept. I, Tübingen, Germany

always correct because some "real tumors" like basal cell carcinoma (BCC), sebaceous gland carcinoma of the eyelids and palpebral or orbital metastases (of breast carcinoma) may be accompanied by tissue loss. Taking the wide definition into account, more than 300 different tumors of the eye and its adnexa can be histologically differentiated [2]. Therefore, the eye region bears by far the greatest tumor variety of the whole human body.

Following the "clinical" tumor definition, there are six main *pathogenic mechanisms for ocular and periocular tumor formation* [3]:

1. *Irreversible, autonomous cell proliferation ("real tumors")*, e.g. retinoblastoma, uveal melanoma; basal cell carcinoma (BCC), sebaceous gland carcinoma and squamous cell carcinoma of the eyelid; seborrheic keratosis, papilloma (Fig. 1), primary acquired melanosis (of the conjunctiva).
2. *Hamartomas and choristomas (developmental tumors)*, e.g. nevus, hemangioma, dermoid cyst (of the eyelid and orbit), limbal dermoid (Fig. 2).
3. *Inflammatory infiltration*, e.g. chalazion (Fig. 3), foreign body granuloma, juvenile xanthogranuloma (JXG), allergic granuloma.
4. *Cyst formation*, e.g. epidermal cyst (of the eyelid), (congenital) iris cyst, (secondary) cyst of the ciliary body in plasmocytoma.
5. *Deposits and exudation*, e.g. proteinaceous deposits in amyloidosis or Urbach-Wiethe Syndrome, choroidal detachment.
6. *Spread of tissue*, e.g. epithelial ingrowth (Fig. 4), or prolapse of orbital fat simulating a conjunctival tumor.

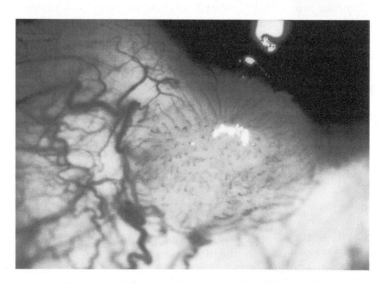

FIGURE 1.   *Sessile conjunctival papilloma at the inferior limbus. Note prominent "feeder vessels" and vascular sprouts within the tumor. Carcinoma of the conjunctival epithelium may have a similar aspect.*

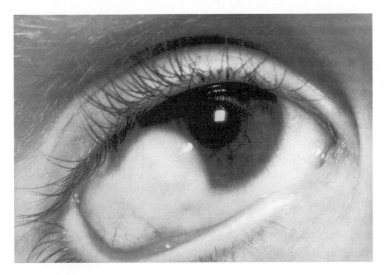

FIGURE 2. *Typical limbal dermoid in Goldenhar's syndrome. This developmental lesion (choristoma) is typically non-growing.*

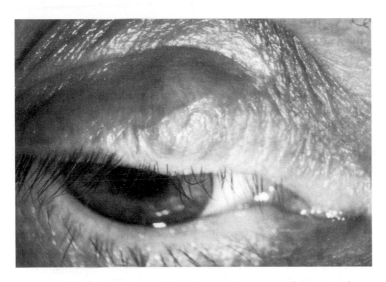

FIGURE 3. *Typical chalazion (chronic granulomatous inflammation because of sebostasis) of the upper eyelid. Differential diagnosis includes sebaceous gland carcinoma!*

It should be remembered that tumors can occur in combination. For example (separate) choroidal nevi are sometimes found in melanoma eyes, and BCC of the eyelid can obstruct sebaceous orifices thus inducing an additional chalazion. Moreover eyelid BCCs and squamous cell carcinoma rarely develop side by side resulting in a "mixed" or "collision tumor".

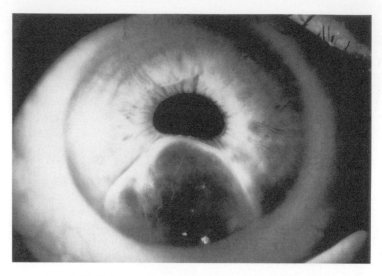

FIGURE 4. *Epithelial ingrowth after "occult" penetrating injury 18 months before. The epithelial cyst covers the iris and the backside of the cornea. Intraocular pressure was normal, and there was no "pseudo-uveitis."*

Ocular tumors may be part of syndromes like

- Limbal dermoid (Fig. 2) (Goldenhar's Syndrome),
- Retinal astrocytoma (Fig. 5) (Bourneville-Pringle's Syndrome),
- Retinal angiomatosis (Hippel-Lindau's Syndrome),
- Optic nerve sheath meningioma and optic nerve glioma (Neurofibromatosis type I),
- Hypertrophy of the retinal pigment epithelium (Familial adenomatous polyposis coli (FAP), and
- Trichilemmomas of the eyelid (Cowden's Syndrome).

The diversity of ocular and periocular tumors finds its explanation in the many different tissues which build up the eye and its adnexa. These are

- Surface epithelium ($\rightarrow$ epidermal tumors),
- Skin appendages ($\rightarrow$ e.g. sebaceous gland carcinoma),
- Mucosa ($\rightarrow$ conjunctival tumors [Fig. 1]),
- Derivates of the mesoderm ($\rightarrow$ fibrous, vascular and muscular tumors),
- Melanocytes of neural crest origin ($\rightarrow$ nevus [Fig. 6], primary acquired melanosis, melanoma),
- Lymphoid tissue ($\rightarrow$ non-Hodgkin's lymphoma),
- Neural tissue (retina, optic nerve) ($\rightarrow$ retinoblastoma, astrocytoma (Fig. 5), optic nerve glioma, optic nerve sheath meningioma, neurofibroma),
- Highly vascularized tissue (choroid) ($\rightarrow$ metastases [Fig. 7]).

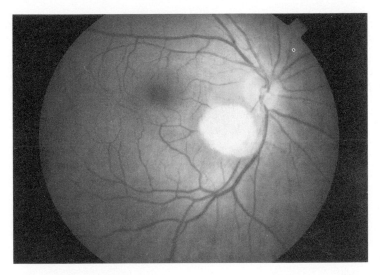

FIGURE 5. *Retinal astrocytoma ("mulberry tumor"). The asymptomatic tumor was detected by chance. There was no evidence of Bourneville-Pringle's Syndrome.*

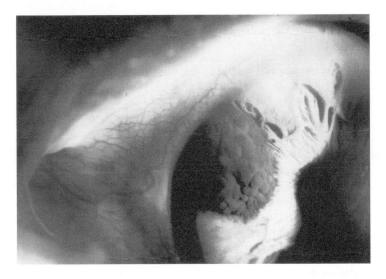

FIGURE 6. *Brown iris tumor, probably nevus. "Waitful watching" was performed without evidence of tumor growth. No therapy was initiated.*

On the other hand the eye is unique in tissues which almost never undergo malignant transformation. In this regard the

- Lens,
- Vitreous,
- Stroma and endothelium of the cornea,

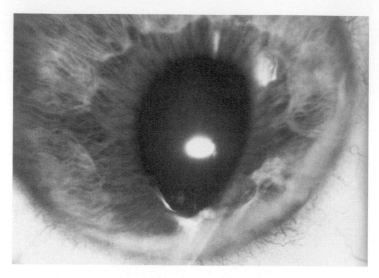

FIGURE 7.   *Iris metastasis of a breast carcinoma with pupil distortion. Chamber angle obstruction caused secondary glaucoma.*

- Endothelium of the trabecular meshwork,
- Sclera,

have to be mentioned. Therefore, the eye allows not only the study of tumorigenesis but also of anti-tumorigenesis.

Diagnosis of (peri-)ocular tumors

New diagnostic tools and growing experience have made the clinical diagnosis of many ocular tumors increasingly safe. For example, false positive diagnoses in eyes enucleated because of (suspected) uveal melanoma have fallen from almost 20% in the sixties and seventies to less than 1% today so that the "pseudo-melanoma problem" is almost completely solved [4—7]. Generally, only few diagnostic steps are required for an adequate diagnosis. These include

- Careful anamnesis,
- Slit lamp microscopy,
- Ophthalmoscopy,
- Ultrasonography (especially for intraocular tumors),
- Computed tomography and magnetic resonance imaging (especially for orbital tumors),
- Fluorescein and indocyanine green angiography,
- Diaphanoscopy (for intraocular and cystic periocular tumors),
- Palpation (of extraocular tumors),
- Medical investigations.

J. M. Rohrbach

The value of positron emission tomography for ocular tumors still awaits clarification. Some tests which were widely performed in the past like radio-phosphorus uptake or immuno-szintigraphy (for uveal melanoma) have been given up because of poor results.

The visible aspect of a tumor allows its classification in many cases without further investigations. Common criteria are:

- Size (most benign tumors stop to grow at a "critical size" so that the maximal diameter is limited),
- Shape (e.g. mushroom shape of some uveal melanomas [Fig. 8], mulberry shape in retinal astrocytoma [Fig. 5], crater shape in keratoakanthoma, dome shape in many tumors of skin appendages),
- Border (e.g. sharp border in most benign tumors, ill-defined border in many malignant tumors),
- Surface (e.g. smooth surface in most subepidermal tumors, rough surface in most epidermal tumors),
- Colour (e.g. brown in pigmented tumors (Fig. 6), reddish in vascular tumors or Merkel's cell carcinoma, yellowish in sebaceous gland carcinoma),

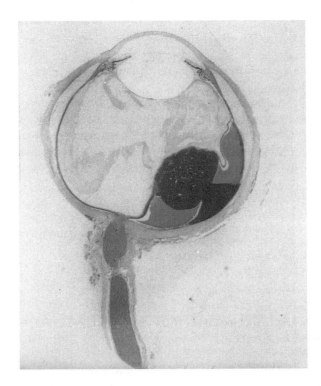

FIGURE 8. *Enucleated melanoma eye. The tumor has penetrated Bruch's membrane so that a typical mushroom shape developed. Exudative retinal detachment besides the dark melanoma. "Stock Collection," University Eye Clinic Tübingen.*

- *Other findings* (e.g. teleangiectasis (in BCC), loss of cilia (in malignant lid tumors), intratumoral cysts (in conjunctival nevus), orange pigment (in uveal melanoma).

Histology is the method with the highest diagnostic safety though it too is not 100% safe. *Biopsy* can be easily performed in most cases of palpebral and conjunctival tumors. However, it becomes increasingly difficult in orbital and especially in intraocular tumors. *Intraocular fine needle aspiration* is performed in few specialized centres only [8].

When a tumor cannot be classified on clinical grounds, and biopsy seems hazardous, a thorough documentation and a "waitful watching" to evaluate tumor growth are indicated (Fig. 6). Quick and radical therapeutic decisions without a clear diagnosis should be avoided.

Growth of (peri-)ocular tumors

Biologically and clinically, *growth characteristics* of a tumor are of essential importance. Tumor growth mostly follows an exponential curve, and about 28 cell doublings are required for a clinically detectable nodule of ca. 5 mm diameter [9].

Because more or less tumor cells undergo apoptosis or do not divide, one cell cycle does not automatically lead to a doubling of tumor cells. Depending on the duration of the cell cycle, many tumors have a subclinical phase of several years.

Tumor growth seems to be quite constant for many tumors but it is irregular with phases of growth acceleration and retardation in others so that the *speed of growth* of an individual tumor is hard to predict. Rapid growth is suspicious but not proving for a malignant neoplasm. Five classes of tumor growth can be differentiated.

1. *Usually rapid growth*:
   - Retinoblastoma,
   - Rhabdomyosarcoma,
   - Merkel's cell carcinoma (of the eyelid),
   - Keratoakanthoma (benign),
   - Pyogenic granuloma (benign).
2. *Usually intermediate growth*:
   - Sebaceous gland carcinoma (of the eyelid),
   - Squamous cell carcinoma (of the eyelid).
3. *Usually slow growth:*
   - Basal cell carcinoma (BCC) (of the eyelid),
   - Most benign tumors (before growth limitation).
4. *Variable growth*:
   - Uveal melanoma (tumor doubling was estimated between 17 and 450 days [10–12]),

J. M. Rohrbach

- Ocular metastases (growth depends on the nature of the primary tumor).
5. *No growth*:
   - Choristomas and some hamartomas,
   - Benign tumors (after growth limitation).

With the exception of uveal melanoma *metastases* occur generally late in ocular tumors [3]. Malignant eyelid and conjunctival tumors first spread via the lymphatics to the preauricular and submandibular lymph nodes. Primary hematogenous spread is very unlikely in these neoplasms. Uveal melanomas form distant metastases via the blood stream with the liver beeing the target in most cases. Death can occur not only because of distant metastases but also because of continuous growth like in retinoblastoma, malignant tumors of the lacrimal gland or malignant neoplasms of the eyelid with orbital invasion.

Clinical signs of (peri-)ocular tumors and masquerade syndromes

The vast majority of palpebral (Fig. 3) and conjunctival tumors (Figs 1 and 2) and some intraocular tumors (Figs 4 and 6) are detected because of a *visible mass.* Most intraocular tumors cannot be seen directly so that they become symptomatic because of *functional impairment* (blurred vision, loss of visual acuity or visual field). Orbital tumors cause *exophthalmus* and eventually motility disorders or optic nerve compression with visual loss. Almost all tumors in the eye region are painless unless painful secondary complications like secondary glaucoma occur. However, *pain* is very typical of adenoid-cystic carcinoma of the lacrimal gland as tumor cells spread along the perineurium.

Growth especially of intraocular tumors can provoke a broad spectrum of *secondary phenomena* which may become prominent so that the tumor is "hidden" and the ophthalmologist is in danger to miss the tumor diagnosis or, less often, to suppose the wrong tumor. The most important of these *"masquerade syndromes"* are the following:

1. *Ulceration (without a mass)*, e.g. in
   - Basal cell carcinoma (BCC),
   - Squamouus cell carcinoma,
   - Sebaceous gland carcinoma,
   - Metastases (of the eyelid).
2. *"False" pigmentation*, e.g. in
   - Pigmented basal cell carcinoma (BCC),
   - Pigmented seborrheic keratosis,
   - Old hemorrhages.
3. *Iris heterochromia*, e.g. in
   - Nevus (iris),

- Melanoma (iris),
- Retinoblastoma,
- Juvenile xanthogranuloma (JXG) [13],
- Medulloepithelioma.

4. *Cataract formation*, e.g. in
   - Uveal melanoma (Fig. 9),
   - Bilateral diffuse uveal melanocytic proliferation (BDUMP) (paraneoplastic syndrome) [14].

5. *Inflammation ("pseudo-uveitis," "pseudo-hypopyon")*, e.g. in
   - Intraocular non-Hodgkin's lymphoma (NHL) (almost all intraocular NHL's are primarily treated as "uveitis" or "vasculitis" so that diagnosis is very often delayed [15−18]),
   - Uveal melanoma (ca. 4−6% of uveal melanomas exhibit a prominent inflammation [19]),
   - Retinoblastoma (ca. 7% of retinoblastoma eyes reveal a prominent inflammation. Especially the diffuse infiltrating variant of retinoblastoma which occurs in older children may lead to a "pseudo-hypopyon" [Fig. 10] [3]),
   - Epithelial ingrowth [20],
   - Juvenile xanthogranuloma (JXG) [13],
   - Metastases (especially of the iris) [3, 21],

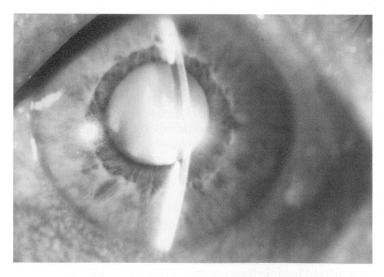

FIGURE 9. *Total lens opacification (mature cataract) and shallowing of the anterior chamber with massive elevation of intraocular pressure. An almost clear lens in the other eye aroused suspicion of an intraocular melanoma which was verified by ultrasonography. Instead of cataract extraction the eye was enucleated. Masquerade Syndrome!*

J. M. Rohrbach

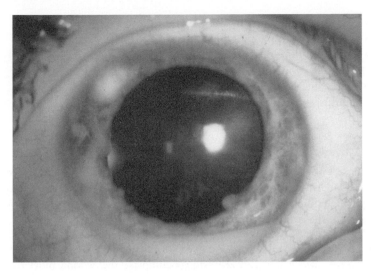

FIGURE 10. *Diffuse infiltrating retinoblastoma in a six-year-old child referred because of "uveitis." Cells of this "liquid" tumor have seeded on the iris surface and at the bottom of the anterior chamber thus forming a "pseudo-hypopyon." Masquerade syndrome!*

- Sebaceous gland carcinoma (lid),
- Fibrosing basal cell carcinoma (lid).
6. *Hemorrhage*, e.g. in
   - Uveal melanoma (ca. 3% of uveal melanomas reveal a prominent hemorrhage [19]),
   - Retinoblastoma,
   - Juvenile Xanthogranuloma (JXG) [13],
   - Metastases (especially of the iris),
   - Varix nodule of the iris [22].
7. *Retinal detachment*
   - Uveal melanoma (almost all uveal melanomas are associated with a at least slight exudative detachment of the retina [Fig. 8] [3]),
   - Retinoblastoma,
   - Choroidal hemangioma,
   - Choroidal metastases [3].
8. *Elevation of intraocular pressure (secondary glaucoma)*, e.g. in
   - Uveal melanoma (3−57% of melanoma eyes reveal secondary glaucoma [3, 23, 24]),
   - Metastases (e.g. iris metastases cause secondary glaucoma in ca. 55−65% of the patients (Fig. 7) [21, 24, 25]),
   - Retinoblastoma (ca. 2−23% of retinoblastoma eyes suffer from secondary glaucoma (Fig. 10) [25, 26]),
   - Epithelial ingrowth (secondary glaucoma occurs in ca. 43−53% of all cases [15, 27]),

- Juvenile xanthogranuloma (JXG) [13],
- Non-Hodgkin's lymphoma,
- Bilateral diffuse uveal melanocytic proliferation (BDUMP) [14].

9. *"Almost nothing"*, e.g. in
   - Fibrosing basal cell carcinoma,
   - Diffuse uveal melanoma.

The frequency of malignant ocular tumors

Though attention of ophthalmologists is primarily drawn on uveal melanoma and retinoblastoma these two tumors represent only a minority of ocular malignant neoplasms. In order of *frequency* ocular and periocular tumors can be listed in the following manner:

- *BCC of the eyelid* is by far the most common malignant tumor.
- *Intra- and periocular metastases* comprise the second most frequent malignant newgrowths in the eye region. Ocular metastases are primarily found in the uveal tract (choroid, ciliary body and iris) (Fig. 7), and second in the orbit. Metastases to the eyelids, to the conjunctiva, retina and to the optic disc are rare. It is nowadays generally accepted that intraocular metastases are much more frequent than uveal melanoma [3].
- *All ocular melanomas (of the uvea, conjunctiva, lids and orbit)* together are only third concerning frequency of ocular malignant neoplasms. The inicidence of uveal melanoma is estimated as 0.5−1/100,000/ year. Intraocular melanomas are ca. 30 times more frequent than extraocular ones [3].
- *All malignant lid tumors* (except BCC) taken together are probably a bit less frequent than melanomas.
- *Rhabdomyosarcoma of the orbit* and *malignant tumors of the lacrimal gland* are more frequent than retinoblastoma.
- *Retinoblastoma* (Fig. 10) occurs in ca. 1 per 15,000−20,000 live births or 9−11 per 1 million children under the age of 5 per year. It represents ca. 2−3% of all childhood malignancies. It is estimated that the ophthalmologist meets only one child with retinoblastoma during lifetime praxis [3].
- *Other malignant tumors of the eye* and its adnexa like carcinoma of the non-pigmented ciliary epithelium, carcinoma of the retinal pigment epithelium, and carcinoma of the lacrimal sac are exceptionally rare, so that larger studies are missing and most ophthalmologists have never seen such patients.

Malignant ocular tumors (except BCC) account for less than 0.5% of the malignant tumors of man [21] so they are not that much important for practical oncology. However, because of the easy visibility and the diversity of its tumors the eye is an excellent object for cancer research, and it thus

J. M. Rohrbach

may deliver important clues for a better understanding of *cancerogenesis* in general.

References

1. Albertini, A. v. (ed.), Histologische Geschwulstdiagnostik. *Systematische Morphologie der menschlichen Geschwülste als Grundlage für die klinische Beurteilung*, 2nd ed., Thieme, Stuttgart, New York, 1974.
2. Zimmerman, L.E., and Sobin, L.H., *Histological typing of tumors of the eye and its adnexa*, World Health Organization, Geneva, Switzerland, 1980.
3. Rohrbach, J.M., and Lieb, W.E. (eds.), *Tumoren des Auges und seiner Adnexe*, Schattauer, Stuttgart, 1998.
4. Chang, M., Zimmerman, L.E., and McLean, I., *Arch. Ophthalmol.* 102: 726–727, 1984.
5. Collaborative Ocular Melanoma Study Group (COMS), *Am. J. Ophthalmol.* 125: 745–766, 1998.
6. Ferry, A.P., *Arch. Ophthalmol.* 72: 463–469, 1964.
7. Shields, J.A., and Zimmerman, L.E., *Arch. Ophthalmol.* 89: 466–471, 1973.
8. Shields, J.A., Shields, C.L., Ehya, H., Eagle, R.C. jr., and de Potter, P., *Ophthalmology* 100: 1677–1684, 1993.
9. Diehl, V., and Lathan, B. in *Die Innere Medizin*, Gross, R., Schölmerich, P. and Gerok, W. (eds.), pp. 1045–1059, Schattauer, Stuttgart, 1996.
10. Friberg, T.R., Fineberg, E., and McQuaig, S., *Arch. Ophthalmol.* 101: 1375–1377, 1983.
11. Guthoff, R., and Chumbley, L., *Spektr. Augenheilkd.* 5: 99–100, 1991.
12. Manschot, W.A., and Peperzeel, H.A. van, *Arch. Ophthalmol.* 98: 71–77, 1980.
13. Rohrbach, J.M., Stübiger, N., Küper, K., and Dopfer, R., *Klin. Monatsbl. Augenheilkd.* 205: 47–49, 1994.
14. Rohrbach, J.M., Roggendorf, W., Thanos, S., Steuhl, K.-P., and Thiel, H.-J., *Am. J. Ophthalmol.* 110: 49–56, 1990.
15. Arocker-Mettinger, E., Huber-Spitzy, V., Stur, M., Haddad, R., Grabner, G., Radaszkiewicz, T., Hawliczek, A., and Neumann, E., *Spektr. Augenheilkd.* 7: 90–96, 1993.
16. Freeman, L.N., Schachat, A.P., Knox, D.L., Michels, R.G., and Green, W.R., *Ophthalmology* 94: 1631–1639, 1987.
17. Ursea, R., Heinemann, M.-H., Silverman, R.H., Deangelis, L.M., Daly, S.W., and Coleman, D.J., *Retina* 17: 118–123, 1997.
18. Whitcup, S.M., de Smet, M.D., Rubin, B.I., Palestine, A.G., Martin, D.F., Burnier, M. jr., Chan, C.-C., and Nussenblatt, R.B., *Ophthalmology* 100: 1399–1406, 1993.
19. Fraser, D.J., and Font, R.L., *Arch. Ophthalmol.* 97: 1311–1314, 1979.
20. Küchle, M., and Green, W.R., *Ger. J. Ophthalmol.* 5: 211–223, 1996.
21. Shields, J.A., Shields, C.L., Kiratli, H., and de Potter, P., *Am. J. Ophthalmol.* 119: 422–430, 1995.
22. Rohrbach, J.M., Eckstein, A., and Schuster, I., *Klin. Monatsbl. Augenheilkd.* 207: 206–207, 1995.
23. Rohrbach, J.M., Steuhl, K.-P., and Thiel, H.-J., *Fortschr. Ophthalmol.* 85: 723–725, 1988.

24. Shields, C.L., Shields, J.A., Shields, M.B., and Augsburger, J.J., *Ophthalmology* 94: 839–846, 1987.
25. Fraumeni, J.F. jr., Devesa, S.S., Hoover, R.N., and Kinlen, L.J., in *Cancer. Principles and Practice of Oncology*, DeVita, V.T. jr., Hellman, S., and Rosenberg, S.A. (eds.), 4th ed., pp. 150–181, Lippincott, Philadelphia, 1993.
26. Yoshizumi, M.O., Thomas, J.V., and Smith, T.R., *Arch. Ophthalmol.* 96: 105–110, 1978.
27. Zagorski, Z., Shresta, H.G., Lang, G.K., and Naumann, G.O.H., *Klin. Monatsbl. Augenheilkd.* 193: 16–20, 1988.

J. WAYNE STREILEIN

Ocular immune privilege and tumors

Abstract

Immune privilege is an active, dynamic process by which certain organs and tissues mold the *induction* and alter the *expression* of immunity in ways that protect those organs and tissues from immune-mediated damage. The anatomic, cellular and molecular strategies known to contribute to immune privilege of the anterior chamber of the eye are described and offered as possible mechanisms by which successful tumors avoid immune detection and destruction.

Keywords: Immune privilege, anterior chamber, immunosuppression, immune deviation

Introduction

The concept of immune privilege originated from studies on the immunological mechanisms responsible for rejection of solid organ transplants. And even though the earliest description of immune privilege in the anterior chamber of the eye in 1873 involved the injection of human tumor cells intraocularly, the idea that tumors and immune privilege might be mechanistically linked was not advanced until the late 1970s by North [1]. Only within the past decade has the linkage of tumors and immune privilege been appreciated by more than a few investigators. Therefore, a workshop devoted to the immunology of tumors arising from and within the eye is particularly timely, if not *avant garde*.

Concerning immune privilege

The phenomenon of immune privilege was first described, albeit not named, by van Dooremaal [2] in 1873 when he discovered that human tumor cells failed to grow at any site he placed them in rabbit organs and tissues—except the anterior chamber of the eye [2]. Since this discovery antedated the discovery of immunity and the development of the field of immunology, the mechanism(s) responsible for intraocular tumor growth were unexplained. This situation changed in the 1940s when Sir Peter Medawar described the immunologic basis for tissue transplant rejection [3]. In the course of his experimental inquiry, he re-discovered van Dooremaal's phenomenon and correctly inferred that the unexpected success of foreign tumors or tissue grafts at certain sites in the body (eye, brain, hamster cheek pouch) was due to a type of immunologic failure [4]. At the time Medawar made his observations, he was aware of the existence of blood tissue barriers in the eye and brain, and he believed that neither of these organs possessed lymphatic drainage pathways. As a consequence, he hypothesized that immune privilege resulted from "immunologic ignorance," i.e. the immune system of animals bearing foreign grafts in immune privileged sites was shielded from detecting antigens on these grafts by vascular barriers.

This hypothesis satisfactorily explained immune privilege until a renaissance of investigation, initiated in the 1970s, produced results that were incompatible with "immune ignorance." First, the number of immune privileged sites began to grow and certain sites, especially the testis, were found to have extensive lymphatic drainage [5]. More recently, the brain and even the eye have been found to display important connections via lymphatic vessels to cervical and other lymph nodes [6–8]. Second, antigens injected into the anterior chamber of the eye were found to escape. Histoincompatible tumor cells injected intracamerally were found within 24 hr in lymph nodes and spleen [9], and ovalbumin similarly injected was found in the blood within a matter of a few minutes [10]. Thus, there is no "barrier" that absolutely prevents antigens or mobile cells placed in privileged sites from escaping into the blood and lymph vasculature. Third, mice and rats were found to make systemic immune responses to foreign grafts and antigens placed in the anterior chamber of the eye and brain, although immune privilege was maintained [11–14]. Observations of this third type formally eliminated "immune ignorance" as the sole explanation for immune privilege. The contemporary view of immune privilege is that it is a dynamic, rather than a static, state in which the immune response to privileged tissues and antigens is molded in directions that are unconventional, and (presumably) related to the physiologic demands of the tissues and organs involved [15,16]. Over the past three decades, a tremendous amount of knowledge had been gained in our quest to understand immune privilege. Mechanisms that contribute to immune privilege can be categorized according to whether they are actively or passively involved. The existence of blood:tissue barriers and the relative absence of lymphatic vessels remain as important to the existence of immune privilege. In the case of the eye, the fact that aqueous humor drains directly intravenously via the trabecular meshwork (rather than via lymphatic vessels) has been found to be important in molding the subsequent immune response. In fact, the spleen (rather than cervical lymph nodes) is the secondary lymphoid organ most important to ocular immune responses of the immune privileged type [17]. Reduced expression of MHC class I and II molecules on immune privileged tissues and sites is also an important factor [18,19]. It is now clear that T lymphocytes recognize foreign antigens in association with these MHC molecules, and that potential target tissues that avoid expression of these molecules can also avoid immune (T cell) destruction. A further important passive feature of immune privilege is the relative deficit of class II MHC-bearing professional antigen presenting cells [20,21]. In the cornea this deficit is absolute, in the iris and ciliary body the deficit is functional, in the sense that bone marrow-derived cells at these sites are unable to function as conventional antigen presenting cells—unless activated by trauma, inflammation or experimental artifice *in vitro* [22–24].

The mechanisms that actively create and maintain immune privilege have captured the attention of the immunologic community. Constitutive expression of molecules such as CD95L, CD59, DAF, MCP on cells of the eye and testis have helped to explain why immune expression is deficient at these sites and tissues. CD95L on corneal cells has been directly implicated in the high level of success of orthotopic corneal allografts, and in the low level of intraocular inflammation found in eyes of certain mice that are infected with herpes simplex virus [25,26]. In addition, Niederkorn has recently demonstrated that the tissues lining the anterior chamber normally express class Ib molecules (Qa-2) which have been implicated in protecting class Ia-negative trophoblastic cells from lysis by NK cells [27]. The constitutive presence in aqueous humor of immunomodulatory molecules has also been found to be crucial to ocular immune privilege [28]. The presence of immunosuppressing cytokines, neuropeptides, and mediators helps to explain why aqueous humor fails to support T cell activation and secretion of lymphokines, and why aqueous humor suppresses activated macrophages and natural killer cells. This bewildering array of molecules is not yet completely described, nor do we completely understand the various ways in which these molecules create and maintain immune privilege.

It is worth pointing out that immune privilege has been attributed to certain tissues and to certain sites in the body [29–35]. Accordingly, there are separate definitions of immune privileged tissues and sites, and relating these definitions is helpful in understanding the possible role of immune privilege in tumors—especially ocular tumors. Immune privileged sites are defined operationally when foreign tissue grafts placed at these sites experience prolonged (often indefinite) survival, whereas similar grafts placed at conventional sites would be promptly rejected. Immune privileged tissues are defined operationally when these tissues are grafted into conventional sites, and experience prolonged/indefinite survival, whereas normal tissues would be summarily rejected. The lists of immune privileged tissues and sites continues to grow. An updated, but by no means complete, list of privileged tissues and sites is presented in Table 1. Tumors have been found to have properties of immune privileged tissues and immune privileged sites.

TABLE 1.

Immune privileged	
Tissues	Sites
Eye (cornea, lens)	Eye (cornea, anterior chamber vitreous cavity, subretinal space)
Cartilage	Brain
Feto-placental unit	Pregnant uterus
Ovary	Ovary
Testis	Testis
Liver	Adrenal cortex
Tumors	Tumors

The eye as a model immune privileged site

Perhaps because of the ease with which it can be manipulated experimentally, the eye—especially the anterior chamber—has been studied extensively as an immune privileged site over the past 30 years. Enough has now been learned so that it is possible to offer distinct mechanistic proposals for how immune privilege "works." There are at least two dimensions to ocular immune privilege: (i) during immune induction to antigens placed in the anterior chamber of the eye, the systemic immune response is modified such that a deviant immunity emerges, (ii) during immune expression in the anterior chamber, local factors prevent certain immune effectors from carrying out their functional programs.

Immune response to eye-derived antigens

The modified immune response elicited by antigen placed in the anterior chamber of the eye has been termed anterior chamber associated immune deviation (ACAID) [36–38]. Recipients of intraocular antigens (a) fail to acquire delayed hypersensitivity and complement fixing antibodies, although they (b) develop primed cytotoxic T cells and non-complement fixing antibodies to the same antigens. The spleens of these mice contain at least three functionally distinct populations of regulatory T cells that suppress the induction of delayed hypersensitivity, the expression of delayed hypersensitivity, and the activation of B cells that secrete complement fixing antibodies [39]. Thus, this deviant response lack some, but not all, antigen-specific immune effectors and as a consequence these animals display concomitant immunity [40].

If the anterior chamber of the eye is altered by trauma, inflammation, or disease so that it loses the capacity to support ACAID induction, immune privilege is also lost [41,42]. Corneal allografts placed orthotopically in such eyes are rejected swiftly, and allogeneic tumor cells are also not able to form progressively growing intraocular tumors. ACAID appears to be physiologically important for the eye. In eyes that lack ACAID-promoting potential, infection of the anterior ocular segment with herpes simplex virus results in a high incidence of stromal keratitis [43]. ACAID has been induced with retinal specific antigens and found to prevent experimental autoimmune uveoretinitis [44–46], and it has been used to prevent corneas grafted into "high-risk" eyes from undergoing acute rejection [47–50]. Therefore, ACAID represents the most important pathway by which immune privilege in the anterior chamber of the eye shapes the immune response following the intraocular introduction of foreign antigens.

Immune expression in the anterior chamber

By now there are numerous examples of the failure of immune effectors to express themselves in the anterior chamber. Cousins et al. reported that it was not possible to elicit delayed hypersensitivity reactions in the anterior chamber of mouse eyes—even if T cells, antigen presenting cells and antigen were provided in the inoculum [51]. Niederkorn demonstrated that injections of immune T cells failed to cause rejection of allogeneic tumor cells in the anterior chamber, except if the T cells were injected at the same time as the tumor cells [52]. More recently, Stuart et al. [53], and Yamagami et al. [54] reported that corneal allografts were protected from immune rejection because the cells expressed CD95L constitutively.

There turn out to be numerous reasons why immune privilege inhibits immune expression in the eye. The existence of a blood:ocular barrier severely limits the egress of effector cells and molecules from the blood from penetrating into the anterior chamber. Aqueous humor contains potent inhibitors of complement activation that act at multiple steps, and that involve both the classical (antibody-dependent) and alternative pathways [55]. TGFβ, VIP and α-MSH suppress T cell activation by antigen [56–59], and CGRP prevents activated macrophages from producing nitric oxide and reactive oxygen intermediates [60]. MIF prevents NK cells from lysing target cells [61,62]. These factors, as well as factors yet to be described, suppress neutrophil activation and release of toxic products. Moreover, effector T cells that have come under the influence of aqueous humor are converted into regulatory T cells—in part, because they begin to secrete TGFβ [63].

Despite the extensive list of regulatory mechanisms, certain types of immune expression are still permitted in the eye. For example, mice bearing a progressively growing allogeneic tumor in one eye, are prevented from accepting another tumor cell inoculum in the contralateral eye [52]. This is a good demonstration of concomitant immunity. The factors that operate in concomitant immunity are not terribly well defined, but they may be related to the observation that cytotoxic T cells that have already acquired their lytic capacity are fully able to lyse target cells in the presence of aqueous humor [28].

TABLE 2. *Features important in immune privilege.*

Microanatomical factors
Blood:tissue barrier
Deficit of lymphatic drainage
Extracellular fluid drains intravascularly
Aberrant/absent antigen presenting cells
Deficit of mast cells

Soluble factors in microenvironment
TGFβ—inhibits T cell activation, alters APC function
α-MSH—alters functional program of effector T cells
VIP—inhibits T cell activation
CGRP—inhibits NO production by activated macrophages
MIF—inhibits NK cell-mediated lysis of target cells
IL-1ra—inhibits IL-1-dependent inflammation
< 1 kD inhibitor of complement activation

Molecules expressed on surface of parenchymal cells
CD59, DAF, CD46—suppress complement activation
CD95 ligand—promotes T cell apoptosis, activates neutrophils
Reduced expression of MHC class I & II
Increased expression of class Ib (atypical) molecules

Similarly, antibodies to HSV-1 can neutralize the virus and prevent infection of target cells in the presence of aqueous humor. It is probably relevant that virus neutralization does not require complement fixing antibodies.

Immune privilege and tumors

If we are to consider the possibilities that (a) tumors may act as privileged tissues, and (b) that tumors may create immune privileged sites, then what has been learned about immune privilege in the eye may be pertinent to tumor immunology. There are at least three categories of factors that make immune privilege possible. In Table 2 these factors are listed according to whether they are microanatomical, soluble factors in the microenvironment, or molecules expressed on the surfaces of cells. Consideration of these factors may prove useful in determining the extent to which a tumor utilizes immune privilege to secure its tenure. More important, strategies to interrupt one or more of these factors may serve to tip the balance of survival away from the tumor and toward the host.

Acknowledgements

Support for some of the experimental work described in this manuscript was provided by USPHS grants EY 05678, and EY 10765.

J. Wayne Streilein

References

1. Spitalny, G.L., and North, R.J., *J. Exp. Med.* 145: 1264–1277, 1977.
2. van Dooremaal, J.C., *Albrecht Von Graefes Arch. Ophthalmol.* 19: 358–373, 1873.
3. Medawar, P.B., *J. Anat. London* 79: 157–168, 1945.
4. Medawar, P., *Br. J. Exp. Pathol.* 29: 58–69, 1948.
5. Head, J.R., Neaves, W.B., and Billingham, R.E., *Transplantation* 35: 91–99, 1983.
6. Cserr, H.F., and Knopf, P.M., *Immunol. Today* 13: 507–510, 1992.
7. Bill, A., *Exp. Eye Res.* 11: 195–206, 1971.
8. Eichhorn, M., Horneber, M., Streilein, J.W., and Lutjen-Drecoll, E., *Invest. Ophthalmol. Vis. Sci.* 34: 2926–2903, 1993.
9. Niederkorn, J.Y., and Streilein, J.W., *J. Immunol.* 128: 2470–2474, 1982.
10. Wilbanks, G.A., and Streilein, J.W., *Reg. Immunol.* 2: 390–398, 1989.
11. Kaplan, H.J., and Streilein, J.W., *J. Immunol.* 118: 809–814, 1977.
12. Kaplan, H.J., and Streilein, J.W., *J. Immunol.* 120: 689–693, 1978.
13. Streilein, J.W., Niederkorn, J.Y., and Shadduck, J.A., *J. Exp. Med.* 152: 1121–1125, 1980.
14. Streilein, J.W., Ksander, B.R., and Taylor, A.W., *J. Immunol.* 158: 3557–3560, 1997.
15. Streilein, J.W. in *Ocular Infection and Immunity*, Pepose, J.W., Holland, G.N. and Wilhelmus, K.R. (eds.), pp. 19–33, Mosby-Year Book, Philadelphia, 1996.
16. Streilein, J.W. in *Encyclopedia of Human Biology*, Dulbecco R. (ed.), Vol. 4, 2 ed., pp. 767–776, Academic Press, San Diego, 1997.
17. Kaplan, H.J., and Streilein, J.W., *Nature* 251: 553–554, 1974.
18. Wang, H.M., Kaplan, H.J., Chan, W.C., and Johnson, M., *Invest. Ophthalmol. Vis. Sci.* 28: 1383–1389, 1987.
19. Abi-Hanna, D., Wakefield, D., and Watkins, S., *Transplantation* 45: 610–613, 1998.
20. Streilein, J.W., Toews, G.B., and Bergstresser, P.R., *Nature* 282: 325–327, 1979.
21. Gillette, T.E., Chandler, J.W., and Greiner, J.V., *Ophthalmology* 89: 700–712, 1982.
22. Williamson, J.S.P., Bradley, D., and Streilein, J.W., *Immunology* 67: 96–102, 1989.
23. Steptoe, R., Holt, P.G., and McMenamin, P.G., *Immunology* 85: 630–637, 1995.
24. McMenamin P.G., and Forrester, J.V. in *Dendritic cells: Biology and clinical applications*, Lotze, M.T. and Thomson, A.W. (eds.), pp. 205–254, Academic Press, San Diego, 1999.
25. Griffith, T.S., Brunner, T., Fletcher, S.M., Green, D.R., and Ferguson, T.A., *Science* 270: 1189–1192, 1995.
26. Griffith, T.S., Yu, X., Harndon, J.M., Green, D.R., and Ferguson, T.A., *Immunity* 5: 7–16, 1996.
27. Li, X.-Y., Niederkorn, J.Y., Chiang, E., Ungchusri, T., and Stroynowski, I. *Invest. Ophthalmol. Vis. Sci.* 40: S861, 1999.
28. Kaiser, C.J., Ksander, B.R., and Streilein, J.W., *Reg. Immunol.* 2: 42–49, 1989.
29. Barker, C.F., and Billingham, R.E., *Adv. Immunol.* 25: 1–54, 1977
30. Niederkorn, J.Y., *Adv. Immunol.* 48: 191–226, 1990.
31. Tompsett, E., Abi-Hanna, D., and Wakefield, D., *Curr. Eye Res.* 9: 1141–1150, 1990.
32. Ksander, B.R., and Streilein, J.W., in *Mechansisms of regulation of immunity chemical immunology*, Granstein, R. (ed.), pp. 117–145, Karger, 1993.
33. Streilein, J.W., *Science* 270: 1158–1159, 1995.
34. Streilein, J.W., *Invest. Ophthalmol. Vis. Sci.* 37: 1940–1950, 1996.

35. Streilein, J.W., Ksander, B.R., and Taylor, A.W., *J. Immunol.* 158: 3557–3560, 1997.
36. Niederkorn, J., Streilein, J.W., and Shadduck, J.A., *Invest. Ophthalmol. Vis. Sci.* 20: 355–363, 1980.
37. Streilein, J.W., Niederkorn, J.Y., and Shadduck, J.A., *J. Exp. Med.* 152: 1121–1125, 1980.
38. Streilein, J.W., *The FASEB Journal* 1: 199–208, 1987.
39. Wilbanks, G.A., and Streilein, J.W., *Immunology* 71: 383–389, 1990.
40. Niederkorn, J.Y., and Streilein, J.W., *J. Immunol.* 131: 2587–2594, 1983.
41. Sano, Y., Ksander, B.R., and Streilein, J.W., *Invest. Ophthalmol. Vis. Sci.* 36: 2176–2185, 1995.
42. Streilein, J.W., Bradley, D., Sano, Y., and Sonada, Y., *Invest. Ophthalmol. Vis. Sci.* 37: 413–424, 1996.
43. McLeish, W., Rubsamen, P., Atherton, S.S., and Streilein, J.W., *Reg. Immunol.* 2: 236–243, 1989.
44. Mizuno, K., Clark, A.F., and Streilein, J.W., *Invest. Ophthalmol. Vis. Sci.* 30: 772–774, 1989.
45. Hara, Y., Caspi, R.R., Wiggert, B., Chan, C.-C., Wilbanks, G.A., and Streilein, J.W., *J. Immunol.* 148: 1685–1692, 1992.
46. Gery, I., and Streilein, J.W., *Curr. Opinion Immunol.* 6: 938–945, 1994.
47. She, S.C., Steahly, L.P., and Moticka, E.J., *Invest. Ophthalmol. Vis. Sci.* 31: 1950–1956, 1990.
48. Niederkorn, J.Y., and Mellon, J., *Invest. Ophthamol. Vis. Sci.* 37: 2700–2707, 1996.
49. Sano, Y., Okamoto, S., and Streilein, J.W., *Curr. Eye Res.* 16: 1171–1174, 1997.
50. Streilein, J.W., in *Uveitis today, Proceedings of the Fourth International Symposium on Uveitis*, S. Ohno *et al.* (eds.), pp. 297–302, Elsevier, Amsterdam, 1998.
51. Cousins, S.W., Trattler, W.B., and Streilein, J.W., *Curr. Eye Res.* 10: 287–297, 1991.
52. Niederkorn, J.Y., and Streilein, J.W., *Invest. Ophthalmol. Vis. Sci.* 25: 336–342, 1984.
53. Stuart, P.M., Griffith, T.S., Usui, N., Pepose, J., Yu, X., and Ferguson, T.A., *J. Clin. Invest.* 99: 396–402, 1997.
54. Yamagami, S., Kawashima, H., Tsuru, T., Yamagami, H., Kayagaki, N., Yagita, H., and Gregerson, D.S., *Transplantation* 64: 1107–1111, 1997.
55. Goslings, W.R.O., Prodeus, A.P., Streilein, J.W., Carroll, M.C., Jager, M.J., and Taylor, A.W., *Invest. Ophthalmol. Vis. Sci.* 39: 989–995, 1998.
56. Granstein, R., Stszewski, R., Knisely, T., Zeira, E., Nazareno, R., Latina, M., and Albert, D., *J. Immunol.* 144: 3021–3027, 1990.
57. Cousins, S.W., McCabe, M.M., Danielpour, D., and Streilein, J.W., *Invest. Ophthalmol. Vis. Sci.* 32: 2201–2211, 1991.
58. Taylor, A.W., Streilein, J.W., Cousins, S.W., *Curr. Eye Res.* 11: 1199–1206, 1992.
59. Taylor, A.W., Streilein, J.W., and Cousins, S.W., *J. Immunol.* 153: 1080–1086, 1994.
60. Taylor, A.W., Yee, D.G., and Streilein, J.W., *Invest. Ophthalmol. Vis. Sci.* 39: 1372–1378, 1998.
61. Apte, R.S., and Niederkorn, J.Y., *J. Immunol.* 156: 2667–2673, 1996.
62. Apte, R.S., and Niederkorn, J.Y., *J. Allergy Clin. Immunol.* 99: S467, 1997.
63. Taylor, A.W., Alard, P., Yee, D.G., and Streilein, J.W., *Curr. Eye Res.* 16: 900–908, 1997.

PURNIMA DUBEY, LISA P. SEUNG AND HANS SCHREIBER

The role of stroma in the growth or rejection of antigenic solid tumors

---

Abstract

In solid tumors, malignant cells are surrounded by stroma (greek: bed) that consists of extracellular matrix and bone-marrow-derived or non-bone-marrow-derived, mobile and sessile cells. We present evidence that tumor stroma can be critical in either preventing or helping tumor rejection. First, tumor cells embedded in stroma, i.e. tumor fragments, are much more tumorigenic than single tumor cells in suspension. Second, mice will reject non-malignant allografts that have antigenic stroma but not malignant allografts that lack antigenic stroma even when both types of allografts express the same antigen. Third, it is sufficient to make the bone-marrow-derived stromal cells antigenic in order to achieve rejection of solid tumor fragments. Fourth, stromal bone-marrow-derived cells attracted by the tumor cells also provide growth factors and stimulate angiogenesis as part of a paracrine stimulatory loop.

Keywords: Tumor antigens, angiogenesis, tumor stroma, paracrine stimulation, stromal barrier, concomitant immunity, allografts

Introduction

The rapidly developing resistance of solid tumors to active immunization shortly after transplantation of tumor cells is a well-known, almost universal phenomenon [1]. Common explanations include: (i) rapid development of peripheral T-cell tolerance to antigens expressed by the tumor cells, (ii) development of systemic immune suppression preventing the development of an effective anti-tumor response, (iii) ignorance, i.e. host failing to recognize antigens on the growing tumor, (iv) clonal exhaustion, i.e. the proliferation of antigen-specific T-cell clones cannot keep up with the rapid expansion of tumor cells, (v) lack of antigens that can lead to tumor

Department of Pathology, The University of Chicago, Chicago,
IL 60637, USA

23

rejection, and (vi) lack of co-stimulatory molecules on the cancer cells that cause apoptosis rather than antigenic stimulation of tumor-specific T cells. In the following, we present evidence that none of these mechanisms (i.e., neither peripheral tolerance, systemic immune suppression, ignorance, clonal exhaustion, nor lack of antigens or co-stimulatory molecules) suffice to explain the progressive growth of antigenic solid tumors in an immuno-competent host. Instead, we show that tumor stroma provides a powerful local device for antigenic cancer cells to both escape immune destruction as well as to acquire the growth factors and nutrients needed for growth.

Materials and methods

Mice   C3H/HeN normal and nude, BALB/cAn and DBA/2 mice, C3H/HeN X 2C F1 mice and K^{216} transgenic mice of C3H/HeN background were used for all experiments [2−5]. The 2C TCR transgenic (anti-L^d) mice were obtained from Dr. D. Loh (Washington University, St. Louis, MO) and backcrossed for over 10 generations to the C57BL/6 background. The K^{216} gene was isolated from the 1591 tumor cell line and it is similar but not identical (three amino acid differences) to K^s (K. Hasenkrug and S. Nathensen, personal communication). Mice were housed in a specific-pathogen-free facility at The University of Chicago and handled according to federal guidelines using protocols approved by the University's Animal User's Committee. Mice were purchased from the National Cancer Institute, Frederick Cancer Research Institute (Frederick, MD).

Tumor cell lines   The tumor cell lines used were of C3H/HeN origin and derived from tumors that were induced by chronic irradiation with ultraviolet light or arose spontaneously in older mice [2]. The K^{216} tumors and L^d transfected tumors were generated as described [3,4]. All cell lines were carefully screened for absence of mycoplasma which does affect the transplantability of cell lines into normal or athymic mice.

Tumor transplantations and full-thickness skin grafting   Solid tumor fragments were obtained from tumors that developed in nude mice or euthymic mice following transplantation. The tumors were minced to 1 mm^3 fragments that were loaded into a 13 gauge trocar for subcutaneous transplantation. Polyurethane sponge matrix grafts 0.5 cm^3 (Future Foam Company, Chicago, IL), were transplanted s.c. as described [5]. Normal organs were transplanted by standard procedures. Rejection of skin grafts was defined as loss of at least 80% of grafted tissue. Fetal gut or heart transplants were placed near the top of the ear to allow easy inspection. Acceptance or rejection of the graft was confirmed 3−5 weeks after transplantation by histology [5].

Treatment of mice with antibodies or irradiation   Granulocytes were depleted by injection of ascites fluid of nude mice bearing the anti-Gr-1 hybridoma antibody RB6-8C5 (a gift from Dr. Robert Coffman). 0.2 ml were given two days before tumor challenge and every three days thereafter until the end of the experiment [6,7]. The anti-CD4 (GK1.5) and anti-CD8 YTS169 antibodies were used as described [3]. Mice were irradiated with a Maxitron X-ray generator at 1.88 Gy/min as described [8].

In vitro *assays*   The chemoattraction assays, co-culture assays and recovery of cells from the peritoneal cavity to measure intraperitoneal growth, as well as the MTT assay have been described in detail [7].

Results

Tumor cells embedded in stroma are more tumorigenic

When tumor cell suspensions are injected subcutaneously, the majority of the injected tumor cells die within the first few days. A tumor is then formed from the remaining few small nests of cancer cells. Tumor cell death is accompanied by a cellular inflammatory response that includes granulocytes, macrophages and other cell types but it is unclear whether this response is the cause or the result of the tumor cell destruction. In any case, the survival of tumor cells in fragments seems to be much superior to a tumor cell suspension, since pieces of tumor that contain far fewer viable tumor cells are nevertheless transplanted much more effectively (Table 1).

TABLE 1   *Increased tumorigenicity of cancer cells in stromal matrices: Tumor cells transplanted as solid tumor fragments or inside a synthetic sponge matrix are more tumorigenic than tumor cells transplanted as cell suspensions.*[1]

Tumor (%)	Host	Form	Number of	
			Tumor cells transplanted	Tumor outgrowth
1591-PRO	Normal	Suspension	50×10^6	0
		Solid tumor	3×10^6	83
		Sponge matrix[2]	10×10^6	90
	Nude	Suspension	1×10^6	100
6134A-PRO	Normal	Suspension	50×10^6	0
		Solid tumor	3×10^6	67
		Sponge matrix	10×10^6	0
	Nude	Suspension	1×10^6	100
6132A-PRO	Normal	Suspension	50×10^6	0
		Solid tumor	3×10^6	90
		Sponge matrix	10×10^6	67
	Nude	Suspension	1×10^6	100
MC-GP	Normal	Suspension	2×10^6	0
		Solid tumor	$2-5 \times 10^6$	74

[1]Modified from [9] and [10], which also provide further details.
[2]Cultured tumor cells were injected into subcutaneously implanted polyurethane sponges.

One explanation may be that tumor cells in fragments have already adapted to growth *in vivo*, whereas cultured cells have not, leading to a higher percentage of growth for tumor fragments. However, enzymatically digested tumor fragments yielded a tumor cell suspension that when injected grew with the same poor efficiency as tumor cells grown *in vitro*, much more poorly than tumor cells embedded in stroma. Alternatively, the non-malignant stromal cells that surround the cancer cells in solid tumors may "protect" the cancer cells from recognition by cellular inflammatory reactions that would otherwise lead to destruction. In order to distinguish between these possibilities, suspended tumor cells were injected into subcutaneous polyurethane sponge implants. Table 1 shows that locating the cultured tumor cells inside a sponge matrix serving as a non-antigenic pseudostroma dramatically increased their tumorigenicity. Since the sponge matrix, or "pseudostroma" *per se* has no cells to influence the immune response, the results may suggest that stroma can act as a barrier to protect tumor cells from immune destruction and, therefore, improve the growth compared to growth of cells injected in suspension. (Suspended tumor cells are indeed eliminated by T-cell-mediated immune attack since much fewer (an order of magnitude) suspended tumor cells are needed to cause tumors in nude mice compared to the number of tumor cells needed to cause tumors in T-cell-competent mice.)

Non-malignant allografts that are rejected and malignant allografts that are accepted differ in the antigenicity of their stroma

Previous work had shown that parental regressor tumors are regularly rejected when transplanted into normal euthymic mice even at the largest possible tumor challenge [2]. However, if the host is immunologically manipulated by concurrent tumor burden of a progressor tumor variant, the regressor will be accepted and continue to grow once established even when the progressor tumor is surgically completely excised [11]. Interestingly, these mice bearing now the established regressor tumor will regularly reject a skin allograft within 10–14 days even though the skin allograft has the same rejection antigen as the tumor cells (Table 2 and [3] and [5]).

A simple explanation would be that the rapid proliferation of the cancer cells was responsible for the escape of the malignant allograft from immunological destruction. However, we think this explanation is probably incorrect since fetal colonic allografts consisting of very rapidly growing epithelial cells were also rejected completely even after forming pseudo-tumors [5].

T-cell exhaustion and systemic anergy do not explain the progressive growth of antigenic solid tumors

MHC Class I alloantigens that we used as model antigens present peptides derived from normal household proteins presented in the context of a syngeneic MHC Class I molecule. It is possible that the cellular concentration and pattern of expression of these peptides may differ between

Purnima Dubey, Lisa P. Seung and Hans Schreiber

TABLE 2. *Animals bearing malignant grafts reject normal grafts that express through gene transfer the same antigen.*

Host	K^{216} tumor burden	Type of tissue	Take of graft (%)	Survival of graft (days)
C3H	Yes	K^{216} tumor	100	—
		K^{216} skin	0	14
		K^{216} fetal heart	0	14
		K^{216} fetal gut	0	14
	No	K^{216} tumor	0	—
		K^{216} skin	0	13
		C57BL/6 skin	0	12
K^{216} C3H	No	K^{216} skin	100	>100
		K^{216} fetal heart	100	>100
		K^{216} fetal gut	100	>100

Modified from [5], which also provides further details.

TABLE 3. *L^d-positive skin is rejected by anti-L^d TCR transgenic mice bearing L^d-positive tumors: Neither T-cell exhaustion nor systemic anergy are responsible for the failure of tumor-bearing animals to reject the established antigenic tumors.*[1]

Host	Anti L^d TCR transgenic	Antibody treatment	L^{d+} tumor burden[2]	Type of tissue	Take of graft	Survival graft (d)
C3Hx2C	Yes	None	yes (early)	L^{d+} skin	0	15
		anti-CD4		L^{d+} skin	0	13
		anti-CD8		L^{d+} skin	100	>24
		None	yes(late)	L^{d+} skin	0	16
C3HxC57BL/6	No	None	yes (early)	L^{d+} skin	0	12

[1]Modified from [3] which also contains further details.
[2]Mice were bearing the L^d transfected AG104A tumor for 13 days at the time the skin was rejected ("early" tumor burden) or were bearing the tumors for 3 or 4 weeks ("late" tumor burden).

normal and malignant allografts. The consequence of such a difference may be that the tumor allografts may tolerize T-cell clones that recognize a certain combination of MHC and peptide prominent in malignant cells, while other T-cell clones that respond to a different MHC peptide combination of the same alloantigen may remain intact. Thus tolerance or exhaustion of T cells that respond to the antigen on tumors may spare the T-cell clones capable of destroying non-malignant allografts in the same host. To exclude this possibility, we used T-cell receptor transgenic mice reactive against a specific peptide presented on L^d as model antigen, because there is one predominant $CD8^+$ TCR clone type in these mice [3]. The results (Table 3) showed that the TCR transgenic mice rejected normal L^d expressing allografts while L^d expressing malignant tumors failed to be rejected. Thus neither exhaustion nor tolerance of the T cells by the malignant allograft seems to be the reason for the failure of the hosts to reject established solid antigenic cancers. We believe, instead, that the lack of antigenicity of the stroma of solid tumors accounts for their ability to grow while antigenic skin grafts are rejected.

Making tumor stroma immunogenic causes solid tumor fragments to be rejected

One of the principle differences between normal and malignant allografts is that the stroma of normal allografts is always antigenic whereas the stroma of cancers consists usually of normal syngeneic non-antigenic cells. In order to explore the possibility that antigenicity of the stroma helps the rejection process, solid cancers that either had allogenic or syngeneic stroma were generated. This could be done by transplanting 1591-PRO progressor tumor cells into either syngeneic mice or transgenic mice that expressed the same alloantigen as a transgene. When solid tumors formed in these mice, they developed either syngeneic or transgenic (antigenic) stroma. Thus, the tumor fragments consisted of malignant cells and stromal cells that expressed the alloantigen or syngeneic non-antigenic stromal cells. When these two types of solid progressor tumors were transplanted, only the tumors expressing the K^{216} antigen in the stroma, were rejected by normal or tumor-bearing immunocompetent mice (Table 4).

TABLE 4. *Antigenic bone-marrow-derived stromal cells can initiate the immunological destruction of antigenic cancer cells in solid tumors.*[1]

Outgrowth[2]		Stroma		1591-PRO tumor incidence[3]	
Host	Tumor burden	Non-bone-marrow-derived ("sessile")	Bone-marrow-derived ("mobile")	Mice with tumors/ mice challenged	(%)
K^{216}C3H	No	K^{216}C3H	K^{216}C3H	14/18	78
C3H		C3H	C3H	22/31	71
		K^{216}C3H	K^{216}C3H	6/38	16
C3H	Yes (late)	C3H	C3H	31/42	74
		K^{216}C3H	C3H	5/17	29
		C3H	K^{216}C3H	1/22	5

[1]Modified from [9] which also contains further details.
[2]Data pooled from four independent experiments.
[3]1591-PRO tumors that had grown in K^{216} and K^{216} chimeric, K^{216} transgenic or regular C3H/Hen mice "adopted" the stroma from these mice during tumor growth as indicated in the Table. In previous experiments, 1591-PRO regularly progresses in about 75% of normal mice upon transplantation of fragments grown in C3H/HeN mice but this tumor is still antigenic since mice can be immunized to reject this tumor.

Purnima Dubey, Lisa P. Seung and Hans Schreiber

In order to determine which part of the stroma, sessile (such as vessels) or mobile (such as bone-marrow-derived cells), would be most efficient, chimeric mice in which the bone marrow was either syngeneic or expressed the alloantigen as a transgene were generated. Solid tumors growing in these mice had therefore a chimeric stroma and were used for transplantation. The results showed that tumor-bearing mice could reject the solid tumor fragments when only the bone-marrow-derived cells in the stroma expressed the alloantigen, even when the sessile stromal components which make up the bulk of the stroma of the entire tumor were non-antigenic [9]. Having only the sessile stroma cells, antigenic also brought down the tumor incidence but less effectively than the bone-marrow-derived antigenic stromal cells.

Stromal cells attracted to tumor cells provide growth factors as part of a paracrine stimulatory loop

Heritable loss of the T-cell-recognized antigen seems to be the mechanism accounting for about one third of the escape variants we have studied, but there seems to be no loss of antigens or the presenting MHC Class I molecules that could explain the progressive nature of the remaining two-thirds of the progressor variants. It was found that each of these antigen-retention variants grew faster than the parental regressor tumors in T-cell-deficient mice [7,12]. Interestingly, escape from B-cell-dependent or NK-cell-mediated immunity is not the reason for the escape of the antigen retention variants since the parental regressor tumors do not grow faster in mice deficient in these cell types [7,12]. In order to determine whether the cell type that was normally restraining the growth of the parental regressor could be destroyed by gamma irradiation, nude mice were irradiated before tumor challenge [8]. Surprisingly, the regressor tumor did not grow faster. Instead, the progressor variant grew as slowly as the RE in unirradiated mice. In further experiments, progressor tumor cells were injected into a site protected from the whole-body X-ray to exclude a so-called tumor-bed-effect (for review see [8]). This name refers to the frequent observation that tumors do not grow well in previously irradiated tissues. Table 5 shows that whole body irradiation impeded the subsequent growth of the progressor tumor cells even when injected into the site (ear) that had been protected from X-ray. Together, these data suggest that a radiation-sensitive circulating component can help the growth of the progressor. Specific elimination of Gr-1-positive cells which include granulocytes by anti-Gr-1 antibody treatment had the same effect as pre-irradiation of mice: PRO tumors grew more slowly. Furthermore, elimination of Gr-1-positive cells lead to the rejection of progressor tumors by euthymic mice. One possible explanation for this result is that elimination of Gr-1-positive cells considerably slowed the growth of the tumor cells *in vivo* so that the normal immune system could eliminate the cancer cells [6]. Further experiments revealed that the progressor tumor variants attracted leukocytes in modified Boyden chambers much more effectively than the parental tumor cells, and growth of the variant cells was

TABLE 5. *Heritable progressor tumor variants that have retained the T-cell-recognized antigens attract bone-marrow-derived cells more effectively and are stimulated by these cells.*

Tumor line	Subcutaneous growth in euthymic mice		Subcutaneous growth in T-cell-deficient mice			Attraction of leukocytes *in vitro*	Stimulation of growth *in vitro* by leukocytes	Intraperitoneal growth		
	untreated	anti-GR-1 treated	No treatment	X-ray (shielded)	anti-GR-1			No Tx	antiGR-1	X-ray
4102-RE	0	0	+	+	+	+ +	−	+ +	+ +	+/−
-PRO	+ +	0	+ + +	+ +	+ +	+ + + +	+ + + +	+ + + +	+ +	+/−
6134A-RE	0	ND	+ +	ND	ND	+/−	+/−	+ +	+	ND
-PRO	+ +	ND	+ +	ND	ND	+ +	+ + + +	+ + +	+	ND

Results modified and compiled from [6–8].

Purnima Dubey, Lisa P. Seung and Hans Schreiber

stimulated in the presence of the leukocytes [7] unless the leukocytes had been activated by bacterial substances to a tumoricidal state. Pretreating mice with the anti-Gr-1 antibody markedly reduced the ability of the progressor variants to grow progressively in the peritoneal cavity of nude mice. Culturing the peritoneal exudate from mice challenged with PRO variants normally revealed large clusters of tumor cells surrounded by a large number of leukocytes while only few leukocytes surrounded the parental regressor.

Discussion

We have provided several lines of evidence indicating that stroma of solid cancers plays a critical role in determining whether antigenic cancers are rejected or grow progressively and kill the host. Loss of MHC Class I antigen expression, lack of co-stimulatory molecules, systemic immune suppression, immunological ignorance, peripheral tolerance, and clonal deletion or exhaustion may certainly contribute to the failure of antigen tumors to be rejected. However, for the tumors we have studied, none of these mechanisms seem to suffice to explain the failure of antigenic tumors to be rejected. Instead, we find that the non malignant stroma which is essential for any solid cancer to grow *in vivo* represents a powerful protector of antigenic cancer cells against immunological destruction. Thus, we think that the lack of antigenicity of the normal stromal components is a major determinant for the lack of rejection of malignant allografts and antigenic syngeneic solid tumors as well [9]. On the other hand, we show that antigenic bone-marrow-derived stromal cells are a powerful inducer of tumor rejection [9], and we also show that even non-antigenic bone-marrow-derived stromal cells can stimulate the growth of cancer cells [6]. Interestingly, others have contended that stromal alloantigen in non-malignant allografts (in particular vessels) is the primary and most important inducer, and target of allograft rejection [13]. At present, we do not know how tight the syngeneic stromal barrier can be to prevent rejection of the most antigenic cancer cells. It is noteworthy that solid tumor fragments of regressor tumors are rejected by normal syngeneic mice at any dose even though the antigenic regressor tumor cells in these fragments are embedded in normal syngeneic stroma. However, it is possible that RE tumor cells would escape immune destruction when situated in a fully vascularized established cancer.

It is tempting to postulate that stroma presents a physical barrier to immune destruction and that antigenic cancer cells can be camouflaged by non-antigenic stromal cells. This possibility is suggested by the finding that antigenic cancer cells injected into non-antigenic synthetic sponges *in vivo* grew more effectively. It is unclear to what extent this camouflage causes a complete ignorance of the host as has been postulated recently [10] and it needs to be examined to what extent mice from which tumors have been removed, either surgically or by tying off the blood supply, develop an immunity. Melanomas may be exceptional tumors with regards to the cytolytic T-cell immunity they can induce and with regards to the regression of individual metastatic lesions which is observed in a small percentage of patients. A reason for regression of melanoma lesions may be that, surprisingly, melanoma cells themselves can make vascular channels [14,15]. Therefore, circulating T cells may be exposed directly to antigenic vasculature similar to what occurs in allografts [13]. Growing melanomas in antigenic stroma experimentally can lead to growth retardation but eventually variants are selected that grow more aggressively [16].

Studies by Wick *et al.* [3] in 1997 showed that highly antigenic (alloantigen-transfected) tumor cells expressing co-stimulatory molecules B7.1 and CD48 failed to be rejected by CD8$^+$ anti-L^d TCR transgenic mice. These mice rejected concurrent non-malignant L^d-positive skin allografts. Rejection of these allografts was observed even in late tumor-bearing animals. This demonstrates clearly the importance of local factors at the tumor site in preventing a strong systemic immunity from destroying established antigenic cancers [16]. Another remarkable example for the failure of established antigenic solid tumors to be destroyed by the immune system is the failure of B7.1 and SV40 T antigen-expressing insulinomas to be rejected [17]. This failure persisted even when the abundance of SV-40-reactive T cells was increased by using anti-SV40-TCR transgenic mice [17]. Similarly, double transgenic mice develop antigenic insulinomas expressing the LCMV glycoprotein as well as SV40 T antigen under control of the insulin promoter; nevertheless, these mice are unable to induce or maintain an activated CD8$^+$ CTL response [18]. Since the antigens are expressed only by the parenchymal β cells, not the stroma (vessels, etc.), the conditions are similar to those of regular tumor cells that also grow in non-antigenic stroma. The malignant state of the tumor cells may not be essential for the local failure of immune destruction since the alloantigen expressed under control of the insulin promoter is also tolerated when expressed on normal β cells [19].

One of the major obstacles to generating an effective rejection response may be the lack of a stromal chemokine/cytokine environment in which destructive T-cell responses can develop. Tumor cells transfected to produce TGF-β fail to be rejected effectively whereas expression of TNFα at the site of alloantigen-expressing β cells "counteracts" the local tolerance and leads to β cell destruction [20]. We show that the presence of antigenic bone-marrow-derived cells, possibly dendritic cells, in the otherwise syngeneic tumor stroma can elicit a destructive T-cell-mediated response [9]. Antigenic stromal bone marrow cells, however, are not sufficient to cause rejection of any malignant cell embedded in such an antigenic stroma because the cancer cells embedded in the stroma must also be antigenic for tumor rejection to occur [9].

Non-antigenic bone-marrow-derived stromal cells not only protect the tumor from the T-cell-mediated responses but also stimulate the growth of solid cancers by several different mechanisms. First, every growing cancer

Purnima Dubey, Lisa P. Seung and Hans Schreiber

cell must establish a vascular supply once it grows beyond a few hundred micrometers in diameter. Macrophages are essential for angiogenesis and granulocytes are the major attractors of macrophages. The importance of Gr-1-positive cells which includes granulocytes and some monocytes in allowing tumor progression is evidenced by rejection of progressor tumors by mice treated with anti-Gr-1 antibody [6]. The number of Gr-1-positive cells in the spleen increases with progressive tumor growth and decreases following surgical tumor removal [21]. However, the role of these Gr-1-positive cells in preventing T-cell destruction of antigenic tumors is still unknown.

Tumor-bearing mice may fail to reject regressor tumors that are normally rejected by tumor-free mice [11,22]. However, even though this failure is obviously caused by a systemic alteration, it has been difficult for us and other groups to show that systemic depression of T-cell functions in these tumor-bearing mice is the main reason for the failure of tumor rejection [11,22,23] even though at later stages of tumor growth, systemic defects in T-cell signaling and function clearly can occur [24−26]. By contrast, B cells and antibodies are not affected and therefore may play an active role in causing the failure of tumor-bearing mice to reject regressor tumors. In particular, immunoglobulin gamma linked to TGF-β in collaboration with the Fc-receptor-positive bone-marrow-derived cell may play a central role in causing the failure of an effective local response [27−29]. In summary, we feel that there are three important goals along the difficult road leading to the immunological therapy of established solid cancers: (i) Identify and remove the cytokines produced by normal stromal cells that attract growth factors and stimulate angiogenesis, (ii) identify and counteract cells and factors that obstruct T-cell activation at the site of the tumor, and (iii) find new approaches to induce a local milieu that is conducive to the attraction of T cells to the tumor and maturation of these T cells at the local site.

Acknowledgement

This work was supported by National Institutes of Health grants RO1-CA-22677, RO1-CA-37516, and PO1-CA74182. The authors also gratefully acknowledge support by a gift from the Passis family.

References

1. Schreiber, H., in *Fund. Immunol.*, 4th ed., Paul, W.E. (ed,), pp 1247 1280, Lippincott Raven Press, New York, 1999.
2. Ward, P.L., Koeppen, H., Hurteau, T., and Schreiber, H., *J. Exp. Med.*, 170: 217−232, 1989.
3. Wick, M., Dubey, P., Koeppen, H., Siegel, C.T., Fields, P.E., Fitch, F.W., Chen, L., Bluestone, J.A., and Schreiber, H., *J. Exp. Med.*, 186: 229−237, 1997.
4. Stauss, H.J., Van Waes, C., Fink, M.A., Starr, B., and Schreiber, H., *J. Exp. Med.*, 164: 1516−1530, 1986.

5. Perdrizet, G.A., Ross, S.R., Stauss, H.J., Singh, S., Koeppen, H., and Schreiber, H., *J. Exp. Med.*, 171: 1205–1220, 1990.

6. Seung, L.P., Rowley, D.A., Dubey, P., and Schreiber, H., *Proc. Natl. Acad. Sci. USA.*, 92: 6254–6258, 1995.

7. Seung, L.P., Seung, S.K., and Schreiber, H., *Cancer Res.*, 55: 5094–5100, 1995.

8. Seung, L.P., Weichselbaum, R.R., Toledano, A., Schreiber, K., and Schreiber, H., *Radiat. Res.*, 146: 612–618, 1996.

9. Singh, S., Ross, S.R., Acena, M., Rowley, D.A., and Schreiber, H., *J. Exp. Med.*, 175: 139–146, 1992.

10. Ochsenbein, A.F., Klenerman, P., Karrer, U., Ludewig, B., Pericin, M., Hengartner, H., and Zinkernagel, R.M., *Proc. Natl. Acad. Sci. USA*, 96: 2233–2238, 1999.

11. Mullen, C.A., Rowley, D.A., and Schreiber, H., *Cell Immunol.*, 119: 101–113, 1989.

12. Pekarek, L.A., Starr, B.A., Toledano, A.Y., and Schreiber, H., *J. Exp. Med.*, 181: 435–440, 1995.

13. Pober, J.S., *Pathol. Biol. (Paris)*, 46: 159–163, 1998.

14. Maniotis, A.J., Folberg, R., Hess, A., Seftor, E.A., Gardner, L.M., Pe'er, J., Trent, J.M., Meltzer, P.S., and Hendrix, M.J., *Amer. J. Pathol.*, 155: 739–752, 1999.

15. Bissell, M.J., *Amer. J. Pathol.*, 155: 675–679, 1999.

16. Mintz, B., and Silvers, W.K., *Cancer Res.*, 56: 463–466, 1996.

17. Ganss, R., and Hanahan, D., *Cancer Res.*, 58: 4673–4681, 1998.

18. Speiser, D.E., Miranda, R., Zakarian, A., Bachmann, M.F., McKall-Faienza, K., Odermatt, B., Hanahan, D., Zinkernagel, R.M., and Ohashi, P.O., *J. Exp. Med.*, 186: 645–653, 1997.

19. Morahan, G., Allison, J., and Miller, J.F., *Nature*, 339: 622–624, 1989.

20. Ohashi, P.S., Oehen, S., Aichele, P., Pircher, H., Odermatt, B., Herrera, P., Higuchi, Y., Buerki, K., Hengartner, H., and Zinkernagel, R.M., *J. Immunol.*, 150: 5185–5194, 1993.

21. Salvadori, S., Martinelli, G., and Zier, K., *J. Immunol.*, 164: 2214–2220, 2000.

22. Mullen, C.A., Urban, J.L., Van Waes, C., Rowley, D.A., and Schreiber, H., *J. Exp. Med.*, 162: 1665–1682, 1985.

23. Radoja, S., Rao, T.D., Hillman, D., and Frey, A.B., *J. Immunol.*, 164: 2619–2628, 2000.

24. Mizoguchi, H., O'Shea, J.J., Longo, D.L., Loeffler, C.M., McVicar, D.W., and Ochoa, A.C., *Science*, 258: 1795–1798, 1992.

25. Horiguchi, S., Petersson, M., Nakazawa, T., Kanda, M., Zea, A.H., Ochoa, A.C., and Kiessling, R., *Cancer Res.*, 59: 2950–2956, 1999.

26. Whiteside, T.L., *Cancer Immunol. Immunother.*, 48: 346–352, 1999.

27. Rowley, D.A., and Stach, R.M., *Int. Immunol.*, 10: 355–363, 1998.

28. Stach, R.M., and Rowley, D.A., *J. Exp. Med.*, 178: 841–852, 1993.

29. Rowley, D.A., and Stach, R.M., *J. Exp. Med.*, 178: 835–840, 1993.

PETER FRIEDL, KERSTIN MAASER[a] AND EVA-B. BRÖCKER

Molecular mechanisms of melanoma cell motility and tissue invasion

———

Abstract

Melanoma invasion and metastasis result from a multi-step cascade involving adhesion receptors for cell motility and force generation as well as to focalized proteolysis of the extracellular matrix and path formation. In collagenous interstitial tissue, a predominant function was shown for $\alpha2\beta1$ integrins mediating melanoma cell attachment and migration, while penetration of basement membrane requires $\alpha6\beta1$ and $\alpha v\beta3$ integrins. CD44 functions are complex and involve both, the interaction with its ligand hyaluronan resulting in promigratory signals and survival as well as the capacity of CD44 to generate a pericellular coat that captures exogenous factors such as matrix proteinases and cytokines. To overcome spatial matrix barriers, melanoma cells express several matrix proteinases such as uPA[1], MMP-2, MMP-9 and MT1-MMP that facilitate matrix remodeling, the shedding of cell surface determinants, and migratory path generation. Consequently, experimental therapeutics comprise a broad spectrum of compounds that target integrin and matrix proteinase functions.

Keywords: Melanoma cell migration, extracellular matrix, adhesion receptors, proteolysis, experimental therapy

[1]The abbreviations used are: 3-D, three-dimensional; α-MSH, α-melanocyte-stimulating hormone; CS, chondroitin sulfate; ECM, extracellular matrix; FITC, fluorescein-isothiocyanate; HA, hyaluronan; LRSC, lissamine-rhodamine sulfonyl chloride; mAb, monoclonal antibody; MMP, matrix-metalloproteinase; MT-MMP, membrane-type matrix-metalloproteinase; PAI, plasminogen activator inhibitor; TGF, transforming growth factor; TIMP, tissue inhibitor of matrix metalloproteinases; tPA, tissue-type plasminogen activator; uPA, urokinase-type plasminogen activator; VEGF, vascular endothelial growth factor.

Cell Migration Laboratory, Department of Dermatology, University of Würzburg, Josef-Schneider-Str. 2, 97080 Würzburg, Germany, Phone: +49-931-2012737; Fax: +49-931-2012700; E-mail: Peter.fr@mail.uni-wuerzburg.de
[a]Present address: Department of Gastroenterology/Infectiology, Benjamin Franklin Clinics, Free University Berlin, Hindenburgdamm 30, 12200 Berlin, Germany

Introduction

Invasion through extracellular matrix (ECM) is part of a complex multi-step process leading to tumor cell motility and metastasis. The paradigm of tumor invasion and migration comprises a cascade of coordinated cell functions resulting in the disintegration of the cells from preexisting junctions, the degradation of tissue barriers such as basement membrane and interstitial tissue, and the generation of migratory force (reviewed in [1–3]). In addition, tumor invasion and survival are supported by angiogenesis induced by tumor-derived factors (reviewed in [4]). These events lead to profound reorganization of the adjacent extracellular matrix including the alignment of fibers and the generation of matrix paths of least resistance. This review will summarize molecular mechanisms established by melanoma cells for invasion and metastasis and highlight some selected experimental anti-invasive therapeutic strategies.

Adhesion receptors in melanoma invasion and metastasis

For interaction with and penetration through basement membranes and interstitial collagenous matrices, melanoma cells utilize different sets of adhesion receptors including integrins [5] and CD44 [6]. Basement membranes are flat layers composed of densely interconnected ECM components, including laminin, type IV collagen, heparin sulfate, entactin, fibronectin, and nidogen. In contrast, interstitial matrix consists of a 3-D fibrillar network build by types I and III collagen and interconnected hyaluronic acid, chondroitin sulfates, and other components. Basement membranes must be penetrated for vertical invasion or may serve as 2-D substrate for horizontal spreading; in contrast, interstitial matrix surrounding the tumor cell is invaded and transmigrated [3].

Integrins

Integrins are a family of $\alpha\beta$ heterodimers binding to extracellular matrix components at the outside of the cell and forming connections to intracellular effector proteins [7]. Integrins are multifunctional receptors mediating not only cell attachment to substrate and immobilization, but also cell spreading and migration [8], induction of gene expression, and the prevention of apoptosis. Upon engagement, integrins cluster at attachment sites and recruit multiple intracellular cytoskeletal proteins, such as α-actinin, talin, and filamin, as well as signaling proteins, including focal adhesion kinase and integrin-linked kinase [7,9,10]. Ultimately, integrins couple attachment complexes to the actin cytoskeleton through direct and indirect interaction with their cytoplasmic tails. Such supramolecular complexes were termed focal adhesions in the case of large and more stationary complexes or focal contacts, if smaller complexes of more

Peter Friedl, Kerstin Maaser and Eva-B. Bröcker

dynamic turn over are present [11]. In many cell types, the formation of focal adhesions or focal contacts is prerequisite for adhesion, spreading (i.e. the dynamic flattening on a ligand-coated surface), and migration on or through ECM ligand [3,12].

In dermal melanoma, integrin α2β1 represents the primary receptor for types I and III collagen, the most abundant ECM components in stromal tissues. Integrin α2β1 is barely expressed on non-neoplastic melanocytes, becomes up-regulated in dermal melanoma in the course of progression and, hence, was proposed as melanoma progression antigen [13]. α2β1 couples to members of the actin cytoskeleton [9,14,15] and is found in focal clusters in migrating melanoma cells [16]. α2β1 is further involved in transducing cytoskeletal action for melanoma cell migration on or through collagenous substrata [17−19] as well as in the contraction and remodeling of collagen lattices [20]. Therefore, α2β1 serves as the principal receptor for penetration of interstitial tissue and migration [3,19]. In melanoma cells, interaction with type I and III collagen can be further provided by integrins α1β1 and, in the case of denatured collagen, by αvβ3 [21], although the contribution of these interactions to migration remains unclear [19].

The penetration of the basement membrane by tumor cells is thought to involve a series of coordinate events [1,22] including receptor-mediated close interaction with the substrate, followed by proteolysis of basement membrane constituents, and migration through the newly formed matrix defect. In melanoma, integrins α3β1, α6β1, and newly expressed α7β1 mediate attachment to major basement membrane constituents laminin and type IV collagen [18,23−25]. The binding epitope recognized by these integrins contains an RGD sequence which is conserved among several extracellular matrix proteins; therefore, RGD-dependent integrin functions may favor an invasive phenotype in different tissue environments. The engagement of β1 integrins at the tip of melanoma cells leads to tyrosine phosphorylation of intracellular effector molecules including Rho-GAP which in turn promote pseudopod protrusion, the formation of "invadopo-dia" [26] and, ultimately, migration [27].

Besides integrins of the β1 family, expression of β3 integrins is predominant at zones of vertical melanoma invasion [28]. In metastatic melanoma lines, αvβ3 integrin is up-regulated by 50- to 100-fold, compared to melanocytes, and greatly favors the attachment to and migration across laminin, fibronectin, vitronectin, and reconstituted basement membrane [29,30]. Furthermore, αvβ3 binds to and activates matrix-degrading matrix metalloproteinase-2 (MMP-2) which in turn contributes to the reorganization of the extracellular matrix in areas of invasion [31]. Because αvβ3 integrins prevent apoptosis in tumor cells and because these integrins are further required for endothelial cell sprouting and tumor-related angiogenesis, αvβ3 is considered as major candidate receptors for adjuvant treatment of melanoma and other tumors [32].

Upon stimulation with autocrine motility factor as well as activation of protein kinase C, integrin αIIbβ3 is up-regulated in melanoma cells. αIIbβ3 mediates adhesion and spreading on fibronectin or vitronectin and enhances the invasion of reconstituted basement membranes [33,34]. Other integrins, most notably $\alpha4\beta1$ and $\alpha5\beta1$ interacting with fibronectin, reduce the tumorigenicity of cultured tumor cells [35,36], presumably by increasing pericellular fibronectin matrix assembly and migration arrest.

The striking multiplicity in integrin—ligand recognition complicates the establishment of a conclusive picture of the invasive cascade in melanoma. In particular, the molecular hierarchy of simultaneously engaged adhesion receptors and the degree of functional compensation by alternative receptor—ligand pairs, once one set of receptors is blocked, require further investigation and will help to establish the relative importance of various integrins at different stages of tumor progression.

CD44

CD44 comprises a multifunctional family of adhesion receptors interacting with hyaluronan as principal ligand and, at lower affinity, to chondroitin sulfate, heparan sulfate, fibronectin, and osteopontin [6,37]. CD44 couples to the actin-based cytoskeleton via ankyrin and members of the ezrin/radixin/moesin family of adapter proteins (reviewed in [38]). Overexpression of alternatively spliced CD44 variants appears to correlate with the aggressiveness and metastasis of various solid tumors [39]. CD44 functions as a signaling receptor inducing cell survival and proliferation. Furthermore, CD44 can capture exogenous cytokines, growth factors, and matrix proteinases favoring cell penetration into the extracellular matrix. A thick pericellular CD44 coat may protect tumor cells from immunological assault as well as anoikis (programmed cell death induced by contact with inappropriate environment, e.g. ECM) [38]. In melanoma, precise information on CD44 function are sparse. *In vitro*, CD44 or CD44v10 interaction with hyaluronan induces melanoma cell motility [40,41], putatively via promigratory signaling or by favoring cell detachment. Similarly CD44-CS, a glycosylated CD44 variant containing chondroitin-6-sulfate residues, collaborates with $\alpha2$ integrins and mediates migration on type I collagen [42], laminin, type IV collagen, and reconstituted basement membrane [43].

Despite these promigratory CD44 functions on isolated ECM substrate, attempts to detect invasion- or motility-promoting CD44 effects in 3-D *in vitro* tissues or *in vivo* models have failed so far. In melanoma cells penetrating 3-D matrices, CD44 is excluded from focal contacts [16] and does not directly contribute to migration [19]; however, CD44 is deposited into cell-derived matrix paths [27] and, hence, may modulate the migration of other cells (C. Mayer and P. Friedl, unpublished). *In vivo* experiments using genetic strategies in lymphosarcoma or pancreatic carcinoma cells have shown that disruption of CD44 function does not diminish tissue penetration and invasion [44,45], while other functions such as survival or proliferation greatly depend on the presence of CD44 [38]. Taking these negative findings into account, CD44 functions are likely to result from

Peter Friedl, Kerstin Maaser and Eva-B. Bröcker

activatory signaling rather than its function as a "classical" adhesion receptor transducing traction force from and to the cytoskeleton.

Other receptors

Carbohydrate receptors expressed by melanoma cells are associated with tumor progression and metastasis, although the mechanism of action remains unclear. Galectin-3 is a cell surface receptor for poly-N-acetyllactosamine carbohydrate residues present in basement membrane components (e.g. laminin). After crosslinking, galectin-3 mediates melanoma cell spreading on laminin [46]. Expression of helix pomatia agglutinin (HPA), which interacts with N-acetyl-galactosamine results in greatly increased invasion of reconstituted basement membrane [47].

Two additional receptors were identified as to favor metastasis formation at the level of transendothelial migration, once the circulation is reached. The CD146 antigen, also designated MUC18 or MCAM, is a member of the immunoglobulin superfamily. The expression of CD146 positively correlates with tumor progression [48]. CD146 mediates cell-cell interaction by binding to an unidentified ligand on endothelial cells [49]. Similarly, ICAM-1 which is expressed at increased levels in metastatic melanoma cells but is also present in benign naevi [50] interacts with LFA-1 expressed on blood vessel endothelium, thereby potentially contributing to distant metastasis.

Invasion and remodeling of the extracellular matrix

The mechanisms of how such different receptor-mediated processes are integrated towards coordinated migratory action and how tumor cells remove tissue barriers without losing adhesive contact to the ECM have been recognized only recently (reviewed in [3]). Tumor cells in conjunction with resident stromal cells express a variety of matrix proteinases required for reconstruction of adjacent normal tissue to allow tumor cell dissemination and neovascularization.

Remodeling of the ECM and generation of matrix paths

In 3-D tissues, this invasion process requires an interplay of matrix fiber traction and remodeling [51], resulting in contact guidance and facilitated directional migration [52,53]. Because the size of tumor cells is frequently larger than the spaces present in the extracellular tissue matrix, cells must develop strategies to generate force as well as weaken the resistance provided by matrix fibers. It now appears that some if not most of the cells established from solid tumors generate pronounced traction and reorganization zones within ECM by pulling fibers at cell extensions towards the cell body (Fig. 1). These interactions are provided by α2β1 integrins coupled to the actin cytoskeleton. In 3-D collagen lattices, the invasion of melanoma cells from solid spheroids leads to the radiary realignment of previously random collagen fibers (Fig. 1, bottom) and the migration of the cells along

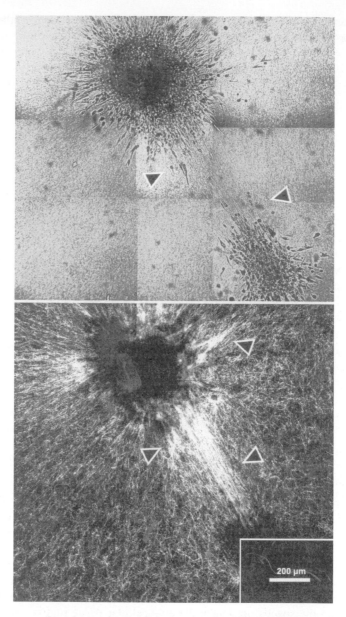

FIGURE 1. *Invasion and migration-associated matrix remodeling in melanoma spheroids cultured in three-dimensional collagen lattices. Highly invasive MV3 melanoma cells were cultured as spheroids and incorporated into 3-D collagen lattices. The extent of invasion was detected by bright field microscopy (top) and confocal reflection contrast microscopy [54]. After 24 hours, migrating MV3 melanoma cells have detachted from the spheroid (top, arrows) accompanied by profound radiary alignment of collagen fibers (bottom, arrowheads). Non-invaded collagen matrix displays lack of fiber traction and random fiber texture. Images are composed of multiple individual frames.*

Peter Friedl, Kerstin Maaser and Eva-B. Bröcker

these bundles (Fig. 1, top). These structural alterations observed in 3-D collagen lattices are reminiscent of reorganized stromal tissue directly adjacent to melanoma invasion zones *in vivo*, as characterized by increased type I collagen fiber density [55]. Such invasion-associated matrix remodeling is consequence of at least three interdependent processes: (1) traction mediated by integrins and cytoskeletal forces, (2) focalized lysis and re-bundling of collagen fibers resulting in tube-like matrix defects, and (3) the deposition of vast amounts of cell surface determinants and secreted ECM components onto fibers bordering these defects [16,27]. All of these events can be blocked by anti-integrin antibodies suggesting that adhesion is interconnected with migration-associated reorganization of the extracellular matrix as prerequisites for tissue penetration and path generation [2].

Function of matrix proteinases

Matrix metalloproteinases are a large family of zink-dependent proteinases, that can act as soluble enzymes but also function as membrane-anchored enzyme-receptor complexes [51,56]. Most MMPs and their physiological endogenous inhibitors TIMPs are secreted as soluble factors. Some MMP (pro)enzymes are then redirected towards the cell surface by specific receptors, including MT-MMPs and integrins. After binding of pro-MMP-2 to a complex of MT1-MMP and TIMP-2 at the cell surface, the ternary MT1-MMP/TIMP-2/MMP-2 complex leads to MMP-2 activation and ECM substrate degradation [57]. Similarly, MMP-2 can be bound and activated by $\alpha v\beta 3$ integrin [31]. The substrate specificity of MMPs includes most if not all ECM components as well as some growth factors and cell surface receptors [51].

In the course of melanoma progression, several MMPs including MMP-1 (collagenase-1), MMP-2 (72 kD gelatinase), MT1-MMP (collagenase-3), MMP-9 (92 kD gelatinase), as well as TIMP-1, -2 and -3 can be expressed at increased levels [58−60]. Most of these enzymes are detected in melanoma cells as well as surrounding stromal cells, in particular fibroblasts and macrophages [58].

MMP-2 appears as a major proinvasive candidate proteinase in melanoma progression [60]. In general, baseline MMP-2 expression in invasive and non-invasive melanoma cell lines can vary from low to high levels [59,61]. In metastatic melanoma cell lines, however, crosslinking and engagement of $\alpha 2\beta 1$ or $\alpha v\beta 3$ integrins by their respective multivalent ligands collagen and vitronectin leads to the up-regulation of MT1-MMP, MMP-2 and TIMP-2 as well as to increased invasiveness through filters coated with reconstituted basement membrane [60−63] and *in vivo* invasion after subcutaneous implantation into nude mice [59]. Similarly, crosslinking of CD44 by mAb (not however the natural CD44 ligand hyaluronan) increases MMP-2 expression and melanoma cell migration through reconstituted basement membrane or collagen [64]. After binding to the cell surface, MMP-2 containing receptor complexes are redistributed to prominent cell edges interacting with ECM, termed invadopodia, promoting the degradation of fibronectin or collagen [65] (K. Wolf and P. Friedl, in preparation). The presence and activation of MMP-2, if expressed at high levels in metastatic cell lines correlates well with increased invasiveness and metastasis after subcutaneous injection into nude mice, as compared to cell lines expressing low MMP-2 levels [59,60]. The importance of the proteolytic function of MMP-2 in melanoma cells is underlined by studies using TIMP-2, the physiological MMP-2 inhibitor. *In vitro*, addition of TIMP-2 to melanoma cells reduces their proteolytic capacity as well as integrin-dependent adhesion and spreading [66], suggesting common pathways between integrins and MMPs. *In vivo*, TIMP-2 overexpression reduces invasion and angiogenesis in murine melanoma [67].

Soluble environmental factors such as cytokines released from tumor cells or the surrounding tumor stroma further contribute to tumor invasion and tissue penetration. TGF-β1 secreted by melanoma cells coordinately up-regulates β1 and β3 integrin expression as well as MMP-9 and also favors a spindle shaped, hence migratory phenotype [68]. Similarly, interleukin-8 leads to the up-regulation and activation of MMP-2, favoring invasion through filters coated with reconstituted basement membrane [69]. ProMMP-1 expressed by melanoma cells is activated by soluble fibroblast-derived MMP-3 or other enzymes to mediate melanoma cell invasion into 3-D type I collagen lattices [70].

In addition to MMPs, various cysteine and serine proteinases promote melanoma progression and metastasis (reviewed in [71,72]). These proteinases comprise, among others, urokinase-type plasminogen activator (uPA) and cathepsins mediating the degradation of extracellular matrix components, including fibronectin and basement membrane components [73]. Furthermore, uPA catalyzes the proteolytic cleavage of plasminogen, which is ubiquitously present in body fluids, to plasmin. In its active form, plasmin is a multifunctional serine proteinase that degrades multiple ECM components including type IV collagen, laminin, and fibronectin [74]. Plasmin activation requires the binding of uPA to its membrane-anchored receptor, uPAR, a mechanism leading to the focalization of matrix-degrading enzymatic activity near the cell surface [72]. Besides mediating tissue degradation, uPA and uPAR also regulate cell adhesion to ECM. The functions of uPA are counteracted by endogenous inhibitors PAI-1 and PAI-2, however their precise role in regulating uPA/uPAR interaction and function remain to be determined.

In cutaneous melanoma the expression of uPA and tissue-type plasmino-gen activator (tPA) are up-regulated, correlating with melanoma-associated degradation of ECM [75] and progression [76]. High level expression and enzymatic function of uPA are further positively correlated with melanoma cell proliferation and growth *in vitro* and *in vivo* [75,77]. A positive effect of uPA was shown for *in vitro* invasion of melanoma cells, such as migration through reconstituted basement membranes [78]. However, in more complex *in vitro* and *in vivo* invasion models, contradictory effects of the uPA/uPAR

Peter Friedl, Kerstin Maaser and Eva-B. Bröcker

system have been reported for melanoma. Both positive as well as negative effects of uPA are present in melanoma invasion into amnionic membrane [79,80] or *in vivo* progression and metastasis [81,82].

Because the net amount of uPA secreted by melanoma cells is not directly correlated with invasion and metastasis [83], the precise mechanism appears to reside in a tightly regulated program in proximity to the cell surface, including both positive and negative regulators. A positive role for uPA in melanoma invasion is underlined by data on melanoma cell invasion and metastasis in mice showing considerable inhibitory effects after transfection of PAI-1 or PAI-2 [81,84], putatively resulting from an induction of a tumor capsule. On the other hand, *in vitro* studies have suggested that PAI favors melanoma cell migration by reducing binding strength to vitronectin [85]. In this model, exogenous soluble uPA can bind to its receptor uPAR and mediate firm attachment on vitronectin, thereby counteracting migration [85].

Recent results from uPA knockout mice indicate that uPA expressed by both melanoma cells themselves and the surrounding stromal cells is important for melanoma metastasis. While local growth and protrusion towards dermal layers occurs independent of uPA, melanoma cell detachment and dissemination towards regionary lymphatic nodes is dependent on uPA expression [86]. UPA was implicated in the initial changes in matrix architecture by degradation of ECM glycoproteins, which then could be degraded more efficiently by MMPs [87]. More indirect functions of uPA such as tumor-induced angiogenesis or the liberation of growth factors may further contribute to *in vivo* invasion [86,88]. In addition, melanocyte-derived cytokines, such as IL-4, can induce the secretion of uPA and matrilysin in neighboring epithelial cells [89]. Because these above findings were established in different models by using melanoma cells from different origin and function, it remains to be established how these putative pro- and anti-invasive uPA/uPAR functions are orchestrated in a given tissue environment to contribute to melanoma progression and metastasis.

Other proteinases such as the gelatinolytic separase can bind $\alpha 3\beta 1$ integrin located at invadopodia of melanoma cells [90]. CD13/aminopeptidase N, a transmembrane proteinase with type IV collagen-degrading activity expressed in melanoma cells, further contributes to the degradation of ECM components [91] and facilitates melanoma cell penetration though reconstituted basement membrane [92].

These and other results strongly suggest that the collaboration of integrins with matrix degrading enzymes at the cell surface result in highly localized and tightly regulated degradation of the extracellular matrix in close proximity to the cell boundary and focal adhesion sites [51].

Melanoma-induced angiogenesis

Cutaneous melanomas are highly vascularized tumors, and the degree of angiogenesis is positively correlated with melanoma progression and metastasis [93]. Melanoma cells secrete various cytokines that induce endothelial cell sprouting, migration, and the formation of new vessels. The sprouting of new vessels requires αv integrins [93] as well as the function of uPA [88] and MMPs, most notably MMP-2 [94]. Angiogenesis-promoting factors released by melanoma cells include IL-8 [69], VEGF [95], and angiogenin [95], the latter two factors particularly after induction by hypoxia. In situ, the expression of IL-8 and angiogenin in primary melanoma as well as lymph node metastasis is located in vicinity to necrotic zones as well as small vessels [95]. Hence, angiogenic factors provide both, close approximation of blood vessels and tumor cells for facilitated spread coupled to an increased delivery of nutrients for melanoma cell survival and proliferation.

Ocular melanoma

In principle, ocular melanoma cells may develop similar invasion and matrix degrading mechanisms as established for cutaneous melanoma. In histopathological sections from uveal melanoma, extensive local invasion is present in more than 80% of the samples; these invasive events include penetration of the Bruch's membrane containing elastic and collagenous fibers (88%) and invasion into the cell-rich retina (50%), vortex veins (9%), and emissary channels (55%) [96].

As a major difference to cutaneous melanoma, no epithelial basement membrane must be traversed by uveal melanoma cells, and laminin receptors are rarely detected [97]. Similar to dermal melanoma, integrins interacting with interstitial ECM are detected in uveal melanoma. In cultured retinal pigment cells, α2β1 integrin is expressed and mediates the contraction of collagen matrices [98], suggesting its function in uveal melanoma. Likewise, plasminogen activators contribute to uveal melanoma metastasis to liver and other organs in a nude mouse model [99]. In humans, the expression of MMP-2 in the cytoplasm of uveal melanoma cells *in vivo* is correlated with poorer prognosis [100], indicating a function of MMP-2 in uveal melanoma dissemination and metastasis.

Experimental therapy

Experimental strategies that target different steps of the invasive process include integrin antagonists, proteinase inhibitors, and adjuvant modulators of proinvasive cofactors. RGD-analogs inhibit integrin-mediated melanoma cell adhesion towards fibronectin and laminin, the *in vitro* invasion and migration through reconstituted basement membrane [101] as well as the spontaneous metastasis in the murine B16 melanoma model [102]. Other anti-adhesive and/or anti-invasive agents include glycosphingolipids [103], protein-bound polysaccharide [104], synthetic YISGR peptide inhibiting melanoma interaction with laminin [105], and a peptide containing amino acids 531−543 from type IV collagen blocking integrin α3β1 function

[106]. Inhibitors of serine proteinases, such as angiostatin which blocks plasmin activation via tPA, inhibit melanoma invasion *in vitro* and *in vivo*, reduce melanoma-induced neovascularization [88,107], and metastasis at distant sites [81,84], although strikingly negative results have been reported as well [82]. Inhibition of plaminogen activators in uveal melanoma using adenovirus gene transfer in nude mice results in greatly reduced overall metastasis and colonization of the liver [99] and suggest a role of uPA in the penetration of tissue barriers. Overexpression of TIMP-2 markedly reduces melanoma growth in the skin of nude mice, although the number of distant metastases is not affected [108]. Similarly, the broad-spectrum MMP inhibitor batimastat does not affect melanoma cell extravasation and spread, but rather inhibits the growth of metastases by impairing angiogenesis [109].

Other compounds were shown to reduce the invasive capacity of melanoma cells by diverse mechanisms. Retinoic acid, a differentiation-inducing agent in dedifferentiated cells, leads to reduced expression of MMPs and uPA [70,110,111]. Furthermore, retinoids increase the expression of β3 integrin vitronectin receptor [112] and TIMP-1 and TIMP-2 [70], favor the formation of stress fibers [113], and reduce melanoma cell motility on ECM substrate [110]. Because stabilization of stress fiber and focal adhesions favor adhesive behavior and counteract motility (reviewed in [3]), retinoic acid may function as adjuvant anti-invasive agent. A similar mechanism was described for adriamycin-induced stabilization of focal adhesions favoring attachment and arresting migration of melanoma cells on laminin, type IV collagen, and reconstituted basement membrane [114].

α-Melanocyte-stimulating hormone (α-MSH) affects melanoma cell adhesion to fibronectin and laminin, reduces the expression of MMP-2 and MMP-9, and inhibits invasion into reconstituted basement membrane [115]. Calmodulin antagonists such as tamixifen or a specific inhibitor, J8, inhibit the invasion of dermal and uveal melanoma cells through a fibronectin layer [116]. Similarly, the calcium-antagonist verapamil disrupts intracellular microfilament assembly and melanoma cell motility, which is accompanied by reduced type IV collagenase expression [117].

While many of these pharmacological interventions function well in two-dimensional migration utilizing isolated receptor-ligand interaction models, it remains to be established how these findings are translated to *in vivo* functions of melanoma cells. In addition, although some *in vitro* and *in vivo* studies have suggested promising anti-invasive and metastasis-inhibiting function of these compounds, no clinical trials on melanoma have been reported so far. In mice bearing epithelial tumors, broad spectrum MMP inhibitors result in potent inhibition of tumor induced angiogenesis, primary tumor growth, and metastasis [118]. Synthetic inhibitors of MMPs have entered the stage of clinical trial in epithelial cancer and preliminary results indicate that these compounds may be effective in slowing tumor growth. To result in efficient treatment, anti-invasive drugs would require application for prolonged time periods coupled to a lack of severe side effects. A conceptual obstacle, however, might reside in the broad spectrum of integrin- and MMP-mediated processes in homeostasis and regeneration, such as immune function and wound healing.

Conclusions

While the function of MMPs and adhesion receptors in tumor invasion are well established, few new promising therapeutic concepts have emerged so far for melanoma. Further investigations will have to dissect mechanisms that distinguish tumor invasion strategies from motility mechanisms utilized by other cells, in particular leukocytes (in the process of immune defense) and fibroblasts (for wound healing). The finding that $\alpha 2\beta 1$ integrin-mediated mechanisms are used by melanoma cells and not, however, by T lymphocytes for migration in 3-D tissue [12,119] may uphold the concept that integrin antagonists might be useful as future anti-metastatic agents without impairing immune cell trafficking and recirculation. Such anti-invasive therapy may be useful in patients undergoing extensive non-curative surgery as well as palliative adjuvant treatment in stage IV melanoma. In conclusion, a combination of integrin antagonists and proteinase inhibitors might emerge as suitable approaches for further therapy of metastasizing tumor disease.

Acknowledgments

The authors thank Kurt S. Zänker, Institute of Immunology, University of Witten/ Herdecke for encouragement and continuous support of these studies. We also thank Katarina Wolf for correction of the manuscript and helpful discussions. The Cell Migration Laboratory is supported by the Deutsche Forschungsgemeinschaft, the Wilhelm-Sander-Foundation, the Bundesministerium für Bildung, Forschung und Technologie, and the Verein für Biologische Krebsabwehr.

References

1. Liotta, L.A., Rao, C.N., and Wewer, U.M., *Annu. Rev. Biochem.* 55: 1037, 1986.
2. Friedl, P., Bröcker, E.B., and Zänker, K.S., *Cell Adhes. Commun.* 6: 225, 1998.
3. Friedl, P., and Bröcker, E.-B., *Cell. Mol. Life Sci.* in press.
4. Hanahan, D., and Folkman, J., *Cell* 86: 353, 1996.
5. Danen, E.H., van Muijen, G.N., ten Berge, P.J., and Ruiter, D.J., *Recent Res. Cancer Res.* 128: 119, 1993.
6. Lesley, J., Hyman, R., English, N., Catterall, J.B., and Turner, G.A., *Glycoconjugate J.* 14: 611, 1997.
7. Yamada, K.M., and Geiger, B., *Curr. Opin. Cell Biol.* 9: 76, 1997.
8. Huttenlocher, A., Sandborg, R.R., and Horwitz, A.F., *Curr. Opin. Cell Biol.* 7: 697, 1997.
9. Reszka, A.A., Hayashi, Y., and Horwitz, A.F., *J. Cell Biol.* 117: 1321, 1992.

10. Schaller, M.D., Otey, C.A., Hildebrand, J.D., and Parsons, J.T., *J. Cell Biol.* 130: 1181, 1995.
11. Burridge, K., and Chrzanowska-Wodicka, M., *Annu. Rev. Cell Dev. Biol.* 12: 463, 1996.
12. Friedl, P., Zänker, K.S., and Bröcker, E.B., *Microsc. Res. Techniq.* 43: 369, 1998.
13. Klein, C.E., Steinmayer, T., Kaufmann, D., Weber, L., and Bröcker, E.B., *J. Invest. Dermatol.* 96: 281, 1991.
14. Haas, T.A., and Plow, E.F., *Protein Eng.* 10: 1395, 1997.
15. Kieffer, J.D., Plopper, G., Ingber, D.E., Hartwig, J.H., and Kupper, T.S., *Biochem. Biophys. Res. Commun.* 217: 466, 1995.
16. Friedl, P., Maaser, K., Klein, C.E., Niggemann, B., Krohne, G., and Zänker, K.S., *Cancer Res.* 57: 2061, 1997.
17. Etoh, T., Thomas, L., Pastel-Levy, C., Colvin, R.B., Mihm, M.C., Jr., and Byers, H.R., *J. Invest. Dermatol.* 100: 640, 1993.
18. Danen, E.H., Van Muijen, G.N., Van de Wiel-van Kemenade, E., Jansen, K.F., Ruiter, D.J., and Figdor, C.G., *Int. J. Cancer* 54: 315, 1993.
19. Maaser, K., Wolf, K., Klein, C.E., Niggemann, B., Zänker, K.S., Bröcker, E.-B., and Friedl, P., *Mol. Biol. Cell* 10: 3067, 1999.
20. Klein, C.E., Dressel, D., Steinmacher, T., Mauch, C., Eckes, B., Krieg, T., Bankert, R., and Weber, L., *J. Cell Biol.* 115: 1427, 1991.
21. Montgomery, A.M., Reisfeld, R.A., and Cheresh, D.A., *Proc. Natl. Acad. Sci. U.S.A.* 91: 8856, 1994.
22. Liotta, L.A., Stetler-Stevenson, W.G., and Steeg, P.S., *Cancer Invest.* 9: 543, 1991.
23. Chelberg, M.K., Tsilibary, E.C., Hauser, A.R., and McCarthy, J.B., *Cancer Res.* 49: 4796, 1989.
24. Kramer, R.H., Vu, M., Cheng, Y.F., and Ramos, D.M., *Cancer Metast. Rev.* 10: 49, 1991.
25. Lauer, J.L., Gendron, C.M., and Fields, G.B., *Biochemistry* 37: 5279, 1998.
26. Nakahara, H., Mueller, S.C., Nomizu, M., Yamada, Y., Yeh, Y., and Chen, W.T., *J. Biol. Chem.* 273: 9, 1998.
27. Friedl, P., and Bröcker, E.-B., in *Extracellular Matrix and Groundregulation System in Health and Disease*, Heine, H. and Rimpler, M. (eds.), pp. 7–18, Gustav Fischer Publ., Stuttgart, 1997.
28. Albelda, S.M., Mette, S.A., Elder, D.E., Stewart, R., Damjanovich, L., Herlyn, M., and Buck, C.A., *Cancer Res.* 50: 6757, 1990.
29. Filardo, E.J., Brooks, P.C., Deming, S.L., Damsky, C., and Cheresh, D.A., *J. Cell Biol.* 130: 441, 1995.
30. Li, X., Chen, B., Blystone, S.D., McHugh, K.P., Ross, F.P., and Ramos, D.M., *Invas. Metast.* 18: 1, 1998.
31. Brooks, P.C., Stromblad, S., Sanders, L.C., von Schalscha, T.L., Aimes, R.T., Stetler-Stevenson, W.G., Quigley, J.P., and Cheresh, D.A., *Cell* 85: 683, 1996.
32. Friedlander, M., Brooks, P.C., Shaffer, R.W., Kincaid, C.M., Varner, J.A., and Cheresh, D.A., *Science* 270: 1500, 1995.
33. Timar, J., Trikha, M., Szekeres, K., Bazaz, R., Tovari, J., Silletti, S., Raz, A., and Honn, K.V., *Cancer Res.* 56: 1902, 1996.
34. Trikha, M., Timar, J., Lundy, S.K., Szekeres, K., Cai, Y., Porter, A.T., and Honn, K.V., *Cancer Res.* 57: 2522, 1997.
35. Qian, F., Vaux, D.L., and Weissman, I.L., *Cell* 77: 335, 1994.

36. Ruoslahti, E., *Kidney Int.* 51: 1413, 1997.
37. Herrlich, P., Sleeman, J., Wainwright, D., Konig, H., Sherman, L., Hilberg, F., and Ponta, H., *Cell Adhes. Commun.* 6: 141, 1998.
38. Knudson, W., *Front. Biosci.* 3: 604, 1998.
39. Sherman, L.S., Sleeman, J., Herrlich, P., and Ponta, H., *Curr. Opin. Cell Biol.* 6: 726, 1994.
40. Goebeler, M., Kaufmann, D., Bröcker, E.B., and Klein, C.E., *J. Cell Sci.* 109: 1957, 1996.
41. Yoshinari, C., Mizusawa, N., Byers, H.R., and Akasaka, T., *Melanoma. Res.* 9: 223, 1999.
42. Faassen, A.E., Mooradian, D.L., Tranquillo, R.T., Dickinson, R.B., Letourneau, P.C., Oegema, T.R., and McCarthy, J.B., *J. Cell Sci.* 105: 501, 1993.
43. Knutson, J.R., Iida, J., Fields, G.B., and McCarthy, J.B., *Mol. Biol. Cell* 7: 383, 1996.
44. Driessens, M.H., Stroeken, P.J., Rodriguez Erena, N.F., Van der Valk, M.A., Van Rijthoven, E.A., and Roos, E., *J. Cell Biol.* 131: 1849, 1995.
45. Sleeman, J.P., Arming, S., Moll, J.F., Hekele, A., Rudy, W., Sherman, L.S., Kreil, G., Ponta, H., and Herrlich, P., *Cancer Res.* 56: 3134, 1996.
46. Van den Brule, F.A., Buicu, C., Baldet, M., Sobel, M.E., Cooper, D.N., Marschal, P., and Castronovo, V., *Biochem. Biophys. Res. Commun.* 209: 760, 1995.
47. Rye, P.D., Fodstad, O., Emilsen, E., and Bryne, M., *Int. J. Cancer* 75: 609, 1998.
48. Johnson, J.P., Rummel, M.M., Rothbacher, U., and Sers, C., *Curr. Top. Microbiol. Immunol.* 213: 95, 1996.
49. Shih, L.M., Hsu, M.Y., Palazzo, J.P., and Herlyn, M., *Am. J. Pathol.* 151: 745, 1997.
50. Hansen, N.L., Ralfkiaer, E., Hou-Jensen, K., Thomsen, K., Drzewiecki, K.T., Rothlein, R., and Vejlsgaard, G.L., *Acta Derm-Venereol.* 71: 48, 1991.
51. Murphy, G., and Gavrilovic, J., *Curr. Opin. Cell Biol.* 11: 614, 1999.
52. Boocock, C.A., *Development* 107: 881, 1989.
53. Barocas, V.H., and Tranquillo, R.T., *J. Biomech. Eng.* 119: 137, 1997.
54. Friedl, P., and Bröcker, E.B., in *Image Analysis and Reconstruction in Biology*, Häder, D.P. (ed.) CRC Press, New York, in press.
55. Van Duinen, C.M., Fleuren, G.J., and Bruijn, J.A., *Histopathology* 24: 33, 1994.
56. Heino, J., *Int. J. Cancer* 65: 717, 1996.
57. Strongin, A.D., Collier, I., Bannikov, G., Marmer, B.L., Grant, G.A., and Goldberg, G.I., *J. Biol. Chem.* 270: 5331, 1995.
58. Airola, K., Karonen, T., Vaalamo, M., Lehti, K., Lohi, J., Kariniemi, A.L., Keski-Oja, J., and Saarialho-Kere, U.K., *Br. J. Cancer* 80: 733, 1999.
59. Hofmann, U.B., Westphal, J.R., Waas, E.T., Zendman, A.J., Cornelissen, I.M., Ruiter, D.J., and Van Muijen, G.N., *Br. J. Cancer* 81: 774, 1999.
60. Hofmann, U.B., Westphal, J.R., Waas, E.T., Zendman, A.J., Becker, J.C., Ruiter, D.J., and Van Muijen, G.N., *J. Pathol.* in press.
61. Kurschat, P., Zigrino, P., Nischt, R., Breitkopf, K., Steurer, P., Klein, C.E., Krieg, T., and Mauch, C., *J. Biol. Chem.* 274: 21056, 1999.
62. Seftor, R.E., Seftor, E.A., Gehlsen, K.R., Stetler-Stevenson, W.G., Brown, P.D., Ruoslahti, E., and Hendrix, M.J., *Proc. Natl. Acad. Sci. U.S.A.* 89: 1557, 1992.
63. Bafetti, L.M., Young, T.N., Itoh, Y., and Stack, M.S., *J. Biol. Chem.* 273: 143, 1998.

64. Takahashi, K., Eto, H., and Tanabe, K.K., *Int. J. Cancer* 80: 387, 1999.
65. Nakahara, H., Howard, L., Thompson, E.W., Sato, H., Seiki, M., Yeh, Y., and Chen, W.T., *Proc. Natl. Acad. Sci. U.S.A.* 94: 7959, 1997.
66. Ray, J.M. and Stetler-Stevenson, W.G., *EMBO J.* 14: 908, 1995.
67. Valente, P., Fassina, G., Melchiori, A., Masiello, L., Cilli, M., Vacca, A., Onisto, M., Santi, L., Stetler-Stevenson, W.G., and Albini, A., *Int. J. Cancer* 75: 246, 1998.
68. Janji, B., Melchior, C., Gouon, V., Vallar, L., and Kieffer, N., *Int. J. Cancer* 83: 255, 1999.
69. Bar-Eli, M., *Pathobiology* 67: 12, 1999.
70. Benbow, U., Schoenermark, M.P., Mitchell, T.I., Rutter, J.L., Shimokawa, K., Nagase, H., and Brinckerhoff, C.E., *J. Biol. Chem.* 274: 25371, 1999.
71. Rabbani, S.A., Xing, R.H., Andreasen, P.A., Kjoller, L., Christensen, L., and Duffy, M.J., *Int. J. Cancer* 72: 1, 1997.
72. Reuning, U., Magdolen, V., Wilhelm, O., Fischer, K., Lutz, V., Graeff, H., and Schmitt, M., *Int. J. Oncol.* 13: 893, 1998.
73. Bjornland, K., Buo, L., Kjonniksen, I., Larsen, M., Fodstad, O., Johansen, H.T., and Aasen, A.O., *Anticancer Res.* 16: 1627, 1996.
74. Hearing, V.J., Law, L.W., Corti, A., Appella, E., and Blasi, F., *Cancer Res.* 48: 1270, 1988.
75. Mueller, B.M., *Curr. Top. Microbiol. Immunol.* 213: 65, 1996.
76. de Vries, T.J., Van Muijen, G.N., and Ruiter, D.J., *Melanoma Res.* 6: 79, 1996.
77. Kirchheimer, J.C., Wojta, J., Christ, G., and Binder, B.R., *Proc. Natl. Acad. Sci. U.S.A.* 86: 5424, 1989.
78. Meissauer, A., Kramer, M.D., Hofmann, M., Erkell, L.J., Jacob, E., Schirrmacher, V., and Brunner, G., *Exp. Cell Res.* 192: 453, 1991.
79. Mignatti, P., Robbins, E., and Rifkin, D.B., *Cell* 47: 487, 1986.
80. Persky, B., Ostrowski, L.E., Pagast, P., Ahsan, A., and Schultz, R.M., *Cancer Res.* 46: 4129, 1986.
81. Alizadeh, H., Ma, D., Berman, M., Bellingham, D., Comerford, S.A., Gething, M.J., Sambrook, J.F., and Niederkorn, J.Y., *Curr. Eye Res.* 14: 449, 1995.
82. Eitzman, D.T., Krauss, J.C., Shen, T., Cui, J., and Ginsburg, *Blood* 87: 4718, 1995.
83. Huijzer, J.C., Uhlenkott, C.E., and Meadows, G.G., *Int. J. Cancer* 63: 92, 1995.
84. Mueller, B.M., Yu, Y.B., and Laug, W.E., *Proc. Natl. Acad. Sci. U.S.A.* 92: 205, 1995.
85. Stahl, A., and Mueller, B.M., *Int. J. Cancer* 71: 116, 1997.
86. Shapiro, R.L., Duquette, J.G., Roses, D.F., Nunes, I., Harris, M.N., Kamino, H., Wilson, E.L., and Rifkin, D.B., *Cancer Res.* 56: 3597, 1996.
87. Montgomery, A.M., De Clerck, Y.A., Langley, K.E., Reisfeld, R.A., and Mueller, B.M., *Cancer Res.* 53: 693, 1993.
88. Min, H.Y., Doyle, L.V., Vitt, C.R., Zandonella, C.L., Stratton-Thomas, J.R., Shuman, M.A., and Rosenberg, S., *Cancer Res.* 56: 2428, 1996.
89. Borchers, A.H., Sanders, L.A., Powell, M.B., and Bowden, G.T., *Exp. Cell Res.* 231: 61, 1997.
90. Mueller, S.C., Ghersi, G., Akiyama, S.K., Sang, Q.X., Howard, L., Pineiro-Sanchez, M., Nakahara, H., Yeh, Y., and Chen, W.T., *J. Biol. Chem.* 274: 24947, 1999.
91. Fujii, H., Nakajima, M., Saiki, I., Yoneda, J., Azuma, I., and Tsuruo, T., *Clin. Exp. Metast.* 13: 337, 1995.

92. Saiki, I., Fujii, H., Yoneda, J., Abe, F., Nakajima, M., Tsuruo, T., and Azuma, I., *Int.J.Cancer* 54: 137, 1993.
93. Brooks, P.C., Clark, R.A., and Cheresh, D.A., *Science* 264: 569, 1994.
94. Hiraoka, N., Allen, E., Apel, I.J., Gyetko, M.R., and Weiss, S.J., *Cell* 95: 365, 1998.
95. Hartmann, A., Kunz, M., Kotlin, S., Gillitzer, R., Toksoy, A., Bröcker, E.B., and Klein, C.E., *Cancer Res.* 59: 1578, 1999.
96. Anonymous *Am. J. Ophthalmol.* 125: 745, 1998.
97. Rohrbach, J.M., Wild, M., Riedinger, C., Kreissig, I., and Thiel, H.J., *Ger. J. Ophthalmol.* 3: 144, 1994.
98. Hunt, R.C., Pakalnis, V.A., Choudhury, P., and Black, E.P., *Invest. Ophthalmol. Vis. Sci.* 35: 955, 1994.
99. Ma, D., Gerard, R.D., Li, X.Y., Alizadeh, H., and Niederkorn, J.Y., *Blood* 90: 2738, 1997.
100. Väisänen, A., Kallioinen, M., von Dickhoff, K., Laatikainen, L., Höyhtya, M., and Turpeenniemi-Hujanen, T., *J. Pathol.* 188: 56, 1999.
101. Komazawa, H., Saiki, I., Aoki, M., Kitaguchi, H., Satoh, H., Kojima, M., Ono, M., Itoh, I., and Azuma, I., *Biol. Pharm. Bull.* 16: 997, 1993.
102. Fujii, H., Nishikawa, N., Komazawa, H., Suzuki, M., Kojima, M., Itoh, I., Obata, A., Ayukawa, K., Azuma, I., and Saiki, I., *Clin. Exp. Metast.* 16: 94, 1998.
103. Helige, C., Smolle, J., Fik-Puches, R., Hofmann-Wellenhof, R., Hartmann, E., Bar, T., Schmidt, R.R., and Tritthart, H.A., *Clin. Exp. Metast.* 14: 477, 1996.
104. Matsunaga, K., Ohhara, M., Oguchi, Y., Iijima, H., and Kobayashi, H., *Invas. Metast.* 16: 27, 1996.
105. Iwamoto, Y., Robey, F.A., Graf, J., Sasaki, M., Kleinman, H.K., Yamada, Y., and Martin, G.R., *Science* 238: 1132, 1987.
106. Lentini, A., Kleinman, H.K., Mattioli, P., Autuori-Pezzoli, V., Nicolini, L., Pietrini, A., Abbruzzese, A., Cardinali, M., and Beninati, S., *Melanoma Res.* 8: 131, 1998.
107. Stack, M.S., Gately, S., Bafetti, L.M., Enghild, J.J., and Soff, G.A., *Biochem. J.* 340: 77, 1999.
108. Montgomery, A.M., Mueller, B.M., Reisfeld, R.A., Taylor, S.M., and DeClerck, Y.A., *Cancer Res.* 54: 5467, 1994.
109. Wylie, S., MacDonald, I.C., Varghese, H.J., Schmidt, E.E., Morris, V.L., Groom, A.C., and Chambers, A.F., *Clin. Exp. Metast.* 17: 111, 1999.
110. Hendrix, M.J., Wood, W.R., Seftor, E.A., Lotan, D., Nakajima, M., Misiorowski, R.L., Seftor, R.E., Stetler-Stevenson, W.G., Bevacqua, S.J., and Liotta, L.A., *Cancer Res.* 50: 4121, 1990.
111. Supino, R., Cecchi, C., Mapelli, E., and Sanfilippo, O., *Melanoma Res.* 4: 251, 1994.
112. Santos, C.L., Giorgi, R.R., Frochtengarten, F., Elias, M.C., Chammas, R., and Brentani, R.R., *Int. J. Clin. Lab. Res.* 24: 148, 1994.
113. Helige, C., Smolle, J., Zellnig, G., Hartmann, E., Fink-Puches, R., Kerl, H., and Tritthart, H.A., *Clin. Exp. Metast.* 11: 409, 1993.
114. Repesh, L.A., Drake, S.R., Warner, M.C., Downing, S.W., Jyring, R., Seftor, E.A., Hendrix, M.J., and McCarthy, J.B., *Clin. Exp. Metast.* 11: 91, 1993.
115. Murata, J., Ayukawa, K., Ogasawara, M., Fujii, H., and Saiki, I., *Invas. Metast.* 17: 82, 1997.

116. Dewhurst, L.O., Gee, J.W., Rennie, I.G., and MacNeil, S., *Br. J. Cancer* 75: 860, 1997.

115. Yohem, K.H., Clothier, J.L., Montague, S.L., Geary, R.J., Winters, A.L., Hendrix, M.J., and Welch, D.R., *Pigm. Cell Res.* 4: 225, 1991.

116. Maekawa, R., Maki, H., Yoshida, H., Hojo, K., Tanaka, H., Wada, T., Uchida, N., Takeda, Y., Kasai, H., Okamoto, H., Tsuzuki, H., Kambayashi, Y., Watanabe, F., Kawada, K., Toda, K., Ohtani, M., Sugita, K., and Yoshioka, T., *Cancer Res.* 59: 1231, 1999.

117. Friedl, P., Entschladen, F., Conrad, C., Niggemann, B., and Zänker, K.S., *Eur. J. Immunol.* 28: 2331, 1998.

D.J. RUITER, T.J. DE VRIES AND G.N.P. VAN MUIJEN

Cellular and molecular mechanisms of metastatic tumor spread in uveal melanoma

Abstract

Key processes in tumor metastasis and proliferation, matrix degradation and migration. The cellular and molecular mechanisms involved in matrix degradation and migration are briefly discussed. Also, the cellular distribution of some relevant molecules expressed in uveal melanomas and their clinical implications are elucidated.

Keywords: Metastasis, proteases, uveal melanoma, immunohistochemistry, adhesion molecules

Introduction

The process of metastasis occurs through a series of complex steps, which include invasive growth into adjacent normal tissue, detachment from the primary tumor and extravasation into lymphatics and blood vessels, transportation through these vascular structures to other organs, and outgrowth to a secondary tumor at these sites. From a cell biological point of view key processes of the metastatic cascade are proliferation, matrix degradation and migration [1]. Interestingly, the same key processes take place during angiogenesis, which suggests a close interrelationship with tumor invasion and metastasis [1]. Much research efforts currently are devoted to unravel the molecular mechanisms of these key processes in order to identify evidence-based strategies for preventive, diagnostic and therapeutic interventions. In this review we will focus on the cellular and molecular mechanisms of matrix degradation and migration and analyze the cellular distribution of relevant molecules studied in uveal melanoma. Where appropriate, possible clinical implications are discussed.

Department of Pathology, University Hospital Nijmegen St Radboud,
P.O. Box 9101, 6500 HB Nijmegen, The Netherlands

53

Matrix degradation

Degradation of extracellular matrix (ECM) components, including basal membranes, is a prerequisite for invasion of the surrounding normal tissues by tumor cells. This is accomplished by proteolytic factors, that can be produced both by tumor cells and adjacent stromal cells such as fibroblasts and macrophages. Tumor cells are thought to induce this production, either by soluble factors or direct cell—cell contact. The proteolyctic factors are involved in a highly complex interplay between (pro-) activators, receptors and inhibitors. The process of ECM degradation may coincide with ECM production, comparable with tissue remodeling and wound healing. In this view the matrix degradation process not only facilitates tumor cell invasion and metastasis, but it also may be inflicted in local stromal reactions to cancer, including desmoplasia and inflammation [2].

Several protease families involved in extracellular proteolysis are currently known: serine proteases, matrix metalloproteinases (MMPs), aspartyl

TABLE 1. *Some properties of protease families.*

Family	Components	Functions
Serine proteases	Plasmin	Degradation of ECM components
	Urokinase-type plasminogen activator (uPA)	Conversion of plasminogen into plasmin
	Tissue-type plasminogen activator (tPA)	Conversion of plasminogen into plasmin
Matrix metallproteases (MMPs)		
—Collagenases	Interstitial collagenase (MMP-1)	Degradation of collangens (amongst others type IV
	Neutrophil collagenase (MMP-8)	collagen, the most important protein in basement
	Collagenase-3 (MMP-13)	membranes) and other
—Membrane-type (MMPs) (1—4)	MMP-14, 15, 16, 17	ECM proteins
—Gelatinases	Gelatinsae A (MMP-2)	
	Galatinase B (MMP-9)	
—Stromelysins	Stromelysin 1 (MMP-3)	
	Stromelysin 2 (MMP-10)	
	Stromelysin 3 (MMP-11)	
	Matrilysin (MMP-7)	
	Enamelysin (MMP-20)	
—MMP-19		
—Metalloelastase	MMP-12	
Aspartyl protease	Cathepsin D	Degradation of ECM components
Cystein protease	Cathepsin B, L and H	Degradation of ECM components

D. J. Ruiter, T. J. de Vries and G. N. P. van Muijen

proteases and cystein proteases. Some properties of these enzyme systems are given in Table 1 [3]. All families are active in the degradation of various ECM components. Each individual protease specifically cleaves one or a few of these components, such as laminin, collagens, fibronectin and proteoglycans. The majority of proteases are secreted as inactive precursor molecules. Activation takes place by cleavage within the peptide chain of the molecule. Some proteolytic systems are known to co-operate with others. For instance, matrix metalloproteinases are activated by plasmin. The nett result of such interaction is proteolysis. Proteolysis may be obstructed by natural inhibitors, that have a specificity per protease family. Most proteases are known to function in a tight balance with receptors and inhibitors. An overview of these molecules is presented in Table 2. *In vitro* degradation of ECM has been shown to be mediated by uPA in highly metastatic human melanoma cell lines xenografted to nude mice. Also, uPAR is expressed by these cell lines. Proteolytic activity of uPA was markedly enhanced after binding to uPAR. Plasminogen activation occurs much more efficiently by cell surface-associated uPA than by secreted tPA. Spontaneous metastasis of human melanoma cell lines is influenced by uPA, uPAR, and remarkably also by PAI-1. Subcutaneous growth and metastasis of these cell lines in nude mice can be suppressed by specific protease inhibitors. The data in the literature suggest an important role for components of the plasminogen activation system in melanoma invasion and metastasis [4,5]. In contrast, activity of MMPs seems to promote melanoma growth in the skin and may not be required for tumor cell dissemination. However, recent work suggests a role of membrane type MMP in melanoma progression [6]. In the past few years proteases have been shown to possess other biological properties than

TABLE 2.   *Protease-related molecules.*

Component	Inhibitors and receptors	Comments
Plasmin	α_2-antiplasmin	Inhibitor of plasmin
UPA, tPA	Plasminogen activation inhibitor type 1 (PAI-1)	Inhibitor of active uPA and tPA
	Plasminogen activation inhibitor type 2 (PAI-2)	Inhibitor of active uPA and tPA
	Receptor for uPA (uPAR)	Activates uPA, focuses proteolytic activity on cell membrane and has nonproteolytic effects
	LRP/α_2-MR, gp600	Clearance and cellular uptake of inactivated proteases
Cathpesin B, L, and D	Cystatins	Inhibitors
MMPs	TIMPs (1−4)	Inhibitors of MMPs
	EMMPRIN	Extracellular inducer of MMPs

proteolysis. For instance, uPAR and PAI-1 interact with vitronectrin, an adhesion receptor on extracellular matrix. Also, evidence exists for a possibly co-ordinately regulated expression of integrin $\alpha v\beta 3$ and uPAR. Therefore, integrins may not only be involved in cell migration, but also in matrix degradation [5].

Migration

Tumor cell migration is defined as transportation of the cells in the interstitial space. Factors involved are active or passive cellular movement and attachment to and detachment from other cells and/or ECM. The latter are mediated by cellular adhesion molecules, of which several families exist: the immunoglobulin superfamily, the integrins, the cadherins, the selectins and CD44 [7]. The immunoglobulin superfamily comprizes a large number of adhesion molecules, all characterized by immunoglobulin-related domains and, usually by fibronectin type III repeats. N-CAM belongs to a group that mediates homophilic (i.e. contact between identical molecules) cell adhesion. ICAM-1 and others bind to $\beta 2$-members of the integrin family.

Integrins form a family of heterodimeric transmembrane receptors. Their α- and β-subunits form glycoproteins with a generally conserved structure, made up of a large extracellular domain, a transmembrane segment, and in general a short cytoplasmic tail. Diversity within the integrin family is generated by a large number of α-subunits that build heterodimers with at least eight different β-subunits. Integrins can bind ECM components or counter receptors on other cells in a divalent cation-dependent way. The members of the $\beta 1$, 2 and 3 subfamilies have been most extensively studied. The $\beta 1$- and $\beta 3$-integrins are mainly involved in ECM interactions whereas $\beta 2$-integrins mediate cell–cell adhesion. Integrins play an important role in cell migration. For instance, $\alpha 4\beta 1$ and $\alpha 5\beta 1$ mediate migration on fibronectin and $\alpha 2\beta 1$ mediates migration on collagen, laminin and tenascin. Concentration of integrins and lineage with the actin filament bundles in focal adhesions are relevant features in cell migration. Integrin aggregation induces clustering of tension and focal adhesion kinase, which can he regarded as the first step in integrin signaling. Clustered integrins in focal adhesions function as a signal transduction unit where cytoskeletal and signaling molecules are concentrated and phosphorylated, ultimately influencing gene expression.

Cadherins are transmembrane molecules that mediate adhesion between cells in a homophilic, Ca^{2+}-dependent manner. Intracellulary, they are lined to the cytoskeleton via a complex of intermediate proteins (e.g. catenins), and these associated molecules are essential for their adhesive function. A large number of different cadherins are known, that all have their own specific pattern of spatial and temporal regulation during embryonic development, and their own pattern of tissue distribution. This suggests that the effect of a certain cadherin is cell-type specific.

D. J. Ruiter, T. J. de Vries and G. N. P. van Muijen

The selectin family consists of three members, i.e. E-, P- and L-selectin. Each is a transmembrane molecule and has a Ca^{2+}-dependent C-type lectin domain, EGF-like repeats, and various repeats with similarity to complement-binding proteins. Selectins are expressed on leukocytes and endothelial cells and mediate adhesion between these cell types.

CD44 is homologous to the cartilage link proteins. Several larger isoforms of the CD44 standard form have been described that are generated by alternative splicing. The CD44 standard molecule is expressed on most cell types, whereas the variants (isoforms) are expressed principally on epithelia and activated leukocytes. Alternative splicing regulates CD44 binding to the ECM components hyaluronic acid, collagen and fibronectin, to the cellular adhesion molecule MadCAM, and to growth factors.

Expression of proteases and adhesion molecules in uveal melanoma

As emergence of uPA, tPA, uPAR, PAI-1 and PAI-2 in advanced primary cutaneous melanoma and melanoma metastasis had been found (reviewed in [8]), De Vries et al. [9] studied their expression in uveal melanoma using immunohistochemistry and antibodies against the different components. The immunohistochemical findings in 45 freshly frozen primary uveal melanomas are summarized in Fig. 1. Focal uPA staining (<5%) of tumor cells as well as staining of fibroblast-like cells was observed in five non-spindle cell tumors. uPA expression correlated with tumor related death: three out of five patients died (total mean follow-up: six years) of disease. All five metastases studied expressed uPA. Focal uPAR immunoreactivity (<5%) was found in 15 tumors, 11 of which were of the non-spindle cell type. Almost all (42 out of 45) tumors expressed tPA, however a moderate to abundant staining (<5% tumor cells, $n = 16$) was mainly present in non-spindle cell type tumors (14/16). No relationship was seen between the percentage of tPA positive cells and tumor related death. All metastases contained tPA. PAI-1 and PAI-2 protein were found in only six and five primary tumors, respectively, and in four and one out of five metastases, respectively. These immunohistohemical findings suggest that uPA expression in uveal melanoma is associated with progression of the disease, and that it may be useful as an additional prognostic marker. Remarkably, far more lesions expressed uPAR than uPA in the melanoma cells, which is in agreement with our findings in a panel of human cutaneous melanoma cell lines [4]. As compared to cutaneous melanoma tPA expression seems more extensively present, especially in metastases. In contrast, expression of uPA, PAI-1 and PAI-2 is much less. Experimental data in an intraocular melanoma model shows that overexpression of PAI-1 could inhibit metastatic spread [9]. Other proteases may play a role in uveal melanoma. To the best of our knowledge no data on their expression in uveal melanoma lesions have been published yet. Cottam et al. [10] however investigated the

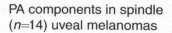

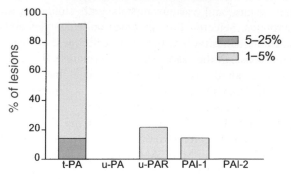

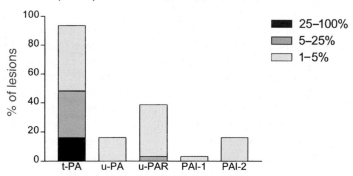

FIGURE 1. *Percentage of immunohistochemically stained tumor cells expressed as percentage of the total number of lesions. Note that expression of t-PA, u-PA, u-PAR and PAI-2 is elevated in non-spindle tumors.*

secretion of MMPs in 15 human melanoma cell lines. They found that all the cell lines secreted MMP-2, and nine of them secreted MMP-9.

Regarding the expression of adhesion molecules in uveal melanoma, NCAM, integrins and CD44 have been studied. Mooy *et al.* [11] found NCAM expression in the majority of primary tumors and metastases using paraplast embedded tissue. Interestingly, they noted an increase in NCAM staining in lesions with non-spindle tumor cells. Furthermore, such an increase was found in a large tumors, in rapidly metastasizing tumors, and in metastases. These findings suggest that NCAM expression is associated with the development of malignant potential in uveal melanoma.

Ten Berge *et al.* [12] studied integrin expression in frozen sections of 32 primary uveal melanomas and 4 metastases using monocloncal antibodies recognizing integrin subunits $\alpha 1-6$, αv, $\beta 1$, $\beta 4$, and integrins $\alpha v\beta 3$ and $\alpha v\beta 5$. As in cutaneous melanoma, $\alpha 4$ expression was rare, whereas most tumors expressed α3 and α6 subunits. In contrast to cutaneous melanoma, where α2 is well expressed in most lesions and α5 is expressed only in a low percentage of primary tumors, in uveal melanoma α2 expression was rare whereas u5 expression was observed in all tumor lesions studied. A major difference was found with regard to the αvβ3 vitronectin receptor. In contrast to cutaneous melanoma, where αvβ3 is expressed in about one-third of primary tumors, αvβ3 could not be detected in any of the primary uveal melanomas studies, irrespective of the thickness or cell type of the tumor. All uveal melanomas expressed αvβ5. A summary of the integrin expression in uveal melanoma is given in Fig. 2. Based on these observations, integrin expression in uveal melanoma cannot be correlated with either cell type or invasiveness, and in contrast to cutaneous melanoma, determination of the integrin expression profile seems not to be useful to subdivide uveal melanomas into low and highly aggressive tumors.

Regarding CD44, all 12 primary uveal melanomas studied by Danen *et al.* [13] strongly stained for the standard portion of the molecule. No expression was found of CD44v7 whereas v5, v6, and v10 were expressed in 2, 5, and 8 tumor lesions, respectively. No correlation was observed between expression of certain splice variants and cell type, tumor diameter, or invasion of the sclera or Bruch's membrane. The three uveal melanoma cell lines Mel 202, 92-I and OCM-1 studied were strongly CD44 positive and expressed low levels of the v6 isoform at the cell surface, whereas CD44v5, v7, and v10 were absent. These observations show that CD44 is strongly expressed in uveal melanoma and that the pattern of CD44 alternative splicing is similar to that observed in cutaneous melanoma. However, in contrast to cutaneous melanoma, in uveal melanoma it does not seem to be related to prognostic parameters.

Future prospects

Regarding proteases, the expression of MMPs, aspartyl proteases and cystein proteinases could be investigated in order to explore a possible relation with tumor progression in uveal melanoma. As the serine proteases now can be demonstrated in paraplast embedded tissue employing antigen retrieval procedures [14] the possible prognostic value of uPA and uPAR should be tested on a large series of cases. In addition, components such as uPAR could be tested in blood samples of patients with uveal melanoma for prognostic purposes, similar to patients with e.g. lung cancer [15]. As proteases play a role in angiogenesis, and discrete vascular patterns have been described in uveal melanoma that had prognostic relevance, it may be interesting to correlate these patterns to the expression of proteases, not only in the melanoma cells, but also in the microvascular cells. This also applies to the integrins αvβ3 and αvβ5, that were shown to be involved in angiogenesis. In addition, it would be worthwhile to study the mechanisms involved in the production of proteases and adhesion molecules in uveal melanoma [16].

Acknowledgements

The authors would like to thank Ms. Anke Vargas for secretarial support.

References

1. Kohn, E.C., and Liotta, L.A., *Cancer Res.*, 55: 1856–1862, 1995.
2. Ohtani, H., *Pathol. Int.*, 48: 1–9, 1998.
3. Ferrier, C.M., Van Muijen, G.N.P., and Ruiter, D.J., *Ann. Med.*, 30: 431–442, 1998.
4. Quax, P.H.A., Van Muijen, G.N.P., Weening-Verhoeff, E.J.D., *et al.*, *J. Cell Biol.*, 115: 191–199, 1991.
5. Seftor, R.E.B., *Am. J. Pathol.*, 153: 1347–1351, 1998.
6. Hofmann, U., Westphal, J.R., Van Muijen, G.N.P., *et al.*, *J. Invest. Dermatol.*, 115: 337–344, 2000.
7. Hart, I.A., Birch, M., and Marshall, J.F., *Cancer Metast. Rev.*, 10: 115–128, 1991.
8. De Vries, T.J., Van Muijen, G.N.P., and Ruiter, D.J., *Melanoma Res.*, 6: 79–88, 1996.
9. Ma, D., Gerard, R.D., Li, X.Y., Alizadeh, H., *et al.*, *Blood*, 90: 2738–2746, 1997.
10. Cottam, D.W., Rennie, I.G., Woods, K., *et al. Invest. Ophthalmol. Vis. Sci.*, 23: 1923–1927, 1992.
11. Mooy, C.M., Luyten, G.P., De Jong, P.T., *et al.*, *Hum. Pathol.*, 26: 1185–1190, 1995.
12. Ten Berge, P.J., Danen, E.H., Van Muijen, G.N., *et al.*, *Invest. Ophthalmol. Vis. Sci.*, 34: 3635–3640, 1993.
13. Danen, E.H.J., Ten Berge, P.J.M., Van Muijen, G.N.P., *et al.*, *Melanoma Res.*, 6: 31–35, 1996.
14. Ferrier, C.M., Van Geloof, W.L., De Witte, H.H., *et al.*, *J. Histochem. Cytochem.*, 46: 469–476, 1998.
15. De Witte, J.H., Pappot, H., Brünner, N., *et al.*, *Int. J. Cancer*, 72: 416–423, 1997.
16. Rennie, I.G., *Eye*, 11: 239– 242, 1997.
17. De Vries, T.J., Mooy, C.M., Van Balken, M.R., *et al.*, *J. Pathol.*, 175: 59–67, 1995.

D. J. Ruiter, T. J. de Vries and G. N. P. van Muijen

DIETER MARMÉ

The pivotal role of VEGF in tumor angiogenesis

Abstract

Angiogenesis is a prerequisite for growth of solid tumors and metastasis formation. The vascular endothelial growth factor (VEGF) is one of the major angiogenic factors produced by the tumor and acting on its receptors at endothelial cells of vessels which are in close contact with or penetrating the tumor. Highly selective expression of VEGF and VEGF receptors in the diseased areas provide a unique possibility for therapeutic intervention. The various mechanisms by which tumor cells and stromal cells enhance the expression of VEGF as well as the mechanisms by which VEGF receptors are up-regulated in endothelial cells will be discussed at the molecular and cellular level. Based on this knowledge, several therapeutic strategies have been worked out which are suited to inhibit the growth of the primary tumor as well as the metastatic spread. One of these strategies is the therapeutic use of soluble VEGF receptors, a second one is the use of specific VEGF receptor tyrosine kinase inhibitors. Both approaches could be shown to be effective in inhibiting the growth of primary tumors and the formation of metastases in appropriate animal models. Phase I clinical studies with a specific inhibitor of the tyrosine-kinases of both VEGF receptors have been started at our clinic.

Keywords: Angiogenesis, VEGF, VEGF receptors, protein kinase inhibitors, tumor therapy

Introduction

Growth of solid tumors and the formation of metastases are dependent on the formation of new blood vessels. This hypothesis was proposed by Judah Folkman more than 25 years ago and has been substantially supported by recent discoveries which unravelled the molecular and cellular processes

Institute of Molecular Medicine, Tumor Biology Center, D-79106 Freiburg, Germany

61

involved in tumor angiogenesis. Clinical data clearly indicate the correlation between vascularization and aggressive tumor growth and metastases formation. Many of the angiogenic factors produced by tumors have been identified and their roles in the formation of new blood vessels have been elucidated [1].

According to our present understanding of cancerogenesis, each tumor originates from a single cell which has been transformed by one or more genetic events. This includes the activation of oncogenes as well as the inactivation of tumor suppressor genes. These cells can grow out to form a cell clone of only a few millimeters in size before the supply of nutrients becomes limited. The tumor clones can remain at this stage for months or years, unless they are eliminated by the immune system or the so-called angiogenic switch is turned on. At the cellular level, the angiogenic switch is defined by the onset of expression and secretion of angiogenic factors. If sufficient of the secreted angiogenic factors reach the neighbouring capillaries of the vasculature by diffusion they initiate the sprouting of new blood vessels from pre-existing ones.

Among the angiogenic factors, the vascular endothelial growth factor (VEGF) plays a pivotal role. Most solid tumors express high levels of VEGF and the VEGF receptors appear predominantly in endothelial cells of vessels surrounding or penetrating the malignant tissue [2, 3]. Thus, VEGF-mediated tumor angiogenesis requiring both, the ligand and its receptors to be in place, seems to be an ideal therapeutic target for cancer therapy. One might expect that the effect of any compound designed to block the VEGF signalling cascade will most likely be restricted to the diseased area. However, the possibility that the presence of other angiogenic mechanisms and/or the loss of antiangiogenic processes should not be neglected. Also, the combination of anti-angiogenic strategies with more conventional therapies such as cytotoxic chemotherapy should be considered.

This article will briefly summarize what we know about the various factors and mechanisms underlying the expression of VEGF in tumors and of the VEGF receptors in tumor endothelial cells. Furthermore, the various experimental approaches undertaken to disrupt the VEGF signalling cascade will be discussed.

Mechanisms of VEGF expression

Expression of VEGF is induced by a variety of factors and growth conditions in normal cells and tumor cells, as well as by genetic changes in tumor cells. Regulation of VEGF expression has been reported to occur on the level of gene transcription, on the level of mRNA stabilization, and on the level of mRNA translation. Transcription of the VEGF gene is enhanced by a variety of growth factors and cytokines including platelet-derived growth factor (PDGF)-BB, basic fibroblast growth factor (bFGF), insulin-like growth factor-1, keratinocyte growth factor, epidermal growth factor, tumor necrosis factor (TNF) α, transforming growth factor (TGF) α, TGFβ1, interleukin-1β, and interleukin 6, in a variety of cultured cells [4−11]. Enhanced VEGF expression has been reported upon activation of protein kinase C by tumor promoters [4,12] and in cells harbouring activated oncogenes, such as ras, raf, and src [13−15], as well as in cells carrying inactivating mutations or deletions of p53, and of von Hippel-Lindau (VHL) tumor suppressor genes, respectively [15−17]. In addition, VEGF expression is markedly elevated in cultured cells by hypoxic conditions and in regions of tumors located near necrotic areas [18, 19].

Recent work has shed some light on the diverse molecular mechanisms involved in enhanced VEGF expression. Sequence analysis of the human VEGF gene promoter [12] revealed several potential binding sites for transcription factors AP-1, AP-2, and Sp-1 which are candidate mediators of VEGF promoter activation. Detailed promoter analyses using reporter gene assays, electrophoretic mobility shift assays and mutagenesis of promoter elements resulted in the identification of a $G + C$-rich region at -50 to -96 relative to the single transcriptional start site to be essential for induction of VEGF by TNFα [20], TGFα [21], and PDGF-BB [22], respectively. This promoter region contains four consensus binding sites for transcription factors Sp-1 and/or Sp-3, two putative binding sites for Egr-1 which are overlapping with the second, third, and fourth Sp-1/Sp-3 sites, respectively, and one AP-2 binding site which is identical to the 5′ Egr-1 site. Ryuto et al. [20] have shown that the four Sp-1/Sp-3 binding sites are essential for basal transcription of the VEGF gene and for TNFα-dependent promoter activation in a human glioma cell line. Deletion of the most 5′ Sp-1/Sp-3 binding site reduced basal transcription and abolished TNFα-responsiveness. Stimulation of the cells with TNFα or bFGF resulted in increased binding of Sp-1 to the promoter element, whereas addition of mithramycin, an inhibitor of Sp-1, inhibited activation of the VEGF gene promoter suggesting Sp-1 as a downstream mediator of TNFα-induced VEGF gene expression. Gille et al. [21] and Finkenzeller et al. [22] found a promoter element covering the second to fourth Sp-1 consensus binding sites necessary and sufficient for VEGF gene promoter activation in PDGF-BB stimulated NIH3T3 fibroblasts and in TGFα stimulated A431 human epidermoid carcinoma cells. Sp-1 and Sp-3 were shown to bind in a constitutive manner to this promoter region. In A431 cells the formation of TGFα inducible DNA binding complex containing AP-2 and Egr-1 transcription factors was observed on this DNA fragment. Transfection of AP-2 and Egr-1 expression vectors revealed AP-2, but not Egr-1, as a transcription factor which activates VEGF gene expression. In NIH3T3 cells mutations within the VEGF promoter element which abolished binding of AP-2 and Egr-1 had no effect on PDGF-responsiveness, whereas mutations which eliminated binding of Sp-1 and Sp-3 impaired PDGF-stimulated transcription of the VEGF gene promoter. Although TNFα, TGFα, and PDGF-BB signalling pathways address different transcription factors or use different modes of their activation, they converge at the proximal promoter region.

Further evidence for the important role of the proximal promoter region for control of VEGF gene expression came from recent findings of Mukhopadhyay *et al.* [23] who identified the −50 and −144 region to mediate transcriptional repression of the VEGF promoter by the VHL gene product. Renal carcinoma cells that either lacked wild-type VHL gene or were transfected with an inactive mutant VHL gene showed deregulated expression of VEGF that was reverted by introduction of wild-type VHL gene [17]. Mukhopadhyay *et al.* [23] now showed that wild-type VHL protein binds to Sp-1 transcription factor and represses Sp-1 mediated activation of the VEGF gene promoter, indicating that VHL regulation of VEGF occurs at least partly at the transcriptional level. Moreover, their results suggest that loss of Sp-1 inhibition may be important in the pathogenesis of VHL disease. Originally, VHL protein was discovered as a negative regulator of the transcriptional elongation factor elongin [24−26]. By binding to the regulatory elongin subunits B and C VHL protein disrupts elongin function. Whether VHL protein is involved in regulation of transcriptional elongation of the VEGF gene remains open so far. Instead, increased VEGF mRNA stabilization, a mechanism that is also driven by hypoxia, has been observed in cells lacking VHL function [27]. Short time hypoxia (3 h) initial induced VEGF mRNA transcription 3−4-fold, whereas continued hypoxia (15 h) resulted in a 810-fold VEGF induction that was the product of both enhanced transcription and an approx. three-fold increased mRNA stability [28]. Both mechanisms have been shown to work *in vivo* in a rat C6 glioma model [29]. Upon subjection of cells to hypoxia formation of RNA-protein complexes on three adenylate-uridylate-rich elements (AREs) in the 3′-untranslated region of the VEGF mRNA was observed which mediate mRNA stabilization [30,31]. AREs destabilize mRNAs and stabilization of labile mRNA is thought to be mediated by specific binding of proteins to AREs that mask the ARE-destabilizing motifs. Formation of these hypoxia-inducible RNA-protein complexes on the VEGF mRNA is constitutively elevated in cells lacking functional VHL protein [31]. As no direct interaction between VHL protein and the hypoxia-inducible complex has been observed to date the molecular mechanism by which the VHL protein mediates constitutive formation of the complex remains to be clarified.

Hypoxia-inducible factor 1 (HIF-1), a heterodimereric basic helix-loop-helix protein that activates transcription of the human erythropoietin gene in hypoxic cells, was shown to be involved in hypoxiainduced VEGF gene transcription and a HIF-1 binding site was identified at −975 of the human gene promoter [32]. An AP-1 transcription factor binding site at −1129 cooperates with the HIF-1 site in the way that this site is unable to confer hypoxia responsiveness on its own, but potentiates hypoxia induction of the human VEGF gene via HIF-1 approx. two-fold [33]. The H-ras oncogene enhances the induction of VEGF by hypoxia via the HIF-1 promoter element [34]. The signalling pathway of H-ras in induction of VEGF expression involves the phosphatidylinositol 3-kinase/Akt pathway whereas the c-raf/mitogen activated kinase and the stress activated kinase pathways appear to be dispensable [35,36]. c-src or src-like kinases have conversely been reported to be involved [37] or not involved [38] in hypoxia-induced VEGF expression.

Recent work of Kevil et al. [39] revealed translational regulation as an important factor for enhanced VEGF expression. Transfection of Chinese hamster ovary cells to overexpress the protein synthesis factor eukaryotic initiation factor 4E increased VEGF secretion up to 130-fold. Eukaryotic initiation factor 4E is a 25 kDa polypeptide that recruits mRNAs for translation by binding to the 7-methylguanosine-containing cap of mRNA. Its overexpression has been observed in metastatic breast carcinomas [40] and transformed cell lines [41] suggesting a contribution to carcinoma progression and survival.

Mechanisms of VEGF receptor expression

In contrast to our knowledge about the regulation of VEGF expression only little is known about the mechanisms which control VEGF receptor expression. A striking observation had been made even before the VEGF receptor genes had been identified: the distribution of high affinity VEGF binding sites revealed a pattern restricted to endothelial cells which had been interpreted as the consequence of cell specific receptor expression [42]. After the identification of the VEGF receptor-1 (FLT-1) gene and VEGF receptor-2 (KDR/FLK-1) gene, in situ hybridization confirmed that the expression of both genes was tightly restricted to endothelial cells and its progenitors [43–45]. Moreover, receptor expression is not only endothelial cell specific but is also down-regulated in quiescent endothelial cells. Up-regulation of both receptors occurs when angiogenesis takes place, as in the case of tumor growth. Two main questions arise from these findings: first—which mechanisms are responsible for the endothelial cell specific expression of both receptors, and second—which mechanisms are responsible for the down-regulation of receptor expression in quiescent endothelial cells and the up-regulation in proliferating endothelial cells?

Whereas almost nothing is known about the molecular basis of endothelial cell specific expression, there is growing evidence for paracrine mechanisms which are involved in the regulation of VEGF receptor expression.

A number of growth factors and cytokines can regulate angiogenesis positively or negatively [46]. Conflicting results have been reported for TNFα, an inflammatory and neoplasia associated cytokine. TNFα promotes angiogenesis in vivo and stimulates the migration of endothelial cells [47] although it has been described as a potent inhibitor of endothelial cell growth in vitro [48]. In a recent publication, Patterson et al. [49] demonstrate the interference of TNFα with the VEGF signalling system of endothelial cells. TNFα blocks the VEGF-stimulated DNA synthesis by significantly lowering the mRNA levels of both VEGF receptors. The underlying molecular mechanisms are not yet fully understood. However, it is likely that transcription is affected since mRNA stability was not influenced by TNFα. TGFβ1 has been reported to down-regulate VEGF receptor-2 (KDR/FLK-1) expression of endothelial cells *in vitro* [50]. Receptor down-regulation has been observed at the mRNA and protein level but the molecular basis is still unclear. An elegant experimental set up for studying the regulation of VEGF receptor expression has been reported by Kremer *et al.* [51]. By using cultured cerebral tissue slices Kremer *et al.* [51] could demonstrate hypoxia-induced VEGF receptor-2 expression. Further analysis revealed that hypoxia-induced VEGF expression in these tissue slices was responsible for enhanced VEGF receptor-2 expression. In other terms: VEGF itself can stimulate the expression of its VEGF receptor-2. Experiments addressing the question of how VEGF receptor-1 expression can be stimulated were published by Barleon *et al.* [52]. Incubation of cultured human umbilical vein endothelial cells (HUVECs) with conditioned medium of various tumor cell lines led to an increase of VEGF receptor-1 expression. As in the case of VEGF receptor-2 up-regulation in brain slices, VEGF itself was identified as the soluble factor produced by the tumor cells and responsible for enhanced VEGF receptor-1 expression. Thus evidence accumulates that VEGF itself is an important paracrine factor which up-regulates the expression of its own receptors *in vivo*.

Hypoxia

The growth of malignant tumors is associated with tissue hypoxia and hypoxia has been described to be a major mechanism leading to the up-regulation of VEGF and its receptors *in vivo*. However, this is not restricted to growing tumors [19] but also occurs in the vasculature of hypoxic lung [53] or skin explants [54]. Conflicting results were coming from experiments where cultured endothelial cells had been exposed to hypoxia. Thieme *et al.* [55] showed an increase in the number of VEGF receptors of bovine retinal and aortic endothelial cells. Studying VEGF receptor expression in hypoxia treated HUVECs we and other failed to demonstrate up-regulation of both VEGF receptors [51,56, Barleon and Marmé, unpublished]. Detmar *et al.* [54] described the up-regulation of VEGF-receptor-1 mRNA and the down-regulation of VEGF-receptor-2 mRNA in dermal microvascular endothelial cells. Meanwhile the promoter regions of both VEGF receptor genes have been cloned [57–59]. Transient transfection of promoter reporter constructs showed a strong transcriptional activation of the VEGF receptor-1 gene under hypoxic conditions while the VEGF receptor-2 activity remained unchanged [60]. The authors could identify the element mediating the hypoxic response as a heptamer sequence matching the consensus sequence of the hypoxia inducible factor-1 (HIF). This element acts like an enhancer and mutation within this HIF consensus binding site led to impaired activation by hypoxia [60]. Thus, the observed hypoxia-mediated expression of both VEGF receptors *in vivo* seems to be regulated by different molecular mechanisms. While direct transcriptional activation mediated by HIF and can up-regulate only VEGF receptor-1 expression. Hypoxia-induced paracrine factors like VEGF are able to activate the expression of both VEGF receptors.

Therapeutic opportunities

Inhibition of the VEGF-mediated signalling cascade has already been shown in various experimental animal models to effectively interfere with tumor vascularization, tumor growth and metastases formation.

Functional inhibition of the mouse VEGF receptor, FLK-1, the mouse homologue of human KDR, by the use of a dominant-negative mutant lacking protein tyrosine kinase, leads to significant inhibition of tumor growth and vascularization. This effect was obtained either by co-injecting a cell line producing retroviruses encoding the dominantnegative mutant together with the glioblastorna cell line, C6, or by local injection of retroviral supernatants [61].

The availability of specific monoclonal antibodies against VEGF made it possible to investigate the role of VEGF in tumor angiogenesis. Nude mice injected subcutaneously with a large variety of human cancer cell lines were treated with anti-VEGF antibodies.

In all cases significant reduction of tumor growth was observed [3,61]. In agreement with the hypothesis that inhibition of tumor growth is due to the inhibition of tumor vascularization, it could be shown that tumors from treated animals had a reduced density of blood vessels [62]. Intravital videomicroscopy techniques revealed almost complete suppression of tumor angiogenesis in tumor bearing nude mice treated with anti-VEGF antibodies [63]. In an orthotopic nude mouse model of liver metastasis, after inoculation with human colon carcinoma, the systemic application of VEGF antibodies resulted in a dramatic decrease of the number and size of metastases [64]. Combination treatment with anti-VEGF monoclonal antibodies and doxorubicin results in a signficant enhancement of the efficacy of either agent alone and led in some cases to a complete regression of tumors derived from MCF-7 breast carcinoma cells in nude mice [3].

VEGF antisense technology was used to explore whether a reduction of VEGF secretion by the tumor cells leads to inhibition of vascularization and tumor growth. In this case, rat C6 glioma cells, secreting VEGF, were stably transfected with a eukaryotic expression vector bearing an antisense-VEGF cDNA. Cell lines with reduced VEGF production were transplanted into nude mice. Substantial reduction of tumor growth, tumor vascularization and significant increase of necrosis was observed [65]. Lowering VEGF expression in tumor cells has also been achieved by blocking EGF-stimulated expression of VEGF in A431 human epidermoid carcinoma cells using an anti-EGF receptor neutralizing antibody. Similar results were reported with an anti-ErbB2/neu monoclonal antibody for SKBR-3 human breast cancer cells [66]. This implicates the potential use of antibodies against growth factor receptors different from VEGF receptors but involved in the control of VEGF expression in tumor cells.

Recently, it was shown that angiogenesis and tumor invasion of malignant human keratinocytes in surface transplants on nude mice could be prevented by using a monoclonal antibody which inhibits the activation of the VEGF receptor-2 [67]. This again demonstrates that interfering with VEGF signalling results in the disruption of the sequence of events involved in tumor progression.

Assuming a substantial redundancy in tumor angiogenesis, i.e. the involvement of several angiogenic factors in the same process as it has been demonstrated for primary breast cancer [68] one might suggest that blocking signalling by one angiogenic factor will not be sufficient. As it will be difficult to estimate in each individual case which angiogenic factors are involved, a cytotoxic approach for endothelial cells involved in tumor angiogenesis might be a therapeutic alternative. By using VEGF-diphtheria toxin conjugates it could be shown that VEGF receptor-2 expressing endothelial cells were affected whereas receptor-negative ovarian cells were not. Furthermore, the conjugate blocked neovascularization in the chick chorioallantoic membrane assay [69].

The inhibition of the VEGF receptor-tyrosine-kinase will certainly be another challenging therapeutic opportunity [70]. Low molecular compounds, penetrating endothelial cells and affecting selectively the activation of the VEGF receptors could be developed. The activity profile of such compounds could be extended to other angiogenic receptor tyrosine kinases if necessary. However, this requires much more work to elucidate the participation of other angiogenic signalling systems in tumor angiogenesis.

References

1. Folkman, J., *Nat. Med.* 1: 27–31, 1995.
2. Marmé, D., *World J. Urol.* 14: 166–174, 1999.
3. Ferrara, N., and Davis-Smyth, T., *Endocr. Rev.* 18: 4–25, 1997.
4. Finkenzeller, G., Marmé, D., Weich, H.A., and Hug, H., *Cancer Res.* 52: 4821–4823, 1992.
5. Brogi, E., Wu, T., Namiki, A., and Isner, J.M., *Circulation* 90: 649–652, 1994.
6. Detmar, M., Brown, L.E., Claffey, K.P., Yeo, K.T., Kocher, O., Jackman, R.W., Berse, B., and Dvorak, H.E., *J. Exp. Med.* 180: 1141–1146, 1994.
7. Pertovaara, L., Kaipainen, A., Mustonen, T., Orpana, A., Ferrara, N., Saksela, O., and Alitalo, K., *J. Biol. Chem.* 269: 6271–6274, 1994.
8. Frank, S., Hubner, G., Breier, G., Longaker, M.T., Greenhalgh, D.G., and Werner, S., *J. Biol. Chem.* 270: 12607–12613, 1995.
9. Li, J., Perrella, M.A., Tsai, J.C., Yet, S.F., Hsieh, C.M., Yoshizurm, M., Patterson, C., Enclege, W.O., Zhou, F., and Lee, M.E., *J. Biol. Chem.* 270: 308–312, 1995.
10. Cohen, T., Nahari, D., Cerem, I.-W., Neufeld, G., and Levi, B.Z., *J. Biol. Chem.* 271: 736–741, 1996.

11. Warren, R.S., Yuan, H., Math, M.R., Ferrara, N., and Donner, D.B., *J. Biol. Chem.* 271: 29483–29488, 1996.
12. Tischer, F., Mitchell, R., Hartman, T., Silva, M., Gospodarowi'cz, D., Fiddes, J.C., and Abraham, J.A., *J. Biol. Chem.* 266: 11947–11954, 1991.
13. Grugel, S., Finkenzeller, G., Weindel, K., Barleon, B., and Marmé, D., *J. Biol. Chem.* 270: 25915–25919, 1995.
14. Rak, J., Mitsuhashi, Y., Bayko, L., Filmus, J., Shirasawa, S., Sasazuki, T., and Kerbel, R.S., *Cancer Res.* 55: 4575–4580, 1995.
15. Mukhopadhyay, D., Tsiokas, L., and Sukhatme, V.P., *Cancer Res.* 55: 6161–6165, 1995.
16. Kieser, A., Weich, H.A., Brandner, G., Marmé, D., and Kolch, W., *Oncogene* 9: 963–969, 1994.
17. Sierneister, G., Weindel, K., Mohrs, K., Barleon, B., Martiny-Baron, G., and Marmé, D., *Cancer Res.* 56: 2299–2301, 1996.
18. Shweiki, D., Itin, A., Soffer, D., and Keshet, E., *Nature* 359: 843–845, 1992.
19. Plate, K.H., Breier, G., Weich, H.A., and Risau, W., *Nature* 359: 845–848, 1992.
20. Ryuto, M., Ono, M., Izumi, H., Yoshida, S., Weich, H.A., Kohno, K., and Kuwano, M., *J. Biol. Chem.* 271: 28220–28228, 1996.
21. Gille, J., Swerlick, R.A., and Caughman, S.W., *EMBO J.* 16: 750–759, 1997.
22. Finkenzeller, G., Sparacio, A., Technau, A., Marmé, D., and Siemeister, G., *Oncogene* 15: 669–676, 1997.
23. Mukhopadhyay, D., Knebelmann, B., Cohen, H.T., Ananth, S., and Sukhatme, V.P., *Mol. Cell. Biol.* 17: 5629–5639, 1997.
24. Duan, D.R., Pause, A., Burgess, W.H., Aso, T., Chen, D.Y.T., Garrett, K.P., Conaway, R.C., Conaway, J.W., Linehan, W.M., and Klausner, R.D., *Science* 269: 1402–1406, 1995.
25. Aso, T., Lane, W.S., Conaway, J.W., and Conaway, R.C., *Science* 269: 1439–1443, 1995.
26. Kibel, A., Iliopoulos, O., DeCaprio, J.A., and Kaelin, W.G. Jr., *Science* 269: 1444–1446, 1995.
27. Iliopoulos, O., Levy, A.P., Jiang, C., Kaelin, W.G. Jr., and Goldberg, M., *Proc. Natl. Acad. Sci. USA* 93: 10595–10599, 1996.
28. Ikeda, E., Achen, M.G., Breier, G., and Risau, W., *J. Biol. Chem.* 270: 19761–19766, 1995.
29. Damert, A., Machein, M., Breier, G., Fujita, M.Q., Hanahan, D., Risau, W., and Plate, K.H., *Cancer Res.* 57: 3860–3864, 1997.
30. Levy, A.P., Levy, N.S., and Goldberg, M.A., *J. Biol. Chem.* 271: 2746–2753, 1996.
31. Levy, A.P., Levy, N.S., and Goldberg, M.A., *J. Biol. Chem.* 271: 25492–25497, 1996.
32. Forsythe, J.A., Jiang, B.H., Iyer, N.V., Agani, F., Leung, S.W., Koos, R.D., and Semenza, G.L., *Mol. Cell. Biol.* 16: 4604–4613, 1996.
33. Damert, A., Ikeda, E., and Risau, W., *Biochem. J.* 327: 419–423, 1997.
34. Mazure, N.M., Chen, E.Y., Yeh, P., Laderoute, K.R., and Giaccia, A.J., *Cancer Res.* 56: 3436–3440, 1996.
35. Mazure, N.M., Chen, E.Y., Laderoute, K.R., and Giaccia, A.J., *Blood* 90: 3322–3331, 1997.
36. Arbiser, J.L., Moses, M.A., Fernandez, C.A., Ghiso, N., Cao, Y., Klauber, N., Frank, D., Brownlee, M., Flynn, E., Parangi, S., Byers, H.R., and Folkman, *J. Proc. Natl. Acad Sci. USA* 94: 861–866, 1997.

37. Mukhopadhyay, D., Tsiokas, L., Zhou, X.M., Foster, D., Brugge, J.S., and Sukhatme, V.P., *Nature* 375: 577−581, 1995.
38. Gleadle, J.M., and Ratcliffe, PJ., *Blood* 89: 503−509, 1997.
39. Kevil, C.G., De Benedetti, A., Payne, D.K., Coe, L.L., Laroux, F.S., and Alexander, J.S., *Int. J. Cancer* 65: 785−790, 1996.
40. Kerekatte, V., Smiley, K., Hu, B., Smith, A., Gelder, F., and De Benedetti, A., *Int. J. Cancer* 64: 27−31, 1995.
41. Miyagi, Y., Sugiyama, A., Asai, A., Okazaki, T., Kuchino, Y., and Kerr, S.J., *Cancer L* 91: 247−252, 1995.
42. Olander, J.V., Connolly, D.T., and DeLarco, J.E., *Biochem. Biophys. Res. Commun.* 175: 68−76, 1991.
43. Quinn, T.P., Peters, K.G., De Vries, C., and Ferrara, N., *Proc. Natl. Acad. Sci. USA* 90: 7533−7537, 1993.
44. Peters, K.G., De Vries, C., and Williams, L.T., *Proc. Natl. Acad. Sci. USA* 90: 8915−8919, 1993.
45. Millauer, B., Wizigmann-Voos, S., Schnurch, H., Martinez, R., MoIler, N.P.H., Risau, W., and Ullrich, A., *Cell* 72: 835−846, 1993.
46. Klagsbrun, M., D'Amore, P.A., *Annu. Rev Physiol.* 53: 217−239, 1991.
47. Frater-Schroder, M., Risau, W., Hallmann, R., and Gautsch, P., *Proc. Natl. Acad. Sci. USA* 84: 5277−5281, 1987.
48. Leibovich, S., Polverini, P., Shepard, H., Wiseman, D., Shively, V., and Nuseir, N., *Nature* 329: 630−632,
49. Patterson, C., PerTella, M.A., Endege, W.O., Yoshizumi, M., Lee, M.-E., and Haber, E., *J. Clin. Invest.* 98: 490−496, 1996.
50. Mandriota, S.J., Menoud, P.-A., and Pepper, M.S., *J. Biol Chem.* 271: 11500−11505, 1996.
51. Kremer, C., Breier, G., Risau, W., and Plate, K.H., *Cancer Res.* 57: 3852−3859, 1997.
52. Barleon, B., Siemeister, G., Martiny-Baron, G., Weindel, K., Herzog, C., and Marmé, D., *Cancer Res.* 57: 5421−5425, 1997.
53. Tuder, R.M., Flook, B.E., and Voelkel, N.F., *J. Clin. Invest.* 95: 1798−1807, 1995.
54. Detmar, M., Brown, L.F., Berse, B., Jackman, R.W., Elicker, B.M., Dvorak, H.F., and Claffey, K.P., *J. Invest. Dermatol.* 108: 263−268, 1997.
55. Thieme, H., Aiello, L.P., Takagi, H., Ferrara, N., and King, G.L., *Diabetes* 44: 98−103, 1995.
56. Brogi, E., Schatteman, G., Wu, T., Kim, E.A., Varticovski, L., Keyt, B., and Isner, J.M., *J. Clin. Inves.* 97: 469−476, 1996.
57. Morishita, K., Johnson, D.E., and Williams, L.T., *J. Biol. Chem.* 270: 27948−27953, 1995.
58. Patterson, C., Perrella, M.A., Hsieh, C.-M., Yoshizumi, M., Lee, M.-E., and Haber, E., *J. Biol. Chem.* 270: 23111−23118, 1995.
59. Ronicke, V., Risau, W., and Breier, G., *Cite Res.* 79: 277−285, 1996.
60. Gerber, H.-P., Condorelli, F., Park, J., and Ferrara, N., *J. Biol. Chem.* 272: 23659−23667, 1997.
61. Millauer, B., Shawver, K.L., Plate, K.H., Risau, W., and Ullrich, A., *Nature* 367: 576−579, 1994.
62. Kim, K.J., Li, B., Winer, J., Armanini, M., Gillett, N., Phillips, H.S., and Ferrara N., *Nature* 362: 841−844, 1993.

63. Borgstrym, P., Hillan, K.J., Sriramarao, P., and Ferrara, N., *Cancer Res.* 56: 4032–4039, 1996.
64. Warren, R.A., Yuan, H., Math, M.R., Gillett, N.A., and Ferrara, N., *J. Clin. Invest.* 95: 1789–1797, 1995.
65. Saleh, M., Stacker, S.A., and Wilks, A.F., *Cancer Res.* 56: 393–401, 1996.
66. Petit, A.M.V., Rak, J., Hung, M.-C., Rockwell, P., Goldstein, N., Fetidly, B., and Kerbel, R.S., *Am. J. Pathol.* 151: 1523–1530, 1997.
67. Skobe, M., Rockwell, P., Goldstein, N., Vosseler, S., and Fusenig, N.E., *Nature Med.* 3: 1222–1227, 1997.
68. Relf, M., LeJeune, S., Scott, P.A.E., Fox, S., Smith, K., Leek, R., Moghaddam, A., Whitehouse, R., Bicknell, R., and Harris, A.L., *Cancer Res.* 57: 963–969, 1997.
69. Ramakrishnan, S., Olson, T.A., Bautch, V.L., and Mohanraj, D., *Cancer Res.* 56: 1324–1330, 1996.
70. Strawn, L.M., McMahon, G., App, H., Schreck, R., Kuchler, W.R., Longhi, M.P., Hui, T.H., Tang, C., Levitzki, A., Gazit, A., Chen, L., Keri, G., Otfi, L., Risau, W., Flamme, L., Ullrich, A., Hirth, K.P., and Shawver, L.K., *Cancer Res.* 56: 3540–3545, 1996.

JERRY Y. NIEDERKORN

Natural killer cells and uveal melanoma

Abstract

Uveal melanoma is the most common and malignant intraocular tumor in adults. Although uveal melanomas and cutaneous melanomas arise from neural crest progenitors, they display markedly different biological properties. Findings from animal models and patients suggest that natural killer (NK) cells might limit the growth and metastasis of intraocular melanomas. Human uveal melanoma cells are sensitive to NK cell-mediated lysis *in vitro* and depletion of NK cells in mice results in a sharp increase in the metastasis of intraocular melanomas. Although NK cells can infiltrate uveal melanomas, intraocular cytokines, such as transforming growth factor-beta (TGF-β) and macrophage migration inhibitory factor (MIF), actively suppress NK cytolytic activity *in situ*. However, once uveal melanoma cells depart from the immunologically privileged confines of the eye, they enter the bloodstream and they eventually extravasate into the liver. Both the bloodstream and the liver express robust NK cell repertoires. However, successful uveal melanoma metastases utilize multiple adaptations to reduce their vulnerability to NK cell-mediated lysis in the bloodstream and in the liver. Dismantling these NK escape mechanisms could have significant impact in the management of uveal melanomas.

Keywords: Natural killer cells, uveal melanoma

Introduction

Melanomas of the uveal tract are the most common intraocular malignancies in adults with an incidence of seven cases per one million adults per year in the western hemisphere [1]. Although cutaneous and uveal melanomas share a neural crest origin, they differ markedly in their epidemiological [2–4], cytogenetic [5], metastatic [6–8], and immunological [6] characteristics. One of the most striking differences between skin and uveal melanomas is in their metastatic behavior. Skin melanoma metastasizes to almost any organ

University of Texas Southwestern Medical Center, 5323 Harry Hines Boulevard, Dallas, TX 75235-9057, USA

in the body and is one of the few cancers that metastasizes regularly to the heart [7]. By contrast, uveal melanoma displays a strong propensity to metastasize to the liver. In fact, liver metastases are present in over 85% of the patients who die from uveal melanoma [8–10]. Not only do uveal and skin melanomas differ in their cell biology, they also arise in anatomical regions with remarkably different immunological and physiological properties. Skin melanomas grow in an environment, which normally permits the full array of immunological functions. By contrast, intraocular melanomas arise in a milieu lacking patent lymphatic drainage and in which many immune processes are stifled.

The notion that the immune system might be capable of recognizing and eliminating neoplasms was first articulated by the eminent microbiologist Paul Ehrlich and later modified by Burnet [11]. In the thirty years since Burnet's proposal of the immune surveillance theory, most research has centered on the role of T cells and cytokines in tumor immunity. However, in addition to T cell-mediated tumor immunity, natural resistance mechanisms may also be important [12]. Natural resistance mechanisms involve macrophages, natural killer (NK) cells, and granulocytes. NK cells seem particularly suited for the surveillance of neoplasms as these cells do not require priming or clonal expansion in order to exert anti-tumor effects. Like T cells, NK cells produce cell-mediated cytotoxicity and secrete a diverse array of cytokines and chemokines. However, unlike B and T cells, NK cell development and function does not require gene rearrangement [12]. Results from animals studies over the past two decades have provided compelling evidence that NK cells play an important role in limiting the growth and metastasis of various rodent tumors, especially skin melanomas. However, the importance of NK cells in the surveillance of human tumors is less clear. Human melanoma cell lines are susceptible to NK cell-mediated cytolysis *in vitro* and *in vivo* [13]. NK cells have been detected within skin melanoma lesions [14] and a positive correlation between NK cell activity and disease-free survival time in cutaneous melanoma patients has been observed [15]. To date, the role of NK cells in uveal melanoma has not been addressed. Therefore, my comments in this chapter will be largely speculative and based on my interpretation of a wide range of *in vitro* and *in vivo* findings from experimental animals and uveal melanoma patients. This discussion should not be viewed as a definitive overview. Instead, I hope that it will be thought-provoking and prompt the reader to explore this topic in greater detail, both in the laboratory and in the literature.

Are uveal melanomas NK-sensitive?

Although numerous studies have demonstrated NK cell-mediated cytolysis of skin melanomas, little is known about the susceptibility of uveal melanomas to NK cells. Our laboratory examined four human uveal melanoma cell lines for their susceptibility to lysis by mouse and human NK

Jerry Y. Niederkorn

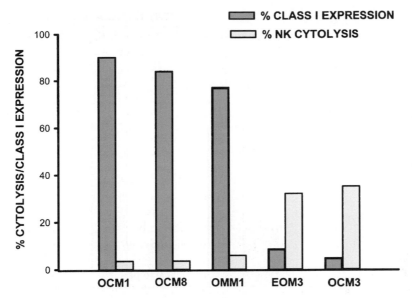

F I G U R E 1 .   *Correlation between MHC class I expression and susceptibility of uveal melanoma cells (OCM1, OCM8 and OCM3) and uveal melanoma metastases (OMM1 and EOM3) to NK cell-mediated cytolysis* in vitro. *Original data were published by Ma and Niederkorn [16].*

cells *in vitro* and found a close correlation between the expression of MIIC class I antigen expression on uveal melanoma cells and reduced susceptibility to NK cell-mediated cytolysis [16,17] (Fig. 1). These findings are in keeping with the "missing self" hypothesis of Kärre and co-workers which proposes that MHC class I molecules on a potential target cell transmit an inhibitory signal to NK cells and thereby prevent cytolysis [18]. However, cells failing to express MHC class I molecules do not send an "off" signal to NK cells, and as a result are killed. Unlike skin melanomas, intraocular melanomas reside in an environment containing a potpourri of factors which might influence MHC class I expression. The aqueous humor in particular is richly endowed with transforming growth factor-β (TGF-β) [19,20], a cytokine noted for its capacity to down-regulate MHC class I expression [21,22]. We have found that uveal melanoma cells incubated in TGF-β display significantly reduced levels of MHC class I molecules and a proportional increase in susceptibility to NK cell-mediated lysis *in vitro* [16] (Fig. 2). Analogous effects were observed with uveal melanomas which constitutively expressed low levels of MIIC class I molecules. Stimulation of class I antigen expression by incubation with interferon-γ (IFN-γ) resulted in a sharp increase in MHC class I expression and a comparable diminution in NK cell-mediated lysis (Fig. 3).

Thus, it appears that human uveal melanomas are indeed susceptible to NK cell-mediated lysis *in vitro*. The capacity of an intraocular cytokine, TGF-β, to down-regulate class I expression and thus, reduce the

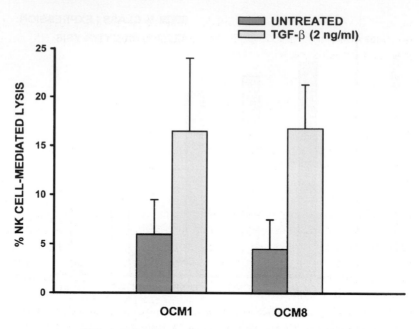

FIGURE 2. *Effect of physiological levels of TGF-β on NK cell-mediated lysis of two human uveal melanoma cell lines. Original data were published by Ma and Niederkorn [16].*

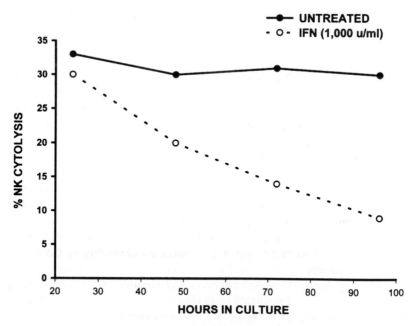

FIGURE 3. *Effect of IFN-γ on NK cell-mediated cytolysis of OCM-3 human uveal melanoma cells. Original data were published by Ma and Niederkorn [16].*

Jerry Y. Niederkorn

vulnerability of melanoma cells to NK-mediated cytotoxicity, suggests that melanomas within the eye might be particularly susceptible to NK cell-mediated surveillance.

Do NK cells enter uveal melanomas?

There is considerable evidence that lymphocytes enter tumor-containing eyes. Lymphocytes have been found infiltrating 7–20% of the uveal melanomas examined [23–25]. However, it is uncertain if the lymphocyte population infiltrating uveal melanomas displays antigen specificity. Nitta and co-workers demonstrated that tumor infiltrating lymphocytes (TIL) present in seven of eight human uveal melanomas expressed the same Vα T cell receptor (TCR) gene suggestive of a melanoma-specific T cell response [25]. By contrast, others have reported that TIL populations from uveal melanomas express a diversity of TCR Vβ genes. Thus, it is not clear if the lymphocytes that infiltrate uveal melanomas are oligoclonal in nature or if they represent a random array of lymphocytes. The former proposition is supported by *in vitro* studies which have demonstrated that TIL from uveal melanoma patients can mediate uveal melanoma-specific cytolysis [26,27]. Much less is known about the presence and functional capacities of NK cells that infiltrate uveal melanomas. In two studies, less than 10% of the TIL in uveal melanomas expressed surface markers indicative of NK cells [28,29]. However, Ksander and co-workers reported that 41% of the TIL population from a choroidal melanoma expressed the CD16 NK cell marker and lysed NK-sensitive K562 target cells *in vitro* [26].

Do NK cells function within the eye?

The immune privilege of the intraocular microenvironment is widely recognized but often misunderstood. It has been known for over a century that the anterior chamber of the eye permits the long term survival of foreign tissue and tumor grafts which are normally rejected at extraocular sites. Multiple mechanisms account for the immunological sanctuary provided by the intraocular milieu; these include: (a) the pervasive expression of Fas ligand (CD95L) within the eye; (b) the presence of aqueous humor cytokines which inhibit lymphocyte proliferation; (c) a putative absence of lymph vessels that drain the interior of the eye; and (d) the active down-regulation of Th1 immune responses to antigens appearing in the anterior segment of the eye.

Until only recently, it was not known if intraocular immune privilege was extended to NK cell-mediated immunity. An important contributor to the immune privilege in the eye is TGF-β a cytokine present within both the anterior and posterior compartments of the eye. TGF-β is a pleiotropic molecule, and among its many functions is its capacity to inhibit T and

B cell proliferation and NK cell-mediated cytotoxicity [30]. *In vitro* studies have demonstrated that the optimal concentration for inhibiting NK cell-mediated cytolytic activity is the same as the normal physiological concentration within the aqueous humor of the eye (i.e., 2 ng/ml) [19,20]. With this in mind, we examined the fate of NK sensitive uveal melanoma cells transplanted into the eyes of athymic nude mice [31]. Although nude mice are deficient in T cell-mediated and T cell-dependent immune responses, they exhibit above normal NK cell-mediated immunity. NK-sensitive human uveal melanomas were promptly rejected following subcutaneous transplantation. The rejection of the subcutaneous tumors was mediated by NK cells because the same tumors grew progressively in hosts whose NK cell population was depleted by systemic treatment with anti-asialo GM1 antibody. By contrast, NK sensitive tumors, which were rejected at subcutaneous sites, grew progressively in the eyes of nude mice, even at doses 50-fold lower than those which were rejected following subcutaneous transplantation [31]. Although NK cells can enter at least some intraocular melanomas, the intraocular milieu stifles the NK cell-mediated cytolytic machinery and allows the tumor to grow progressively.

What is the basis for NK cell immune privilege in the eye?

According to the "missing self" hypothesis, cells failing to express nominal quantities of MHC class I molecules are susceptible to NK cell-mediated cytolysis [18]. In this regard, it is noteworthy that the corneal endothelium expresses infinitesimal quantities of classical MHC class I molecules [32], and the lens epithelium fails to even express class I transcripts [33]. Moreover, corneal endothelial cells are highly susceptible to NK cell-mediated cytolysis *in vitro* [34], yet there is no compelling evidence to date indicating that the intact corneal endothelium is damaged by NK cells under normal or disease conditions. Accordingly, we wondered if constituents of the aqueous humor inhibited NK cell-mediated cytolytic activity. As mentioned earlier, TGF-β is a major component of the aqueous humor (AH) and has been shown to inhibit NK cell-mediated cytolytic activity *in vitro* [30]. *In vitro* studies confirmed that AH inhibited NK cell-mediated cytolysis *in vitro* (Fig. 4); however, unlike TGF-β which requires 18–20 hours to exert its inhibitory effect, AH produced an immediate diminution of NK cell activity [34,35]. Moreover, treating AH with anti-TGF-β antibody did not remove its NK inhibitory activity. Gel filtration chromatography of rabbit AH revealed that a single 10–12 kDa protein fraction was responsible for the immediate inhibitory effect on NK cell-mediated cytolytic activity. Amino acid sequence analysis of this fraction indicated that the molecule shared >90% amino acid homology with macrophage migration inhibitory factor (MIF). Further *in vitro* studies demonstrated that recombinant MIF produced an immediate inhibition of NK cell-mediated cytolysis similar to that produced by rabbit AH.

Jerry Y. Niederkorn

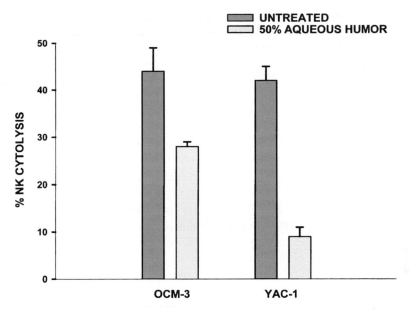

F I G U R E 4 .   *Effect of aqueous humor on NK cell-mediated cytolysis of OCM-3 human uveal melanoma cells and YAC-1 murine lymphoma cells. Original results were published by Apte* et al. *[31].*

These results begged the obvious question "How do AH and MIF inhibit NK cell-mediated cytotoxicity?" In order for NK cells to lyse a potential target cell, three processes must be satisfied. First, the NK cell and the target cell must bind to form cell−cell conjugates. Second, activation molecules on the NK cell membrane, such as the recently described immunoreceptor tyrosine based activation motif (ITAM), must engage their receptors on the target cells. Third, the NK cell must release its cytolytic perforin granules onto the target cell membrane. *In vitro* analysis of MIF indicted that it did not impair NK-target cell conjugate formation or affect the expression of killer activation receptors (e.g., 2B.4) or killer inhibitor receptors (ITIM; 5E6) on the NK cell surface. However, AH produced a steep reduction in the exocytosis of perforin from NK cells [35]. It is noteworthy that this inhibitory effect appears to spare the action of cytotoxic T lymphocytes (CTL) because incubation of allospecific CTL in AH has no demonstrable effect on the cytolysis of allogeneic target cells [34]. Thus, the inhibitory effect of MIF appears to be specific for NK cells and acts at the terminal stage of the NK cell-mediated cytolytic process (Table 1). It bears noting that not only is MIF present in the AH, but the MIF gene is also expressed by cells in the cornea, lens, iris, and ciliary body [36−38]. Moreover, we have recently found that some cell lines from uveal melanomas and their metastases produce MIF *in vitro* (unpublished findings). Thus, intraocular melanomas reside in a milieu that shields them from NK

TABLE 1.   *Effect of aqueous humor and MIF on NK cell activity.*

Property	Effect
Cytolysis of NK sensitive targets	Inhibited
Effect on allospecific CTL	No effect
Viability of NK cells	No effect
NK/Target cell conjugate formation	No effect
Expression of activation molecules	No effect
Expression of inhibitory molecules	No effect
Induction of NK inhibition	Induced in less than 4 hrs
NK perforin granule release	Inhibited

cell-mediated destruction. The capacity of uveal melanoma cells to constitutively secrete MIF suggests that metastases arising from some uveal melanomas are preadapted to escape NK cell-mediated assault once they leave the sanctuary of the eye.

Do NK cells influence the development of uveal melanoma metastases?

A sizable body of evidence from prospective studies indicates that NK cells inhibit tumor metastasis in mice. Circumstantial evidence from clinical studies suggests a similar role for NK cells in limiting the spread of skin melanoma in humans. A positive correlation between NK cell activity and disease-free survival time has been reported in patients with skin melanoma [15]. Although the intraocular milieu provides relief from NK cell-mediated attack, once metastatic uveal melanoma cells leave the eye, they must evade NK cells within the bloodstream and within the parenchyma of the liver—two sites of intense NK activity. For example, studies in mice have shown that *in vivo* depletion of NK cells with anti-asialo GM 1 antibody results in a 200-fold increase in liver metastases in mice challenged intravenously with B16 melanoma cells [39]. If NK cell-mediated immune surveillance plays a significant role in controlling uveal melanoma metastases, one might predict that successful metastases must be endowed with properties which inhibit NK cell activity outside of the immunologically privileged confines of the eye. Two possibilities come to mind. First, the expression of MHC class I molecules is known to protect tumor cells from NK cell-mediated lysis and might be an effective strategy for metastases to escape destruction in the bloodstream and liver. A second strategy is for the melanoma cells to create their own immune privileged nidus by secreting NK inhibitory factors such as TGF-β and MIF. Two studies on human melanoma patients offer support for the hypothesis that MHC class I antigen expression favors the development of uveal melanoma metastases. Verbik and co-workers demonstrated that only 4% of the tumor cells from a primary uveal melanoma expressed MHC class I molecules; by

Jerry Y. Niederkorn

contrast, the incidence of class I expression was nine times higher in melanoma cells isolated from four different liver metastases in the same patient [40]. Further support for this hypothesis comes from studies by Blom and co-workers who examined 30 primary uveal melanomas and found a significant correlation between the expression of MHC class I molecules and poor prognosis [41].

Corneal endothelial and lens epithelial cells express little or no MHC class I antigen, yet do not experience NK cell-mediated destruction within the eye, presumably due to the presence of NK inhibitory molecules in the AH which bathes the cells lining the anterior chamber. Moreover, both lens epithelial cells and corneal endothelial cells produce MIF [37, 38]. We suspected that metastatic uveal melanoma cells might adopt a similar strategy for shielding themselves from NK cell-mediated lysis once they depart from the eye. Preliminary results from our laboratory indicate that at least some uveal melanoma cell lines produce MIF which protects them from NK cell-mediated lysis. Interestingly, the most potent inhibitor effect was found with supernatants from a cell line established from a uveal melanoma metastasis. It remains to be seen if these preliminary findings can be confirmed, but if they are, it would help explain the capacity of uveal melanomas to escape NK cell-mediated elimination in the bloodstream and in the liver.

One can only speculate as to whether activation of NK cells will be an effective adjunct therapy for uveal melanoma patients. The profound inhibitory effect of TGF-β and MIF within the eye casts doubt on the feasibility of activating NK cells as a means of eradicating primary uveal melanomas. Likewise, NK cells might be faced with an insurmountable task if liver metastases express high MHC class I and secrete MIF (and perhaps other inhibitor molecules such as TGF-β). Efforts to utilize NK cells to treat liver metastases should consider strategies for dismantling these barriers and thereby allowing NK cells to perform their role in immune surveillance.

References

1. Mooy, C., and De Jong, P.T.V.M., *Surv. Ophthalmol.* 41: 215−228, 1996.
2. Mahoney, M., Burnett, W.S., Majerovics, A., and Tanenbaum, H., *Ophthalmology* 97: 1143−1147, 1990.
3. Roberts, D., *Clin. Exp. Dermatol.* 15: 406− 409, 1990.
4. Schwartz, Sm. W.N., *Int. J. Cancer* 41: 174−177, 1988.
5. McCarthy, J.M.R.J., Horsman, D., and White, V.A., *Surv. Ophthalmol.* 37: 377−386, 1993.
6. Niederkorn, J., *Progr. Retinal Eye Res.* 14: 505−526, 1995.
7. Vijayasaradhi, S., and Houghton, A.N., *Adv. Pharmacol.* 32: 343−374, 1995.
8. Char, D., *Am. J. Ophthalmol.* 86: 76−80, 1978.
9. Donoso, L., Berd, D., Augsburger, J.J., Mastrangelo, M.J., and Shields, J.A., *Arch. Ophthalmol.* 103: 796−798, 1985.
10. Rajpal, S., Moore, R., and Karakousis, C.P., *Cancer* 52: 334−340, 1983.
11. Burnet, F., *Progr. Exp. Tumor Res.* 13: 1−27, 1970.

12. Ortaldo, J., and Longo, D.L., *J. Natl. Cancer Inst.* 80: 999−1009, 1988.
13. Hill, L., Perussia, B., McCue, P.A., and Korngold, R., *Cancer Res.* 54: 763−770, 1994.
14. Kornstein, M., Stewart, R., and Elder, D.E., *Cancer Res.* 47: 1411−1412, 1987.
15. Hersey, P., Edwards, A., Milton, G.W., and McCarthy, W.H., *Br. J. Cancer* 37: 505−513, 1978.
16. Ma, D., and Niederkorn, J., *Immunology* 86: 263−269, 1995.
17. Ma, D., and Niederkorn, J.Y., *Invest. Ophthalmol. Vis. Sci.* 39: 1067−1075, 1998.
18. Ljunggren, H., and Kärre, K., *Immunol. Today* 11: 237−244, 1990.
19. Jampel H, Roche N, Stark, W.J., and Roberts, A.B., *Curr. Eye Res.* 9: 963−969, 1990.
20. Cousins, S., McCabe, M., Danielpour, D., and Streilein, J.W., *Invest. Ophthalmol. Vis. Sci.* 32: 2201−2211, 1991.
21. Krueger, J., Krane, J., Carter, D., and Gottlieb, A., *J. Invest. Dermatol.* 94: 135, 1990.
22. Orcl, P., Bielakoff, J., and De Vernejoul, M.D., *J. Cell Physiol.* 142: 293, 1990.
23. De La Cruz, Jr. P., Specht, C.S., and McLean, I.W., *Cancer* 65: 112−115, 1990.
24. Durie, F., Campbell, A.M., Lee, W.R., and Damato, B.E., *Invest. Ophthalmol. Vis. Sci.* 31: 2106−2110, 1990.
25. Nitta, T., Oksenberg, J.R., Rao, N.A., and Steinman, L., *Science* 249: 672−674, 1990.
26. Ksander, B., Rubsamen, P., Olsen, K., Cousins, S., and Streilein, J.W., *Invest. Ophthalmol. Vis. Sci.* 32: 3198−3208, 1991.
27. Ksander, B., Geer, D.C., Chen, P.W., Salgaller, M.L., Rubsamen, P., and Murray, T.G., *Curr. Eye Res.* 17: 165−173, 1998.
28. Meecham, W., Char, D.H., and Kaleta-Michaels, S., *Ophthalmol. Res.* 24: 20−26, 1992.
29. De Waard-Siebinga, I., Hlders, C.G.J.M., Hansen, B.E., van Delft, J.L., and Jager, M.J., *Graefe's Arch. Clin. Exp. Ophthalmol.* 234: 34−43, 1996.
30. Rook, A., Kehrl, J.H., Wakefield, L.M., Roberts, A.B., Sporn, M.B., Burlington, D.B., Lane, H.C., and Fauci, A.S., *J. Immunol.* 136: 3916−3920, 1986.
31. Apte, R., Mayhew, E., and Niederkorn, J.Y., *Invest. Ophthalmol. Vis. Sci.* 38: 1277−1282, 1997.
32. Fujikawa, L., Colvin, R., Bhan, A., Fuller, T., and Foster, C., *Cornea* 1: 213, 1982.
33. Shaughnessy, M., and Wistow, G., *Curr. Eye Res.* 11: 175−181, 1992.
34. Apte, R., and Niederkorn, J.Y., *J. Immunol.* 156: 2667−2673, 1996.
35. Apte, R., Sinha, D., Mayhew, E., Wistow, G.J., and Niederkorn, J.Y., *J. Immunol.* 160: 5693−5696, 1998.
36. Wistow, G., Shagnessy, M.P., Lee, D.C., Hodin, J., and Zelenka, P.S., *Proc. Natl. Acad. Sci. USA* 90: 1272−1275, 1993.
37. Matsuda, A., Kotake, S., Tagawa, Y., Matsuda, H., and Nishihira, J., *Immunol. Lett.* 53: 1−5, 1996.
38. Matsuda, A., Tagawa, Y., Matsuda, H., and Nishihira, J., *FEBS Lett.* 385: 225−228, 1996.
39. Wiltrout, R., Herberman, R.B., Zhang, S.-R., Chirigos, M.A., Ortaldo, J.R., Green, Jr., K.M., and Talmadge, J.E., *J. Immunol.* 134: 4267−4275, 1985.
40. Verbik, D., Murray, T.G., Tran, J.M., and Ksander, B.R., *Int. J. Cancer* 73: 470−478, 1997.
41. Blom, D.-J., Luyten, G.P.M., Mooy, C., Kerkviet, S., Zwinderman, A.H., and Jager, M.J., *Invest. Ophthalmol. Vis. Sci.* 38: 1865−1872, 1997.

Jerry Y. Niederkorn

Specific immune response against tumor antigens defined by cytotoxic T lymphocytes (CTL)

Abstract

Tumor-associated antigens recognized by cellular or humoral effectors of the immune system represent attractive targets for antigen-specific cancer therapy. Different groups of cancer-associated antigens have been identified inducing cytotoxic T lymphocyte (CTL) responses *in vitro* and *in vivo*: (1) "Cancer Testis" (CT) antigens, which are expressed in different tumors and normal testis, (2) melanocyte differentiation antigens, (3) point mutations of normal genes, (4) antigens that are overexpressed in malignant tissues, and (5) viral antigens. Clinical studies with peptides derived from these antigens have been initiated to study the induction of specific CTL responses *in vivo*. Immunological and clinical parameters for the assessment of peptide-specific reactions have been defined, i.e. delayed-type hypersensitivity (DTH)-, CTL-, autoimmune-, and tumor regression responses. Early results show that tumor-associated peptides alone induce specific DTH- and CTL responses and tumor regression after intradermal administration. GM-CSF was used as an adjuvant to enhance peptide-specific immune reactions by amplification of dermal peptide-presenting dendritic cells. Complete tumor regressions have been observed in the context of measurable peptide-specific CTL. However, in single cases with disease progression after an initial tumor response, either a loss of the respective tumor antigen targeted by CTL or of the presenting MHC class I allele was detected suggesting immunization-induced immune escape. Based on these observations, cytokines to modify antigen- and MHC class I expression *in vivo* are being tested to prevent immunoselection. Recently, a new CT antigen, NY-ESO-1, has been identified with a strategy utilizing spontaneous antibody responses to tumor-associated antigens (SEREX). NY-ESO-1 is regarded as one of the most immunogenic antigens known today inducing spontaneous immune responses in 50% of patients with NY-ESO-1 expressing cancers. Clinical studies with antigenic constructs to induce both humoral and cellular immune responses will show whether these are more effective for immunotherapy of cancer.

Keywords: Tumor antigens, cytotoxic T cells, immunoselection

Introduction

Five groups of human tumor antigens have been identified so far that can be recognized by autologous and allogeneic CTL restricted by different MHC class I molecules. The first group, "Cancer Testis" (CT) antigens, includes the MAGE-gene family, BAGE, GAGE, and NY-ESO-1, antigens that are expressed in melanomas and some other tumors, but not in normal tissues except testis [1—4]. The second group of antigens represents melanocyte differentiation antigens that are expressed in melanomas and normal melanocytes [5—8]. Several peptide epitopes derived from these antigens, i.e. Melan A/MART-1, tyrosinase, gp100/Pmel17, and gp75 have been identified as targets for CTL and tumor infiltrating lymphocytes (TIL) in the context of HLA-A2.1 and other MHC class I molecules [6—9]. The third group of antigens caused by point mutations has been shown to generate potent CTL responses in individual human tumor systems [10,11]. The fourth category includes constitutive self-antigens, such as HER2/neu, p53 etc, that can become relevant tumor rejection antigens in case they are overexpressed in malignant tissues [12]. The fifth group of antigens includes viral antigens, that can be expressed by virus-associated malignancies, i.e. HPV in cervical cancer, HBV in hepatocellular carcinoma, and EBV in Burkitt's lymphoma [13—15].

Antigens expressed in tumor tissues and recognized by CTL are attractive targets for immunotherapeutic interventions to inhibit tumor growth. After adoptive transfer of tumor-infiltrating lymphocyte (TIL) lines recognizing epitopes derived from gp100/Pmel17, tyrosinase, and gp75, objective tumor regressions in single melanoma patients have been observed [6,16,17]. Active immunization with melanoma associated peptides derived from Melan A/MART-1 and tyrosinase has been shown to induce peptide-specific CTL responses *in vivo* [18,19]. In the presence of peptide-specific CTL, partial regression of antigen-positive tumors was observed. On the other hand, progressing melanoma lesions were observed in single patients in the presence of strong antigen-specific CTL responses [20]. Different mechanisms accounting for this phenomenon of immune escape have been identified in single patients.

CTL-mediated regression of metastatic melanoma—dependence on homogeneity of antigen- and MHC class I expression

In two clinical phase I studies using HLA-A2 restricted peptides derived from Melan A, tyrosinase, and gp100 for immunization in patients with metastatic melanoma, four objective remissions (two complete, two partial remissions) were observed in a collective of 26 treated patients [18,19]. The retrospective analysis of melanoma specimens biopsied before immunization showed, that responding patients had a strong and homogenous expression of both the target antigens and MHC class I in the autologous tumor tissues. Patients who developed progressive disease under treatment showed either a weak, heterogenous, or a lack of expression of either single melanoma-associated antigens, or MHC class I. These observations made in a small group of patients warrant further exploration with respect to additional tumor-associated antigens and different methods of assessment for antigen- and MHC class I expression. Since antigen-specific monoclonal antibodies have become available for immunohistochemical staining, tumor specimens can be analyzed for the intensity and heterogeneity of antigen expression on the cellular level. This way, the tissue distribution of antigens expressed is better reflected compared to RT-PCR analysis [21].

Evolution of antigen- and MHC class I expression under antigen-specific immunotherapy

On the basis of clinical development of single patients under antigen-specific immunotherapy, we were provided with new insights in mechanisms of escape from antigen-specific CTL recognition *in vivo*. Two examples are presented in Figs 1 a and b to illustrate the significance of CTL interaction with tumor cells expressing the respective antigens for both tumor regression and the selection of antigen loss variants. The first example (patient NW16) shows the regression of a tyrosinase-positive lesion after induction of a tyrosinase-specific CTL response *in vivo*, and a further progression of a tyrosinase-negative metastasis simultaneously. Subsequent tumor biopsies taken at 3- and 6-month intervals show an unchanged pattern of antigen expression in both lesions in the presence of a stable tyrosinase-specific CTL reactivity. Over a period of six months, a clinical complete regression of the tyrosinase-positive metastasis was noticed. Another biopsy taken from the original metastatic area confirmed this result histologically. A second patient (NW14) with Melan A-positive axillary lymph node metastases received immunotherapy with Melan A peptide to induce a specific CTL response *in vivo*. Over a period of 3 months, a stabilization of the lesion was confirmed. A second biopsy, however, revealed a weaker expression of Melan A by RT-PCR compared to the pre-study status. Under continued immunization, the Melan A-specific CTL response was maintained. After 6 months of immunization, the patient was diagnosed with rapid disease progression in the original lesion and with new liver-, spleen-, and lung metastases. Biopsies taken from all tumor sites showed a complete loss Melan A, whereas the Melan A-specific CTL reactivity persisted. These clinical examples suggest, that (1) antigen-specific CTL induced by peptide-immunization can mediate the regression of tumors expressing the respective antigens, and (2) antigens targeted by specific CTL may become

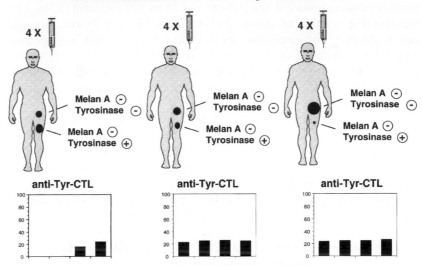

Immunoselection in vivo - Tyrosinase

FIGURE 1(A).   *The clinical course of disease of melanoma patient NW16, who had a Melan A, tyrosinase-negative metastasis in the left inguinal region, and a Melan A-negative, tyrosinase-positive lesion in the thigh. A tyrosinase-specific CTL response was induced under immunization with the HLA-A2 restricted tyrosinase-leader peptide (MLLAVLYCL) and maintained under continued immunization. The tyrosinase-positive metastasis decreased in size, whereas the tyrosinase-positive metastasis progressed under treatment.*

down-regulated under continued immunotherapy as one possible mechanism of immune escape.

In a larger collective of melanoma patients immunized with peptides derived from Melan A, tyrosinase, and gp100, we observed additional mechanisms of escape from antigen-specific CTL recognition. Of five patients immunized, four showed objective responses to treatment and progressed subsequently, one patient showed progressive disease initially. In responding patients, an increase of peptide-specific CTL reactivitiy was observed, that was maintained in the later state of disease progression. However, tumor biopsies taken at the time of tumor progression and analyzed by immunohistochemistry revealed that not only single target antigens, but also MHC class I alleles, as well as the MHC class I complex were down-regulated in single cases [21].

Loss of expression of tumor-associated antigens and MHC class I molecules—implications for antigen-specific immunotherapy

The results of the first clinical phase I studies on immunization using peptides derived from tumor-associated antigens in melanoma patients show

E. Jäger, D. Jäger and A. Knuth

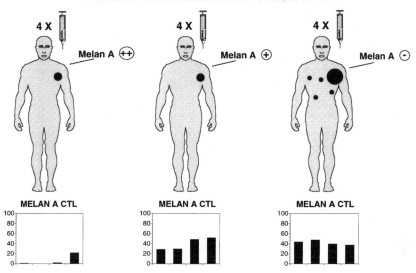

Immunoselection in vivo - Melan A

FIGURE 1(B). *The effects of immunization with the HLA-A2 restricted Melan A peptide (EAAGIGILTV) in melanoma patient NW13, who had a Melan A-positive axillary lymph node metastasis. Melan A-specific CTL were induced under immunization, and the metastastic lesion remained stable. However, Melan A expression seemed to decrease in the presence of Melan A-specific CTL. Under continued immunization, the patient developed rapid progression of the disease. The assessment of Melan A expression in the original and new lesions showed a complete loss of expression at all progressive sites.*

that tumor regressions can be observed in single cases. Tumor regression correlates closely to 2 parameters, (1) measurable increase of peptide-specific CTL response, and (2) homogeneous expression of the target antigen and MHC class I in the autologous tumor. Factors accompanied with tumor progression were a lack of peptide-specific CTL reactivitiy and/or a lack of expression of the respective target antigen and/or MHC class I. Retrospective large-scale reviews of metastatic melanoma tissues revealed that the differentiation antigens Melan A, tyrosinase, and gp100 were expressed in 75–85%, whereas MHC class I was expressed only in 64% of the samples. Furthermore, it was noticed that both antigen and MHC class I were expressed highly heterogenously in >50% of all tissues. For future studies on antigen-specific immunotherapy it seems essential to establish standards for the immunohistochemical assessment of defined antigens and MHC class I molecules that describe the pattern of antigen expression (homogeneous/heterogeneous) and the intensity on a cellular level. Subsequent clinical trials will then show, whether these qualitative and quantitative aspects of antigen- and MHC class I expression represent prognostic parameters for response to antigen-specific immunotherapy, and whether antigen and MHC class I expression can be modulated by concurrent treatments, i.e. cytokines (interferons), to prevent CTL-dependent immunoselection *in vivo*.

References

1. Boel, P., Wildman, C., Sensi, M.L., Brasseur, R., Renauld, J.C., Coulie, P., Boon, T., and Van der Bruggen, P., *Immunity* 2: 167−175, 1995.
2. Chen, Y.-T., Scanlan, M.J., Sahin, U., Türeci, Ö, Gure, A.O., Tsang, S., Williamson, B., Stockert, E., Pfreundschuh, M., and Old, L.J., *Proc. Natl. Acad. Sci. USA* 94: 1914−1918, 1997.
3. Van den Eynde, B., Peeters, O., De Backer, O., Gaugler, B., Lucas, S., and Boon, T., *J. Exp. Med.* 182: 689−698, 1995.
4. Van der Bruggen, P., Traversari, C., Chomez, P., Lurquin, C., De Plaen, E., Van den Eynde, B., Knuth, A., and Boon, T., *Science* 254: 1643−1647, 1991.
5. Anichini, A., Maccalli, C., Mortarini, R., Salvi, S., Mazzocchi, A., Squarcina, P., Herlyn, M., and Parmiani, G., *J. Exp. Med.* 177: 989−998, 1993.
6. Bakker, A.B., Schreurs, M.W.J., De Boer, A.J., Kawakami, Y., Rosenberg, S.A., Adema, G.J., and Figdor, C.G., *J. Exp. Med.* 179: 1005−1009, 1994.
7. Brichard, V., Van Pel, A., Wölfel, T., Wölfel, C., DePlaen, E., Lethe, B., Coulie, P., and Boon, T., *J. Exp. Med.* 178: 489−495, 1993.
8. Coulie, P.G., Brichard, V., Van Pel, A., Wölfel, T., Schneider, J., Traversari, C., Mattei, S., DePlaen, E., Lurquin, C., Szikora, J.-P., Renauld, J.-C., and Boon, T., *J. Exp. Med.* 180: 35−42, 1994.
9. Kawakami, Y., Eliyahu, S., Delgado, C.H., Robbins, P.F., Rivoltini, L., Topalian, S.L., Miki, T., and Rosenberg, S.A., *Proc. Natl. Acad. Sci. USA* 91: 3525−3519, 1994.
10. Coulie, P.G., Lehmann, F., Lethe, B., Herman, J., Lurquin, C., Andrawiss, M., and Boon, T., *Proc. Natl. Acad. Sci. USA* 92: 7976−7980, 1995.
11. Wölfel, T., Hauer, M., Schneider, J., Serrano, M., Wölfel, C., Klehmann-Hieb, E., DePlaen, E., Hankeln, T., Meyer zum Büschenfelde, K.-H., and Beach, D., *Science* 269: 1281−1284, 1995.
12. Disis, M.L., and Cheever, M.A., *Curr. Opinion Immunol.* 8: 637−642, 1996.
13. Feltkamp, M.C., Smits, H.L., Vierboom, M.P., Minnaar, R.P., De Jongh, B.M., Drijfhout, J.W., Ter Schegget, J., Melief, C.J., and Kast, W.M., *Eur. J. Immunol.* 23: 2242−2249, 1993.
14. Murray, R.J., Kurilla, M.G., Brooks, J.M., Thomas, W.A., Rowe, M., Kieff, E., and Rickinson, A.B., *J. Exp. Med.* 176: 157−168, 1992.
15. Rehermann, B., Fowler, P., Sidney, J., Person, J., Redeker, A., Brown, M., Moss, B., Sette, A., and Chisari, F.V., *J. Exp. Med.* 181: 1047−1058, 1995.
16. Kawakami, Y., Eliyahu, S., Delgado, C.H., Robbins, P.F., Sakaguchi, K., Appella, E., Yannelli, J.R., Adema, G.J., Miki, T., and Rosenberg, S.A., *Proc. Natl. Acad. Sci. USA* 91: 6458−6462, 1994.
17. Robbins, P.F., El-Gamil, M., Kawakami, Y., and Rosenberg, S.A., *Cancer Res.* 54: 3124−3126, 1994.
18. Jäger, E., Bernhard, H., Romero, P., Ringhoffer, M., Arand, M., Karbach, J., Ilsemann, C., Hagedorn, M., and Knuth, A., *Int. J. Cancer* 66: 162−169, 1996.

E. Jäger, D. Jäger and A. Knuth

19. Jäger, E., Ringhoffer, M., Dienes, H.-P., Arand, M., Karbach, J., Jäger, D., Ilsemann, C., Hagedorn, M., Oesch, F., and Knuth, A., *Int. J. Cancer* 67: 54–62, 1996.
20. Jäger, E., Ringhoffer, M., Karbach, J., Arand, M., Oesch, F., and Knuth, A., *Int. J. Cancer* 66: 470–476, 1996.
21. Jäger, E., Ringhoffer, M., Karbach, J., Arand, M., Oesch, F., Jäger, D., and Knuth, A., *Int. J. Cancer* 71: 142–147, 1997.

M.A. LÓPEZ-NEVOT, L. RAMAL, T. CABRERA,
F. RUIZ-CABELLO AND F. GARRIDO

HLA and cancer: β_2-Microglobulin mutations and malignant melanoma

Abstract

It is well documented that human and experimental tumours loose MHC class I molecules during tumor progression. These altered MHC phenotypes provides the tumour with an important immune escape mechanism from T cell responses. Multiple molecular mechanisms are responsible for these HLA alterations and any step required for the synthesis of an active HLA class I molecule can be the target for these genetic lessions. For instance, β_2 microglobuline gene mutations, loss of heterozigocity (LOH) associated with chromosome 6, mutations of particular HLA alleles, transcriptional defects . . . ect. are frequently found in tumors derived from different tissues, including melanoma. The HLA defective class I expression frequently found in human tumors must be seen as a crucial step happening during tumor progression and not just an obstacle to performe T cell based immunotherapy.

Keywords: HLA, tumour, escape, melanoma, T cell

Introduction

HLA class I molecules, which are constitutively expressed on most nuclear cells, play a basic role in the presentation of antigenic peptides to CD8-positive cytotoxic lymphocytes [1]. At the end of the 1970s it was discovered that tumors lost the expression of HLA class I molecules; this loss was interpreted as a mechanism of escape from antitumoral responses of the immune system [2]. Recently, much work has centered on the characterization of tumoral antigens and on the use of antitumoral vaccines with one or more antigenic peptides expressed by the tumor and presented to cytotoxic T lymphocytes by HLA class I molecules (HLA restriction). These studies have demonstrated the importance of determining the HLA

Laboratorio de Análisis Clínicos e Inmunología, Hospital Virgen de las Nieves,
Avda. Fuerzas Armadas 2, 18014 Granada, Spain

phenotype of the tumor to optimize the selection of appropriate patients and evaluate the efficacy of vaccination [3].

Alterations in HLA expression in human tumors

Anti-HLA class I monoclonal antibodies (mAbs) show different patterns of reaction: (1) monomorphic, i.e., recognizing an epitope common to all HLA class I molecules; (2) locus-specific, i.e., recognizing only HLA-A or HLA-B loci (isotypic); and (3) polymorphic, i.e., recognizing only one allele. Findings obtained with anti-HLA class I mAbs in cryostatic sections of human tumors, and with flow cytometric analyses of human tumoral cell lines, have suggested that these tumors can be divided into five phenotypes [4] (Fig. 1).

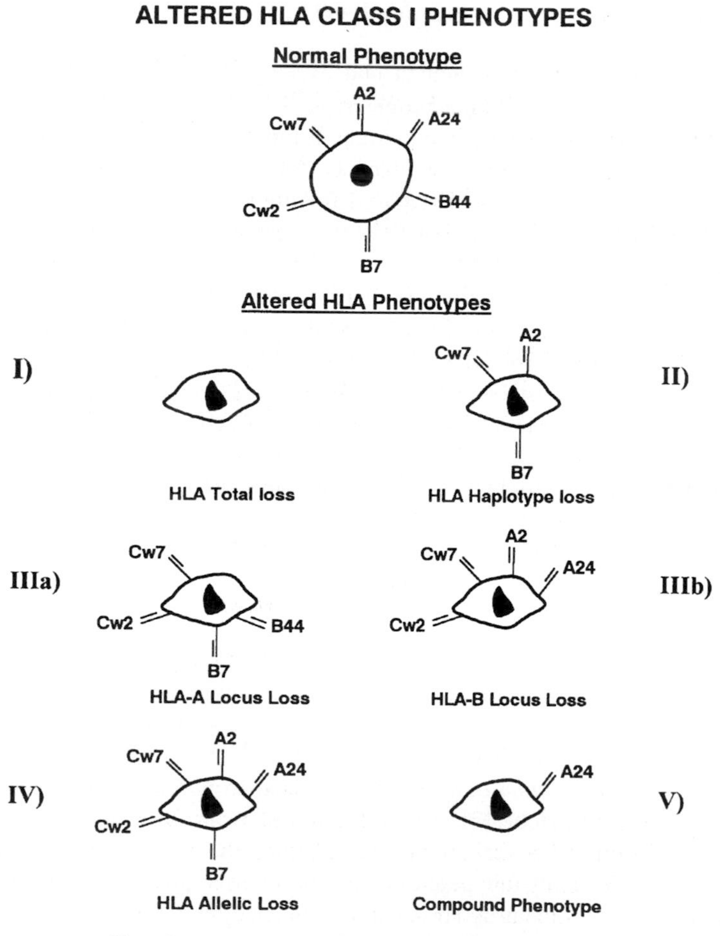

FIGURE 1. *Classification of HLA phenotypes in human tumors.*

- *Phenotype I* is characterized by total loss of expression of HLA class I molecules. No reaction is seen with W632 (anti-HLA class I) or anti-β2-microglobulin mAbs. In some tumors HLA class I heavy chain is detected with mAb HC-10 [5,6].
- *Phenotype II* shows loss of one HLA class I haplotype which comprises one HLA-A, one HLA-B, and one HLA-C allele. Staining with monomorphic and locus-specific anti-HLA class I mAbs is positive, but polymorphic anti-HLA class I mAbs specific for each allele of the haplotype are negative [7,8].
- *Phenotype III* is characterized by the loss of one HLA class I locus. Locus-specific mAbs and polymorphic anti-HLA-A and anti-HLA-B mAbs are negative [9,10].
- *Phenotype IV* shows the selective loss of one allele. Only mAbs specific for that allele are negative [11].
- *Phenotype V* is a complex phenotype in which HLA class I alterations characteristic of phenotypes II and III are combined, giving rise to a tumor that expresses only one HLA-A or HLA-B allele [12].

Alterations in the expression of HLA class I molecules appear in most human tumors, and are frequently variable. The use of polymorphic mAbs in immunohistological analyses, although not yet available for all allelic variants of the HLA class I molecule, has considerably increased the frequency with which altered HLA phenotypes are detected in human tumors [13]. The type of tumor in which alterations in HLA class I expression are found most frequently is breast cancer (88%) [14], followed by prostate (85%) [15], larynx (79%) [16] and colon cancer (65%) [17]. In cutaneous melanoma, 51% of the tumors show alterations in HLA class I expression, with phenotype IV being more frequent (25%) than phenotype I (16%) [18].

Decreased expression of HLA class I molecules correlates with a greater likelihood of tumoral progression. HLA class I-negative cutaneous melanomas show greater local growth, and reach higher scores for Breslow thickness and Clark level [19]. Moreover, loss of HLA class I is more frequent in metastases from cutaneous melanomas than in primary cutaneous melanomas. In other tumors such as breast, larynx or cervical cancer, loss of HLA class I expression also correlates with greater tumor aggressiveness [13].

Molecular basis for the loss of HLA class I expression

HLA class I expression is a dynamic process that occurs continuously in human nuclear cells. The HLA class I and class II molecules are characteristic attributes that identify the cell to the immune system as belonging to a human being, an individual, and a certain tissue. The peptide load in different HLA class I alleles indicates the type of tissue a given human cell is from, its functional status (quiescent or proliferative), whether it is infected by a virus or an intracellular microorganism, and whether it has undergone malignant transformation.

The presentation of antigenic peptides by HLA class I molecules triggers recognition by and activation of CD8-positive lymphocytes, which remove virally-infected and neoplastic cells. Because of the importance of HLA class I molecules for the immune system, their expression is coordinated in such a way that if any of its components (β_2-microglobulin, heavy chain or peptide) fails, expression is blocked [4]. Loss of expression of HLA class I molecules can result from alterations in the following three components:

Heavy chain

Three HLA class I loci—A, B and C—have been identified on the short arm of chromosome 6. They code for heavy chains of the classic HLA class I molecules, and are characterized by a high degree of polymorphism, and by their joint transmittal as part of the HLA class I and II gene haplotype [20].

The expression of genes for HLA class I heavy chain depends on the presence of transcription factors that act on their promoters and enhancers to induce the transcription of messenger RNA [21]. In some human tumors and human tumor cell lines, the absence of transcription factors leads to total loss of expression of HLA class I molecules (phenotype I) [22,23].

In other tumors such as colon cancer, the loss of expression of HLA locus B (phenotype III) results from the absence of a B-locus-specific transcription factor [24]. In cell lines derived from human cutaneous malignant melanoma, increased expression of the c-*myc* oncogene selectively inhibits the expression of the HLA-B locus, a phenomenon that has also been found in neuroblastoma cell lines [25]. In contrast, no such association has been confirmed for tumoral cell lines derived from lung cancer; this difference between types of cancer suggests that the antagonistic action of c-*myc* on the HLA-B locus is somehow conditioned by the histological origin of the tumor [26].

Phenotype II arises as a result of genomic instability of the tumor, a defect that leads to deletion of the entire chromosome 6, or of the fragment containing the HLA haplotype. Microsatellite analyses of the 6q and 6p regions is highly useful in mapping loss of heterozygosity (LOH) for chromosome 6 [27,28].

Phenotype IV is the result of point mutations, deletions or aberrant splicing of pre-mRNA of a specific allele [29].

Antigenic peptide processing

Antigenic peptides are generated in the cytosol by the proteolytic action of the proteasome that contains the LMP2 and LMP7 subunits, which are coded by genes in the HLA class II region. The peptides are transported to the endoplasmic reticulum by TAP1 and TAP2, where they bind to the heavy chain [30]. Any alteration in the processing or transport of the antigenic peptide leads to the appearance of so-called empty HLA molecules, which present only the heavy chain and β_2-microglobulin (B2M). These defective molecules are unstable and have a high turnover; as a result, HLA class I expression on the cell membrane is reduced [31,32].

Human cutaneous melanoma is the type of tumor which most frequently shows decreased TAP1 expression (down-regulation) (56%), followed by cervical and breast cancer. Loss of TAP1 expression has been found more frequently in metastases than in primary tumors [33].

Down-regulation of TAP1 leads to an incomplete decrease in HLA class I expression, which is more marked for HLA-B than for HLA-A. This reflects the existence of peptides independent of TAP1 and TAP2, which in the endoplasmic reticulum show greater binding affinity for HLA-A than for HLA-B [34].

The down-regulation of LMP2 alone leads to only a moderate reduction in HLA class I molecule expression. In some tumors the expression of TAP and LMP can be recovered by IFN-γ treatment, which achieves the re-expression of HLA class I molecules as long as the genes that code for the heavy chain or B2M are not altered [32].

β_2-microglobulin

The gene that codes for B2M contains four exons, is located in the 15q21-22 region, and is not polymorphic [35]. The role of B2M is to stabilize the folding of the heavy chain to maintain the groove between the α_1 and α_2 domains, where the peptide will bind [36].

The lack of B2M expression leads to loss of expression of all classic HLA class I molecules (A, B and C) (phenotype I), because without B2M the heavy chains become denatured and are not exported to the cytoplasmic membrane [37]. β_2-microglobulin-negative tumors do not react with monomorphic anti-HLA mAbs, often display intracytoplasmic HLA class I heavy chain, show normal TAP expression, and do not respond to induction with IFN-γ [38]. Different mutations and deletions of the B2M gene have been described in tumor cell lines from colon carcinoma and cutaneous malignant melanoma [39]. Mutations of the B2M gene are located in exon 1 and exon 2 [40]. One hot spot has been identified in exon 1 between codons 13 and 15, in which mutations have been found in three cell lines derived from three different colon cancers and two different melanomas [41,42]. In the start codon (ATG) two different substitutions have been reported: one in a Daudi cell line and one in a melanoma cell line [43,44]. In exon 2 the mutations are distributed randomly [45].

HLA phenotype in tumors of patients treated with peptide-based immunotherapy

We recently studied HLA expression in two patients (LB1622 and BB74) with cutaneous malignant melanoma who failed to respond to treatment with peptides MAGE-1 and MAGE-3 [46]. Metastatic tumor tissue was analyzed with immunohistological methods, and the homologous tumor cell lines LB1622-MEL and BB74-MEL were established.

Immunohistological studies showed that metastases from both patients showed phenotype I (total HLA class I loss). Flow cytometric studies

PATIENT BB74

T C A C G T C A T C
40

DNA OF PBL

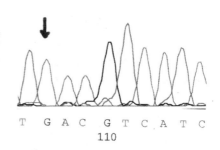

T G A C G T C A T C
110

cDNA OF TUMOR CELL LINE

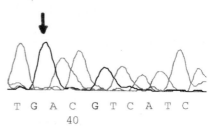

T G A C G T C A T C
40

DNA OF TUMOR CELL LINE

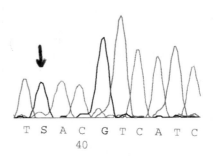

T S A C G T C A T C
40

DNA OF TUMOR TISSUE

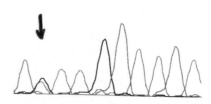

FIGURE 2.   *Continued*

M. A. *López-Nevot* et al.

showed that the alteration in the corresponding cell lines was also phenotype I. The main difference between the metastases and the cell lines was that LB1622 expressed intracytoplasmic heavy chain (HC-10-positive), whereas BB74 did not.

Neither cell line responded to induction with IFN-γ in terms of plasma membrane expression of HLA class I, although intracytoplasmic heavy chain was detected in line BB74-MEL after IFN-γ treatment. The pattern of reaction to anti-HLA and anti-B2M mAbs, and the lack of response to

PATIENT LB1622

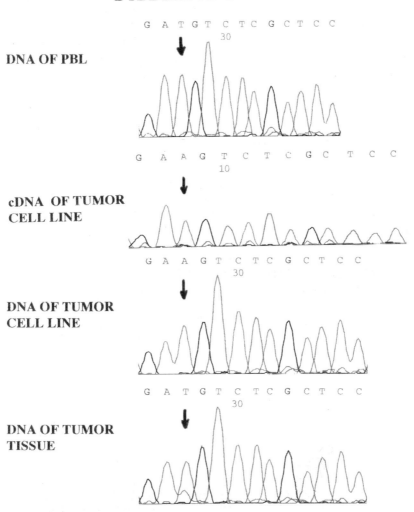

FIGURE 2. *Sequence data of DNA samples from patients BB74 (a) and LB1622 (b). Arrows indicate the mutations found in tumor cells.*

IFN-γ, suggest that an alteration in B2M was responsible for the appearance of phenotype I in these metastases.

Transcripts of the B2M gene were found with reverse transcriptase PCR in cDNA from both cell lines. Sequencing of cDNA revealed a different substitution in each line. In LB1622-MEL an A was substituted for a T in the start codon (AAG instead of ATC); this blocked the translation of mRNA into protein. In line BB74-MEL a G was substituted for a C in codon 31; this led to a premature stop codon and a nonfunctional truncated protein [44] (Figs. 2a and b).

Sequencing of the genomic DNA in both cell lines confirmed the results obtained with cDNA, and no normal sequences were seen. This result suggested that the other B2M allele had been deleted. Analyses with microsatellites which delimit the B2M locus confirmed that in both cell lines an allele of the B2M gene had been lost. When the B2M gene from the metastases was studied, the normal sequence appeared together with the mutated one in both lines; we interpreted this as evidence of contamination with normal cells from the inflammatory infiltrate.

In both cutaneous melanomas we found total loss of expression of HLA class I molecules, resulting from the deletion of one B2M allele and a mutation in the other allele which impeded the normal translation of mRNA. This situation would explain the failure of treatment with peptides MAGE-1 and MAGE-3.

Conclusions

The use of immunohistological techniques together with an extensive panel of anti-HLA mAbs has made is possible to detect increasing numbers of

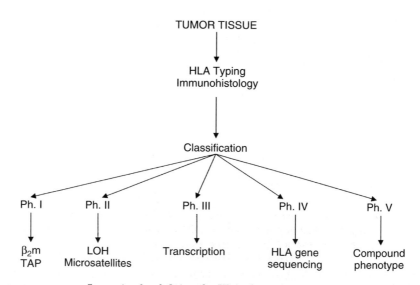

FIGURE 3. *Strategies for defining the HLA phenotype in human tumors.*

M. A. López-Nevot et al.

tumors with altered expression of HLA class I molecules. Molecular biology techniques, DNA sequencing, and microsatellite analysis have established the causes of the different phenotypes of HLA alterations. The HLA alterations should be analyzed in detail in patients who are to undergo peptide immunotherapy for tumors. The tumor to be treated should satisfy two conditions in these patients: it must express (1) the immunizing tumoral antigen, and (2) the HLA molecule that presents the immunogenic tumoral peptide. Figure 3 is a general summary of suitable strategies for investigating the HLA phenotype of human tumors.

References

1. York, I.A., and Rock, K.L., *Annu. Rev. Immunol.* 14: 369–396, 1996.
2. Garrido, F., Cabrera, T., Concha, A., Glew, S., Ruiz-Cabello, F., and Stern, P., *Immunol. Today* 14: 491–493, 1993.
3. Ruiz-Cabello, F., and Garrido, F., *Immunol. Today* 19: 539–542, 1998.
4. Garrido, F., Cabrera, T., López Nevot, M.A., and Ruiz-Cabello, F., *Adv. Cancer Res.* 67: 155–195, 1995.
5. Momburg, F., Degener, T., Bacchus, E., Modenhauer, G., Hammerling, G.J., and Moller, P., *Int. J. Cancer* 37: 179–184, 1986.
6. Ruiter, D.J., Mattijssen, V., Broecker, E.B., and Ferrone, S., *Semin. Cancer Biol.* 2: 35–45, 1991.
7. López Nevot, M.A., Esteban, F., Ferron, A., Ruiz-Cabello, F., and Garrido, F., *Br. J. Cancer* 59: 221–226, 1989.
8. Ruiz-Cabello, F., Pérez-Ayala, M., Gomez, O., Redondo, M., Concha, A., Cabrera, A., and Garrido, F., *Int. J. Cancer* 6: S123–130, 1991.
9. Torres, M., Ruiz-Cabello, F., Skoudy, A., Berrozpe, G., Serrano, A., Jimenez, P., Real, F.X., and Garrido, F., *Tissue Antigens* 47: 372–381, 1996.
10. Marincola, F.M., Shamamian, P., Alexander, R.B., Gnarra, J.R., Turetskaya, R.L., Nedospasov, S.A., Simonis, T.B., Taubenberger, J.K., Yannelli, J., et al., *J. Immunol.* 153: 1225–1237, 1994.
11. Wang, Z., Seliger, B., Mike, N., Momburg, F., Knuth, A., and Ferrone, S., *Cancer Res.* 58: 2149–2157, 1998.
12. Real, L.M., Jimenez, P., Cantón, J., Kirkin, A.F., García, A., Abril, E., Zeuthen, A., Ruiz-Cabello, F., and Garrido, F., *Int. J. Cancer* 75: 317–323, 1998.
13. Garrido, F., Ruiz-Cabello, F., Cabrera, T., Perez-Villar, J.J., Lopez-Botet, M.A., Duggan-Keen, M., and Stern, P., *Immunol. Today* 18: 89–95, 1997.
14. Cabrera, T., Sierra, A., Fernandez, M.A., Herruzo, A., Fabra, A., and Garrido, F., *Hum. Immunol.* 50: 127–134, 1996.
15. Blades, R.A., Keating, P.J., McWilliam, L.J., George, N.J., and Stern, P.L., *Urology* 46: 681–686, 1995.
16. Esteban, F., Concha, A., Huelin, C., Sanchez Rozas, F., Pedrinaci, S., Ruiz-Cabello, F., and Garrido, F., *Int. J. Cancer* 43: 436–442, 1989.
17. Browning, M.J., Petronzelli, F., Bicknell, D.C., Krausa, P., Rowan, A., Tonks, S., Murray, N., and Bodmer, W.F., *Tissue Antigens* 47: 364–371, 1996.
18. Ferrone, S., and Marincola, F.M., *Immunol. Today* 16: 487–494, 1995.
19. López Nevot, M.A., García, E., Romero, C., Oliva, M.R., Serrano, S., and Garrido, F., *Exp. Clin. Immunogen.* 5: 203–212, 1988.

20. Trowsdale, J., Raggousis, J., and Campell, R.D., *Immunol. Today* 12: 443–446, 1991.
21. Singer, D.S., and Maguire, J.E., *Crit. Rev. Immunol.* 10: 235–237, 1990.
22. Henseling, U., Schmidt, W., Scholer, H.R., Grus, P., and Hatzopoulos, A.K., *Mol. Cell Biol.* 10: 4100–4109, 1990.
23. Blanchet, O., Bourge, J.F., Zinszer, H., Tatari, Z., Degos, L., and Paul, P., *Int. J. Cancer* 6 (Suppl.): 138–145, 1991.
24. Soong, T.W., and Hui, K.M., *J. Immunol.* 149: 2008–2014, 1992.
25. Peltenburg, L.T.C., and Schrier, P.I., *Immunogenetics* 40: 54–61, 1994.
26. Redondo, M., Ruiz-Cabello, F., Concha, A., Cabrera, T., Pérez, M., Oliva, M.R., and Garrido, F., *Cancer Res.* 51: 2463–2468, 1991.
27. Jiménez, P., Cantón, J., Collado, A., Cabrera, T., Serrano, A., Real, L.M., García, A., Ruiz Cabello, F., and Garrido, F., *Int. J. Cancer* 83: 91–97, 1999.
28. Feenstra, M., Veltkamp, M., Van Kuik, J., Wiertsema, S., Slootweg, P., Van den Tweel, J., De Weger, R., and Tilanus, M., *Tissue Antigens* 54: 235–245, 1999.
29. Wang, Z., Marincola, F.M., Rivoltini, L., Parmiani, G., and Ferrone, S., *J. Exp. Med.* 2: 205–215, 1999.
30. Parmer, E., and Cresswell, P., *Annu. Rev. Immunol.* 16: 323–358, 1998.
31. Cromme, F.V., Airley, J., Heemels, M.T., Ploegh, H.L., Keating, P.J., Stern, P.L., Meijer, C.J., and Walboomers, J.M., *Int. J. Cancer* 179: 335–340, 1994.
32. Seliger, B., Maeurer, M.J., and Ferrone, S., *Immunol. Today* 18: 292–299, 1997.
33. Hicklin, D.J., Marincola, F.M., and Ferrone, S., *Mol. Med. Today* 5: 178–186, 1999.
34. Salter, R.D., and Cresswell, P., *EMBO J.* 5: 943–949, 1986.
35. Gussow, D., Rein, R., Ginjaar, I., Hochstenbach, F., Seeman, G., Kottman, A., and Ploegh, H.L., *J. Immunol.* 139: 3132–3138, 1987.
36. Bjorkman, P.J., Saper, M.A., Samorui, B., Bennet, W.S., Strominger, J.L., and Wiley, D.C., *Nature* 329: 506–512, 1987.
37. Hicklin, D.J., Dellaratta, D.V., Kishore, R., Liang, B., Kageshita, T., and Ferrone, S., *Melanoma Res.* 7: S67–S74, 1997.
38. Chen, H.L., Gabrilovich, D., Virmani, A., Ratnani, I., Girgis, K.R., Nadaf-Rahrov, S., Fernandez-Viña, M., and Carbone, P., *Int. J. Cancer* 67: 756–763, 1996.
39. Wang, Z., Cao, Y., Albino, A.P., Zeff, R.A., Houghton, A., and Ferrone, S., *J. Clin. Invest.* 91: 684–692, 1993.
40. D'Urso, C.M., Wang, Z., Cao, Y., Tatake, R., Zeff, R.A., and Ferrone, S., *J. Clin. Invest.* 87: 284–290, 1991.
41. Bicknell, D.C., Rowan, A., and Bodmer, W.F., *Proc. Natl. Acad. Sci. U.S.A.* 91: 4751–4755, 1994.
42. Perez, B., Benitez, R., Fernandez, M.A., Oliva, M.R., Soto, J.L., Serrano, S., López Nevot, M.A., and Garrido, F., *Tissue Antigens* 53: 569–572, 1999.
43. Rosa, F., Berissi, H., Weissenbach, J., Maroteaux, L., Fellous, M., and Revel, M., *EMBO J.* 2: 239–243, 1983.
44. Benitez, R., Godelaine, D., Lopez Nevot, M., Brasseur, F., Marchand, M., Cabrera, T., van Baren, N., Andry, G., Jimenez, P., Landry, C., Ruiz-Cabello, F., Boon, T., and Garrido, F., *Tissue Antigens* 52: 520–529, 1998.
45. Gattoni-Celli, T., Kirsch, K., Timpane, R., and Isselbacher, K.J., *Cancer Res.* 52: 1201–1204, 1992.
46. Boon, T., Cerottini, J.C., Van den Eyden, B., Van der Bruggen, P., and Van Pel, A., *Annu. Rev. Immunol.* 12: 337–365, 1994.

M. A. López-Nevot et al.

H. MONIQUE H. HURKS, LUC R.H.M. SCHURMANS,
JESSICA A.W. METZELAAR-BLOK, DERK J.R. BLOM AND
MARTINE J. JAGER

HLA antigens of ocular melanoma

Abstract

Human leucocyte antigens (HLA) play a crucial role in the immunological defense against tumor cells. Down-regulation of HLA expression is a common feature in many different types of cancer and may have serious consequences for tumor elimination by cytotoxic T cells and natural killer (NK) cells. In uveal melanoma, a low expression of HLA-A and HLA-B in primary tumors was correlated with a better patient survival, suggesting a protective role for NK cells in the development of metastatic disease. HLA allele-specific down-regulation may be mechanism for uveal melanoma cells to avoid killing by both cytotoxic T cells and NK cells. Alterations of HLA class I phenotype may complicate the development of immunotherapy.

Keywords: HLA, NK cells, melanoma

Human leucocyte antigens (HLA)

Human leucocyte antigens (HLA) play a central role in immune recognition. HLA class I molecules are expressed on the cell surface of all nucleated cells and platelets and can be divided into HLA-A, HLA-B and HLA-C. Each of these loci show a large polymorphism, mainly caused by differences in the α1- and α2-domains of the class I heavy chain [1]. The α-domains form a groove in which endogenously derived peptides, e.g. melanoma-associated antigens, can be presented to CD8$^+$ (cytotoxic) T cells. The peptide binding specificity is different for each particular HLA allele. In addition to CD8$^+$ T cells, HLA class I expression is also important for the function of natural killer (NK) cells. In general, low expression of HLA renders a cell susceptible for NK cell-mediated lysis. However, during the last few years it has been discovered that NK cells also express killer inhibitory and killer activatory receptors (KIRs and KARs) that recognize specific HLA alleles (reviewed in Colonna [2] and Moretta et al. [3]).

Department of Ophthalmology, Leiden University Medical Center,
Leiden, The Netherlands

HLA class II molecules, encoded by the HLA-D locus, are predominantly expressed on professional antigen presenting cells such as dendritic cells, B cells, Langerhans cells and on activated T lymphocytes. They can be subdivided in HLA-DR, HLA-DQ and HLA-DP. In contrast to HLA class I, HLA class II polymorphism is mainly located in the β-chain [4]. HLA class II molecules generally present peptides derived from endocytosed exogenous antigens to $CD4^+$ (helper) T cells, which in turn give help to cytotoxic T cells and stimulate antibody production by B cells.

HLA expression and malignancy

HLA expression plays a crucial role in the recognition of tumor cells by the immune system. Both $CD4^+$ and $CD8^+$ T cells can only be activated when they recognize tumor-specific antigens, e.g. MAGE, MART-1 and gp100, in association with the appropriate HLA molecules. Therefore, alteration of the HLA phenotype of the tumor may have serious consequences for the hosts defence against tumor growth and the development of metastatic disease. Down-regulation of HLA class I expression has been demonstrated in many different types of cancer, including cutaneous and uveal melanoma [5–10]. In general, loss of HLA class I expression in tumors originating from HLA class I positive epithelia is only apparent after the tumors become invasive [11]. The relation between HLA expression and prognosis is not always clear. In cutaneous melanoma and primary breast carcinoma, loss of HLA-A, HLA-B and HLA-C expression was correlated with a worse patient survival [12,13]. However, studies on colorectal cancer, non-small cell lung carcinoma and prostate cancer failed to demonstrate a significant prognostic influence of HLA class I expression [14–16]. Remarkably, in uveal melanoma low expression of HLA-A and HLA-B was correlated with a better patient survival.[1] The implications of this finding will be discussed later (see "Locus-specific HLA class I expression").

Alteration of tumor HLA class II expression usually concerns class II positive tumors originated from class II negative tissues [17–19]. Remarkably, premalignant lesions often show a higher HLA class II expression than the malignant lesions [19–21]. For cutaneous melanoma, an association between HLA class II expression and progression of malignancy has been described [19, 20]. In primary uveal melanoma, only 0–35% of the tumor cells are HLA class II positive and no correlation with patient survival has been found [7].

HLA class I expression and uveal melanoma

Monomorphic HLA class I expression

The expression of HLA class I antigens on uveal melanoma has been extensively investigated using immunohistochemistry on paraffin and cryostat tissue sections. Application of monomorphic monoclonal antibodies (moAb), i.e. moAb W6/32 recognizing HLA-A,B,C and moAb BBM1 directed to the β2-microglobulin of the class I heavy chain, demonstrated that all primary uveal melanomas showed a high level of HLA class I expression [7]. No associations were observed between HLA class I expression and prognostic markers such as tumor diameter, prominence and scleral invasion. On the other hand, a positive correlation was found between the expression of monomorphic HLA class I determinants and the presence of tumor infiltrating $CD3^+$ and $CD4^+$ T cells and $CD11b^+$ monocytes/macrophages. The correlation with $CD8^+$ T cells did not reach significance [22]. The prognostic significance of tumor-infiltrating lymphocytes in uveal melanoma is unclear, both positive and negative associations with patient survival have been found [23–25].

The data of De Waard-Siebinga et al. [7] showed that total HLA class I down-regulation is not a common feature in primary uveal melanoma. In contrast, other tumor types frequently exhibit a complete loss of expression of HLA antigens, ranging from 9% in larynx carcinoma to 52% in breast carcinoma [26]. In primary lesions of cutaneous melanoma, down-regulation of HLA-A + B + C has been observed in 16% of the tumors. In metastatic lesions this percentage is increased to 58% (Table 1) [21,29–31,33].

TABLE 1. *Frequency of monomorphic and locus-specific HLA class I down-regulation in uveal and cutaneous melanoma.*

Specimen	HLA class I determinant								
	monomorphic			A locus			B locus		
	n	%	ref	n	%	ref	n	%	ref
Uveal melanoma									
Primary	0/23	0	7	10/30	33	5	12/30	40	5
Metastases	0/4[1]	0	27	0/4[1]	0	27	0/4[1]	0	27
Cell lines[2] −IFN	0/6	0	28	1/6	17	28	4/6	67	28
+IFN	0/6	0	28	1/6	17	28	1/6[3]	17	28
Cutaneous melanoma									
Primary	66/414	16	29[4]	1/10	10	32	1/10	10	32
Metastases	287/495	58	29[4]	2/6	33	32	2/6	33	32
				0/6	0	34	5/6	83	34
Cell lines[5] −IFN	4/13[6]	31	35	0/24	0	34	10/22	45	34
+IFN	nd			nd			0/22	0	34

[1] Metastases were all derived from one patient; HLA-A and HLA-B expression of the primary tumor was high.

[2] Cell lines were derived from five primary uveal melanomas and one uveal melanoma metastasis.

[3] Cell line derived from an uveal melanoma metastasis in the skin.

[4] Data are adapted from Ferrone and Marincola [29] and based on references 21,30–33.

[5] Cell lines were derived from cutaneous melanoma metastases.

[6] Some cell lines were obtained from lesions of patients who had received interleukin-2 immunotherapy.

Lack of monomorphic HLA class I expression may result from defects in the β2-microglobulin synthesis [10,36], TAP (transporters associated with antigen processing) defects [10,37] or structural defects in MHC genes [26]. However, as all primary uveal melanoma lesions were stained by moAb directed to HLA-A,B,C and β2-microglobulin, such defects do not seem to play a role in uveal melanoma.

Locus-specific HLA class I expression

The locus-specific HLA class I expression in primary uveal melanoma has been extensively analyzed by Blom *et al.* [5]. The moAb HCa2 and HC10 were used to stain respectively HLA-A and HLA-B antigens on 30 paraffin sections of uveal melanoma. Expression levels of HLA-A and -B were significantly correlated. Large variations in expression were observed between different uveal melanomas. Complete loss of HLA-A was observed in 10 tumors (33%), whereas HLA-B expression was absent in 12 tumors (40%). A high expression of HLA-B was related to the presence of prognostically unfavourable non-spindle cells. No significant correlations were observed between HLA-A or -B expression and other prognostic parameters such as largest tumor diameter, Mib-1 score or mitotic rate. The most important finding of this study was the relation between locus-specific HLA expression and patient survival. High expression of HLA-A and HLA-B molecules was significantly correlated with death from metastases (Fig. 1). Multiple regression analysis showed that the contribution of HLA-A expression to survival exceeded that of tumor diameter and Mib-1 score.

The finding that expression of HLA-A and HLA-B is a marker of poor prognosis is unique for uveal melanoma. In general, the opposite correlation is expected because down-regulation of HLA expression may lead to tumor escape from cytotoxic T cells. In some tumors, including cutaneous melanoma, this also has been found [12,13]. The findings in uveal melanoma support a protective role for NK cells in the development of metastatic disease, as NK cells can attack target cells more efficiently in the absence of HLA class I molecules. This hypothesis is strengthened by the study of Ma *et al.* [38], who found that the development of hepatic metastases in mice injected with uveal melanoma cells was inversely correlated with the degree of NK cell mediated lysis. In addition, patients with advanced metastatic disease often show abnormal NK cell function and/or number [39]. Finally, since uveal melanoma metastases spread hematogeneously, especially NK cell lysis may be an important first line of defence. In most other types of cancer spreading occurs mainly lymphatically, suggesting a more crucial role for cytotoxic T cells.

The frequency of locus-specific down-regulation in primary uveal melanoma is very high, 33% and 40% for HLA-A and -B respectively. In other tumors, frequencies of only 3–19% (HLA-A) and 5–19% (HLA-B) were documented [26]. In cutaneous melanoma, 10% of primary lesions showed a locus-specific down-regulation, whereas in 0–83% of metastatic

H. M. H. Hurks et al.

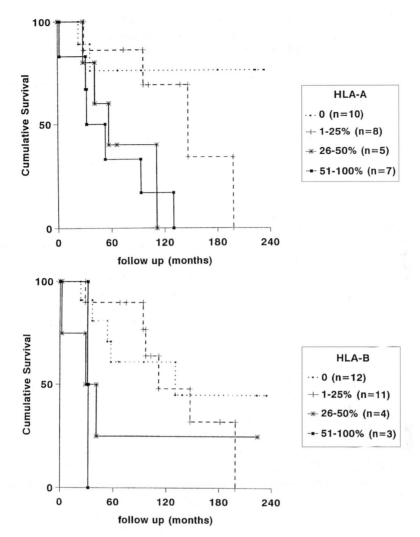

FIGURE 1. *HLA-A (top) and HLA-B (bottom) expression were determined by immunohistology on sections of uveal melanoma, and the percentage of positively-stained tumor cells was determined. Patients were divided into four categories on the basis of the number of stained cells, and the tumor-related survival was calculated. Cumulative survival of uveal melanoma patients is shown in percentages. Reproduced from Blom* et al. *[5]*

lesions HLA-A or HLA-B antigens were absent (table 1A) [29,32,34,40]. Abrogation of HLA-B expression has been reported to be correlated with an increased expression of the c-myc oncogene, which is strongly involved in the control of cell proliferation and can interfere with HLA-B transcription [40,41]. Comparable with cutaneous melanoma, also in uveal melanoma such an inverse correlation has been found [42]. Activation of c-myc in cutaneous melanoma is considered to be a tumor escape mechanism, based on its properties to stimulate cell proliferation and to down-regulate HLA-B expression [40]. In contrast, c-myc activation in uveal melanoma may have a beneficial effect, i.e. increased susceptibility to NK cell lysis related to a decreased expression of HLA-B antigens. However, expression of c-myc in uveal melanoma has been reported to be an independent prognostic parameter of poor prognosis [43], which is in line with the involvement of c-myc in maintaining cell proliferation.

Locus-specific down-regulations can be transcriptionally-mediated or caused by genetic defects [26,29]. Immunohistochemical methods can not easily discriminate these two possibitities. Analysis of HLA expression using cell lines may give more information, as transcriptionally-mediated down-regulations can often be restored by cytokine treatment [44,45]. We found that in two out of six uveal melanoma cell lines no expression of HLA-B was detectable at the cell surface, intracellularly and at the mRNA level (Schurmans, unpublished data). Treatment of the cells with interferon-γ (IFNγ) could up-regulate the expression of HLA-B molecules of one cell line (MEL-202). In contrast, the metastatic cell line OMM-1 showed a complete lack of IFNγ responsiveness, implicating the occurrence of a genetic defect. Marincola *et al.* [34] observed HLA-B locus-specific down-regulations in 10/22 cell lines derived from cutaneous melanoma metastases (Table 1), but in all cases IFNγ treatment could induce the expression of HLA-B antigens.

Allele-specific HLA class I expression

Analysis of the expression of HLA class I allospecificities has been hampered by the limited availability of allele-specific moAb. Therefore, the frequency of allele-specific abnormalities described in literature is probably underestimated. Most studies have focussed on the expression of HLA-A2 because of its high frequency in the Caucasian population and the availability of A2-specific antibodies. In cutaneous melanoma, loss of HLA-A2 expression has been found in 25% of primary lesions and in 31% of metastatic lesions (Table 2) [29,46,47]. In tissue sections of six uveal melanoma patients with an HLA-A2 positive HLA-typing, we did not find a specific loss of HLA-A2 expression [7].

We flowcytometrically analyzed the allele-specific HLA class I surface expression on six uveal melanoma cell lines (five derived from a primary tumor and one cell line obtained from a skin metastasis), using a broad panel of allele-specific moAb [28]. In order to up-regulate HLA expression, cells were cultured with IFNα or IFNγ. In general, the expression of the HLA-A alleles was high and could be further up-regulated by both IFNα and IFNγ. However, in one cell line, IFNγ treatment resulted in a significant HLA-A expression, while IFNα had no effect. The expression of the HLA-B alleles was low or even negative and variable effects were observed after IFN treatment. In three cell lines, the expression of one B allele could not be restored by IFNα and IFNγ, whereas the other B allele showed an enhanced expression level upon IFN

TABLE 2. *Frequency of allele-specific[1] HLA class I down-regulation in uveal and cutaneous melanoma.*

Specimen	Uveal melanoma			Cutaneous melanoma		
	n	%	ref	n	%	ref
Primary (only HLA-A2)	0/6	0	7	9/36	25	47
Metastases (only HLA-A2)	1/4[2]	25	27	12/39	31	46
Cell lines −IFN	5/6[3]	83	28	3/24[4,5]	13	34
+IFN	3/6	50	28	3/24[6]	13	34
				10/37[4]	27%	48

[1] In primary and metastatic lesions only HLA-A2 expression was examined, in the cell lines more allospecificities were determined.
[2] Metastases were all derived from one patient. HLA-A2 expression in the primary tumor was high.
[3] Cell lines were derived from five primary uveal melanomas and one uveal melanoma metastasis.
[4] Cell lines were derived from cutaneous melanoma metastases.
[5] Only HLA-A2 and A29 were examined.
[6] Loss of full haplotype.

stimulation (Table 3). Finally, in conjunction with the finding of Schurmans *et al.* (unpublished data), the metastatic cell line OMM-1 showed a structural lack of expression of both B alleles, indicating an HLA-B locus-specific loss.

In our study, three of the five (60%) cell lines derived from a primary uveal melanoma showed a structural loss of one HLA-B allele. Geertsen *et al.* [48] studied allele-specific HLA expression in short-time cultures derived from primary and metastatic cutaneous melanomas. They found HLA-B allele-specific losses in only one of 11 (9%) primary cultures and in eight of 37 (22%) metastatic cultures (Table 2). Selective loss of HLA-A alleles (A2) was found in only two cultures (both derived from metastases), which corresponds to 5% of the total cultures and 12% of the cultures derived from HLA-A2 positive patients. This is in agreement with the study of Marincola *et al.* [34], who noted loss of allelic expression in two of 14 (14%) HLA-A2 positive cell lines originated from cutaneous melanoma metastases. In our study, the two HLA-A2 positive cell lines (one primary and one metastatic) showed no lack of HLA-A2 expression. It should be noted that it is difficult to compare different studies analyzing allelic HLA expression. First, in tissue sections it is not possible to discriminate between structural HLA defects and down-regulations which can be restored. Secondly, the social geographic background of the patient group determines the frequency of specific alleles in a group and may thus influence the observed frequency of a specific HLA defect. Finally, the availability of allele-specific moAb may be a limiting factor, especially for the staining of tissue sections.

Allele-specific down-regulation of HLA class I expression may have serious consequences for the immunological defence against uveal melanoma.

TABLE 3. *Allele-specific down-regulation of HLA class I expression in uveal melanoma cell lines determined by FACS analysis[1].*

Cell line[2]	HLA alleles recognized by moAb[3]	Treatment[4]		
		–	IFNα	IFNγ
92-1	A2	12.0[5]	53.7	42.0
	A3	18.5	133	116
	B5	5.8	50.8	60.0
	B44	**1.2[6]**	**3.3**	**2.7**
OCM-1	A11	9.3	14.5	18.0
	A24	32.0	59.2	66.2
	B15	**1.3**	**1.4**	**1.3**
	B15 + B35	15.9	36.0	47.7
MEL-202	A1	9.0	29.7	41.7
	A3	14.5	49.3	65.7
	B5	**1.2**	**1.2**	**1.4**
	B5 + B38	**1.6**	10.2	29.0
OMM-1	A2	35.3	67.6	84.7
	B27	**1.2**	**1.3**	**1.3**
	B40	**2.0**	**2.1**	**2.2**
EOM-3	A10	**1.3**	**2.0**	9.3
	B18	**3.2**	11.0	24.3
OCM-3	A11	37.0	47.5	48.8
	B40	**1.8**	11.3	23.0

[1] Data are derived from Hurks *et al.* [28].

[2] Cell lines were derived from five primary uveal melanomas and one uveal melanoma metastasis (OMM-1).

[3] Human allele-specific moAb were obtained from the SVM Foundation, Bilthoven, The Netherlands. The alleles reflect the HLA-genotype of the cell lines.

[4] Cell culture with 200 U/ml IFNα or IFNγ during 48 hours.

[5] Data are expressed as multiplication of the background (non-stained cells) fluorescence.

[6] HLA down-regulations are presented in bold.

By down-regulating one or more HLA alleles, tumor cells can avoid recognition by a specific population of cytotoxic T cells. On the other hand, normal expression of the remaining alleles can inhibit NK cell mediated lysis. This bilateral escape mechanism may be one of the answers to the question why cytotoxic T cells do not adequately react to HLA class I expressing metastatic uveal melanoma cells. Furthermore, if the frequency of allele-specific HLA loss, without the capacity of recovery, is as high *in vivo* as we found *in vitro*, it may complicate the development of immunotherapy for uveal melanoma (see "HLA expression and immunotherapy").

Allelic loss may result from defects in the HLA class I genes, such as point mutations, partial deletions, chromosomal breakage or somatic recombination [26]. We examined 20 paraffin sections of primary uveal melanomas for the presence of loss of heterozygosity (LOH) on three different loci of chromosome 6p [49]. LOH at chromosome 6p, where the HLA genes are located, has been observed in many human neoplasms [50–52]. In our study, we found that 65% of the tumors displayed LOH at least at one locus on chromosome 6p. We did not find a correlation between LOH and the expression of HLA-A and HLA-B. Allele-specific staining of the paraffin sections was not possible because suitable antibodies were not available.

HLA class I expression in uveal melanoma metastases

Although the expression of monomorphic and polymorphic HLA class I determinants in primary uveal melanoma has been analyzed in several studies, data on HLA expression of uveal melanoma metastases are scarce. In a study of Blom *et al.* [27], HLA expression was determined in tissue sections of a primary uveal melanoma and four of its metastases (adrenal gland, skin, liver and heart). Monomorphic HLA expression (HLA-A,B,C and β2-microglobulin) and the expression of HLA-B was high (75–100% positive cells) in the primary tumor as well as in all metastases. HLA-A expression was high in the primary tumor, slightly reduced in the skin metastasis and significantly decreased in the metastasis of the liver (26–50% positive cells). The HLA-A2 expression in the liver was severely down-regulated to less than 5% HLA-A2 positive cells. HLA-Bw4 expression was low in all lesions. The HLA-B genotype of this patient is B*05 and B*44, both associated with Bw4. In the cell line 92-1 derived from the primary tumor, we found an allele-specific defect of HLA-B44 (Table 2), which is in agreement with the low HLA-Bw4 expression in the tissue sections.

HLA expression and immunotherapy

Although many treatment modalities have been developed for the primary uveal melanoma, no effective therapy is yet available for the treatment or prevention of uveal melanoma metastases. Immunotherapy is regarded as a promising tool in human cancer therapy. During the last decade, a great number of tumor-associated antigens has been identified, such as MAGE, MART-1 and gp100 for melanoma [53–55]. Immunodominant peptides derived from, or DNA encoding for, these tumor antigens can be used for the generation of cytotoxic T cells with great anti-tumor potency [56,57]. In patients with cutaneous melanoma-derived metastases, several immunotherapy trials, e.g. cytokine treatment, vaccination with melanoma-specific peptides or dendritic cells presenting tumor-specific antigens, adoptive transfer of tumor-specific cytotoxic T cells and treatment with cytokine gene-modified tumor cells, already have been performed [58–66]. These immunotherapies produce response rates of 10% to 42%, but the number of durable remissions is low. One of the underlying causes of these limited responses may be a down-regulated surface expression of HLA class I antigens on the tumor cells.

In uveal melanoma, the number of immunotherapy trials is limited. Mitchell *et al.* [67] reported that, in an elderly patient with a primary choroidal melanoma, repeated administration of cutaneous melanoma cell lysates caused a significant regression of the tumor. Two groups have treated metastatic uveal melanoma patients with a chemotherapy regimen combined with IFNα administration and reported partial response rates in approximately 20% of the patients [68,69]. INFα has been shown to induce a broad spectrum of immunomodulatory and anti-proliferative effects in a variety of malignancies [60]. We have shown that IFNα, like IFNγ, can stimulate HLA class I expression in uveal melanoma cells [28,70]. However, for patients that display constitutive HLA defects, cytokine treatment with the purpose to stimulate HLA class I expression will be ineffective. Gene (transfer) therapy may be an alternative for these patients. Several animal and human studies have reported positive results, e.g. increased levels of HLA class I expression, decreased tumorigenicity and decreased metastatic spread, after tumor cell transfection with (allogeneic) MHC class I genes [35,71].

An alternative approach is not to aim at an improvement of the cytotoxic T cell response, but to enrich particular NK cell subsets that attack tumor cells [57,72]. Our finding that high expression of HLA-A and HLA-B was correlated with a poor prognosis suggests that NK cells play a crucial role in the protection against metastatic disease [5]. Furthermore, we found that all the allele-specific down-regulations in the uveal melanoma cell lines concerned an HLA-B allele [28]. Therefore, enrichment of NK cell clones bearing HLA-B restricted KIRs, e.g. p70 recognizing HLA-Bw4, might be a promising strategy. In order to recommend a specific immunotherapy for the treatment or prevention of uveal melanoma metastases, it is necessary to establish the frequency and nature of HLA expression deficiencies in uveal melanoma metastases *in vivo*.

HLA-G expression

The nonclassical class I antigen HLA-G is expressed selectively on trophoblast cells and has been shown to play an important role in the foetomaternal tolerance [73]. The HLA-G molecule can inhibit NK cell function by interaction with KIRs that belong to the C-type lectin or the Ig superfamily [74]. The existence of numerous common features, such as high mitotic rate, invasive capacity, expression of growth factors, growth factor receptors and proto-oncogenes, between trophoblast cells and neoplastic cells, has raised the question whether HLA-G is also expressed on malignant cells [75]. Tumor HLA-G expression would be an additional mechanism by which tumor cells can escape immunosurveillance by NK cells.

Two studies have demonstrated high levels of HLA-G mRNA and protein in cutaneous melanoma cell lines and *ex vivo* biopsies [75,76]. Moreover, they showed that HLA-G expression protected melanoma cells from NK cell lysis. However, in uveal melanoma we could not detect HLA-G expression (preliminary data). We did not find HLA-G mRNA in 15 uveal melanoma cell lines, nor did we observe positive staining on 12 frozen uveal melanoma tissue sections.

Summary

Downregulation of HLA expression is a common feature in many different types of cancer and may have serious consequences for the immune recognition of tumor cells by cytotoxic T cells and NK cells. In contrast with cutaneous melanoma, monomorphic HLA class I defects are very rare in uveal melanoma. On the other hand, a high frequency of locus and allele-specific down-regulations has been found in uveal melanoma tissue sections and cell lines. A low expression of HLA-A and HLA-B in primary uveal melanoma was correlated with a better patient survival, suggesting a protective role for NK cells in the development of metastatic disease. The occurrence of allele-specific defects may be a mechanism for uveal melanoma cells to escape immunosurveillance by both cytotoxic T cells and NK cells. Constitutive HLA class I defects may complicate the development of immunotherapy in uveal melanoma. In this view, it is important to establish the frequency and the nature of HLA deficiencies in uveal melanoma metastases.

References

1. Evans, G.A., Margulies, D.H., Shykind, B., Seidman, J.G., and Ozato, K., *Nature* 300: 755–757, 1982.
2. Colonna, M., *Immunol. Rev.* 155: 127–133, 1997.
3. Moretta, A., Biassoni, R., Bottino, C., Pende, D., Vitale, M., Poggi, A., Mingari, M.C., and Moretta, L., *Immunol. Rev.* 155: 105–117, 1997.
4. Shackelford, D.A., Kaufman, J.F., Korman, A.J., and Strominger, J.L., *Imm. Rev.* 66: 133–187, 1982.
5. Blom, D.J.R., Luyten, G.P.M., Mooy, C.M., Kerkvliet, S., Zwinderman, A.H., and Jager, M.J., *Invest. Ophthalmol. Vis. Sci.* 38: 1865–1872, 1997.
6. Browning, M., Petronzelli, F., Bicknell, D., Krausa, P., Rowan, A., Tonks, S., Murray, N., Bodmer, J., and Bodmer, W,, *Tissue Antigens* 47: 361 371, 1996.
7. De Waard-Siebinga, I., Houbiers, J.G.A., Hilders, C.G.J.M., De Wolff-Rouendaal, D., and Jager, M.J., *Ocul. Immunol. Inflamm.* 4: 1–14, 1996.
8. Garrido, F., Cabrera, T., Lopez-Nevot, M.A., and Ruiz-Cabello, F., *Adv. Cancer Res.* 67: 155–195, 1995.
9 Keating, P.J., Cromme, F.V., Duggan-Keen, M., Snijders, P.J.F., Walboomers, J.M.M., Hunter, R.D., Dyer, P.A., and Stern, P.L., *Br. J. Cancer* 72: 405–411, 1995.
10. Wang, Z., Margulies, L., Hicklin, D.J., and Ferrone, S., *Tissue Antigens* 47: 382–390, 1996.
11. Garrido, F., Cabrera, T., Concha, A., Glew, S., Ruiz-Cabello, F., and Stern, P.L., *Immunol. Today* 14: 491–499, 1993.
12. Concha, A., Esteban, F., Cabrera, T., Ruiz-Cabello, F., and Garrido, F., *Cancer Biol.* 2: 47–54, 1991.

13. Van Duinen, S.G., Ruiter, D.J., Bröcker, E.B., van der Velde, E.A., Sorg, C., Welvaart, K., and Ferrone, S., *Cancer Res.* 48: 1019–1025, 1988.
14. Levin, I., Klein, T., Kuperman, O., Segal, S., Shapira, J., Gal, R., Hart, Y., and Klein, B., *Cancer Detect. Prev.* 18: 443–445, 1994.
15. Möller, P., Momburg, F., Koretz, K., Moldenhauer, G., Herfarth, C., Otto, H.F., Hammerling, G.J., and Schlag, P., *Cancer Res.* 51: 729–736, 1991.
16. Passlick, B., Izbicki, J.R., Simmel, S., Kubuschok, B., Karg, O., Habekost, M., Thetter, O., Schweiberer, L., and Pantel, K., *Eur. J. Cancer* 30(A): 376–381, 1994.
17. Momburg, F., Degener, T., Bacchus, E., Moldenhauer, G., Hämmerling, G.J., and Möller, P., *Int. J. Cancer* 37: 179–184, 1986.
18. Natali, P.G., Giacomini, P., Bigitti, A., Imai, K., Nicotra, M.R., and Ferrone, S., *Cancer Res.* 43: 660–668, 1983.
19. Ruiter, D.J., Bergman, W., Welvaart, K., Scheffer, E., Van Vloten, W.A., Russo, C., and Ferrone, S., *Cancer Res.* 44: 3930–3935, 1984.
20. Bröcker, E.B., Suter, L., Bruggen, J., Ruiter, D.J., Macher, E., and Sorg, C., *Int. J. Cancer* 36: 29–35, 1985.
21. Ruiter, D.J., Mattijssen, V., Broecker, E.B. and Ferrone, S., *Semin. Cancer Biol.* 2: 35–45, 1991.
22. De Waard-Siebinga, I., Hilders, C.G.J.M., Hansen, B.E., Delft, J.L., and Jager, M.J., *Graefe's Arch. Clin. Exp. Ophthalmol.* 234: 34–42, 1996.
23. De la Cruz, P.O., Specht, C.S., and McLean, I.W., *Cancer* 65: 112–115, 1990.
24. Kremer, I., Gilad, E., Kahan, E., Derazne, E., and Bar-Ishak, R., *Acta Ophthalmol.* 69: 347–351, 1991.
25. Lang, J.R., Davidorf, F.H., and Baba, N., *Cancer* 40: 2388–2394, 1977.
26. Garrido, F., Ruiz-Cabello, F., Cabrera, T., Perez-Villar, J.J., Lopez-Botet, M., Duggan-Keen, M., and Stern, P.L., *Immunol. Today* 18: 89–95, 1997.
27. Blom, D.J.R., Schurmans, L.R.H.M., De Waard-Siebinga, I., De Wolff-Rouendaal, D., Keunen, J.E.E., and Jager, M.J., *Br. J. Ophthalmol.* 81: 989–993, 1997.
28. Hurks, H.M.H., Mulder, A., Claas, F.H.J., and Jager, M.J., *Int. J. Cancer* in press.
29. Ferrone, S., and Marincola, F.M., *Immunol. Today* 16: 487–494, 1995.
30. Carrel, S., Dore, J.F., Ruiter, D.J., Prade, M., Lejeune, F.J., Kleeberg, U.R., Rumke, P., and Brocker, E.B., *Int. J. Cancer* 48: 836–847, 1991.
31. Kageshita, T., Nakamura, T., Yamada, M., Kuriya, N., Arao, T., and Ferrone, S., *Cancer Res.* 51: 1726–1732, 1991.
32. Kageshita, T., Kimura, T., Yoshi, A., Hirai, S., Ono, T., and Ferrone, S., *Int. J. Cancer* 56: 370–374, 1994.
33. Lopez-Nevot, M.A., Garcia, E., Romero, C., Oliva, M.R., Serrano, S., and Garrido, F., *Exp. Clin. Immunogenet.* 5: 203–212, 1988.
34. Marincola, F.M., Shamamian, P., Alexander, R.B., Gnarra, J.R., Turetskaya, R.L., Nedospasov, S.A., Simonis, T.B., Taubenberger, J.K., Yannelli, J., Mixon, A., *et al.*, *J. Immunol.* 153: 1225–1237, 1994.
35. Restifo, N.P., Marincola, F.M., Kawakami, Y., Taubenberger, J., Yanelli, J.R., and Rosenberg, S.A., *J. Natl. Cancer Inst.* 88: 100–108, 1996.
36. D'Urso, C.M., Wang, Z.G., Cao, Y., Tatake, R., Zeff, R.A., and Ferrone, S., *J. Clin. Invest.* 87: 284–292, 1991.
37. Cromme, F.V., Airey, J., Heemels, M.T., Ploegh, H.L., Keating, P.J., Stern, P.L., Meijer, C.J., and Walboomers, J.M., *Exp. Med.* 179: 335–340, 1994.
38. Ma, D., Luyten, G.P.M., Luider, T.M., and Niederkorn, J.Y., *Invest. Ophthalmol. Vis. Sci.* 36: 435–441, 1995.

H. M. H. Hurks et al.

39. Whiteside, T.L., Herberman, R.B., *Clin. Diag. Lab. Immunol.* 74: 777–779, 1994.
40. Versteeg, R., Kruse-Wolters, K.M., Plomp, A.C., *et al.*, *J. Exp. Med.* 170: 621–635, 1989.
41. Peltenburg, L.T.C., and Schrier, P., *Immunogenetics* 40: 54–61, 1994.
42. Blom, D.J.R., Mooy, C.M., Luyten, G.P.M., Kerkvliet, S., Ouwerkerk, I., Zwinderman, A.H., Schrier, P.I., and Jager, M.J., *J. Pathol.* 181: 75–79, 1997.
43. Mooy, C.M., Luyten, G.P.M., De Jong, P.T.V.M., Luider, T.M., Stijnen, T., Van de Ham, F., Van Vroonhoven, C.C.J., and Bosman, F.T., *Am. J. Pathol.* 147: 1097–1104, 1995.
44. Schrier, P.I., Versteeg, R., Peltenburg, L.T., Plomp, A.C., Van't Veer, L.J., and Kruse-Wolters, K.M., *Semin. Cancer Biol.* 2: 73–83, 1991.
45. Versteeg, R., Peltenburg, L.T., Plomp, A.C., and Schrier, P.I., *J. Immunol.* 143: 4331–4337, 1989.
46. Kageshita, T., Wang, Z., Calorini, L., Yoshii, A., Kimura, T., Ono, T., Gattoni-Celli, S., and Ferrone, S., *Cancer Res.* 53: 3349–3354, 1993.
47. Natali, P.G., Nicotra, M.R., Bigotti, A., Venturo, I., Marcenaro, L., Giacomini, P., and Russo, C., *Proc. Natl. Acad. Sci. USA* 86: 6719–6723, 1989.
48. Geertsen, R.C., Hofbauer, G.F.L., Yue, F.Y., Manolio, S., Burg, G., and Dummer, R., *J. Invest. Dermatol.* 111: 497–502, 1998.
49. Metzelaar-Blok, J.A.W., Jager, M.J., Hanifi Moghaddam, P., Van der Slik, A.R., and Giphart, M.J., *Human Immunol.* in press.
50. Kisseljov, F., Semionova, L., Samoylova, E., Mazurenko, N., Komissarova, E., Zourbitskaya, V., Gritzko, T., Kozachenko, V., Netchushkin, M., Petrov, S., Smirnov, A., and Alonso, A., *Int. J. Cancer* 69: 484–487, 1996.
51. Merlo, A., Gabrielson, E., Mabry, M., Vollmer, R., Baylin, S.B., and Sidransky, D., *Cancer Res.* 54: 2322–2326, 1994.
52. Saitoh, Y., Bruner, J.M., Levin, V.A., and Kyritsis, A.P., *Gene Chromosome Canc.* 22: 165–170, 1998.
53. De Plaen, E., Arden, K., Traversari, C., Gaforio, J.J., Szikora, J.P., De Smet, C., Brasseur, F., Van der Bruggen, P., Lethé, B., Lurquin, C., Brasseur, R., Chomez, P., De Backer, O., Cavenee, W., and Boon, T., *Immunogenetics* 40: 360–369, 1994.
54. Kawakami, Y., Eliyahu, S., Delgado, C.H., Robbins, P.F., Rivoltini, L., Topalian, S.L., Miki, T., and Rosenberg, S.A., *Proc. Natl. Acad. USA* 91: 3515–3519, 1994.
55. Kawakami, Y., Eliyahu, S., Delgado, C.H., Robbins, P.F., Sakaguchi, K., Apella, E., Yanelli, J.R., Adema, G.J., Miki, T., and Rosenberg, S.A., *Proc. Natl. Acad. USA* 91: 6458–6462, 1994.
56. Irvine, K.R., Rao, J.B., Rosenberg, S.A., and Restifo, N.P., *J. Immunol.* 156: 238–245, 1996.
57. Rosenberg, S.A., *Immunol. Today* 18: 175–182, 1997.
58. Chang, A.E., Aruga, A., Cameron, M.J., Sondak, V.K., Normolle, D.P., Fox, B.A., and Shu, S., *J. Clin. Oncol.* 15: 796–807, 1997,
59. Jaeger, E., Bernhard, H., Romero, P., Ringhoffer, M., Arand, M., Karbach, J., Ilsemann, C., Hagedorn, M., and Knuth, A., *Int. J. Cancer* 66: 162–169, 1996.
60. Legha, S.S., *Semin. Oncol.* 24: 24s–31s, 1997.
61. Möller, P., Sun, Y., Dorbic, T., Alijagic, S., Makki, A., Jurgovsky, K., Schroff, M., Henz, B.M., Wittig, B., and Schadendorf, D., *Br. J. Cancer* 77: 1884–1892, 1998.
62. Nestle, F.O., Alijagic, S., Gilliet, M., Sun, Y., Grabbe, S., Dummer, R., Burg, G., and Schadendorf, D., *Nat. Med.* 4: 328–332, 1998.

63. Rosenberg, S.A., Yannelli, J.R., Yang, J.C., Topalian, S.L., Schwartzentruber, D.J., Weber, J.S., Parkinson, D.R., Seipp, C.A., Einhorn, J.H., and White, D.E., *J. Natl. Cancer Inst.* 86: 1159–1166, 1994.

64. Rosenberg, S.A., Yang, J.C., Schwartzentruber, D.J., Hwu, P., Marincola, F.M., Topalian, S.L., Restifo, N.P., Dudley, M.E., Schwarz, S.L., Spiess, P.J., Wunderlich, J.R., Parkhurst, M.R., Kawakami, Y., Seipp, C.A., Einhorn, J.H., and White, D.E., *Nat. Med.* 4: 321–327, 1998.

65. Sun, Y., Jurgovsky, K., Moller, P., Alijagic, S., Dorbic, T., Georgieva, J., Wittig, B., and Schadendorf, D., *Gene Ther.* 5: 481–490, 1998.

66. Villikka, K., and Pyrhönen, S., *Ann. Med.* 28: 227–233, 1996.

67. Mitchell, M.S., Liggett, P.E., Green, R.L., Kan-Mitchell, J., Murphree, A.L., Dean, G., Spears, L., and Walonker, F., *J. Clin. Oncol.* 12: 396-401, 1994.

68. Nathan, F.E., Berd, D., Sato, T., Shield, J.A., Shields, C.L., De Potter, P., and Mastrangelo, M.J., *J. Exp. Clin. Cancer Res.* 16: 201–208, 1997.

69. Pyrhönen, S., *Eur. J. Cancer* 34: S27–S30, 1998.

70. De Waard-Siebinga, I., Creyghton, W.M., Kool, J., and Jager, M.J., *Br. J. Ophthalmol.* 79: 847–855, 1995.

71. Stopeck, A.T., Hersh, E.M., Akporiaye, E.T., Harris, D.T., Grogan, T., Unger, E., Warneke, J., Schluter, S.F., and Stahl, S., *J. Clin. Oncol.* 15: 341–349, 1997.

72. Porgador, A., Mandelboim, O., Restifo, N.P., and Strominger, J.L., *Proc. Natl. Acad. Sci. USA* 94: 13140–13145, 1997.

73. Kovats, S., Main, E.K., Librach, C., Strubblebine, M., Fisher, S.J., and De Mars, R., *Science* 249: 220–223, 1990.

74. Pazmany, L., Mandelboim, O., Vales-Gomez, M., Davis, D.M., Reyburn, H.T., and Strominger, J.L., *Science* 274: 792–795, 1996.

75. Paul, P., Rouas-Freiss, N., Khalil-Daher, I., Moreau, P., Riteau, B., Le Gal, F.A., Avril, M.F., Dausset, J., Guillet, J.G., and Carosella, E.D., *Proc. Natl. Acad. Sci. USA* 95: 4510–4515, 1998.

76. Cabestre, F.A., Lefebvre, S., Moreau, P., Rouas-Friess, N., Dausset, J., Carosella, E.D., and Paul, P., *Semin. Cancer Biol.* 9: 27–36, 1999.

Abbreviations

HLA   human leukocyte antigen
IFN   interferon
KAR   killer activatory receptor
KIR   killer inhibitory receptor
LOH   loss of heterozygosity
moAb   monoclonal antibody
NK   natural killer
TAP   transporters associated with antigen processing

H. M. H. Hurks et al.

M.J. JAGER, D.J.R. BLOM, W.R.O. GOSLINGS,
J.A.W. METZELAAR-BLOK AND H.M.H. HURKS

Antigen expression on uveal melanoma

Abstract

Cell-surface molecules have a multitude of functions, and while some help to protect malignant cells from attack, others can be used as targets for immunotherapy. On cutaneous and uveal melanoma, melanocyte differentiation antigens are expressed, which can function as targets for cytotoxic T cells. On the other hand, regulators of complement may inhibit tumor-cell lysis by blocking complement activation after antibody binding, and multidrug resistance proteins may block the function of chemotherapeutic agents that are being tried against uveal melanoma metastases. Finally, cell surface molecules may affect the metastatic behaviour of the tumor cells themselves, and determine their sensitivity to environmental factors. Studies on cell surface molecules expressed on uveal melanomas contribute greatly to our understanding of the behaviour of this malignancy.

Keywords: Uveal melanoma, tumor-specific antigens, regulators of complement, multidrug resistance, EGF-receptor

Introduction

Tumor cells may express a wide range of antigens with different functions. Such antigens can be recognized by various methods, including the application of monoclonal antibodies (MoAbs), biochemical methods, or functional assays. A subdivision is made between differentiation antigens, that are expressed on malignant cells as well as on normal cells of the same lineage, and tumor-associated antigens, such as the MAGE or BAGE antigens, that have been found on some other non-malignant tissues as well. Other antigens include hormone receptors, regulatory molecules that play a role in the inhibition of complement, or transport molecules that are expressed on the cell surface. Expression of some of the cell surface molecules plays a role in the

Department of Ophthalmology, Leiden University Medical Center,
2300 RC Leiden, The Netherlands

clinical behaviour of the tumor, such as the development of metastases, or in the resistance against immuno- or chemotherapy.

Although attempts have been made to identify uveal melanoma-specific antigens, no specific antigens have so far been recognized. Most often, antigens were first identified on skin melanoma or on non-malignant dermal pigmented cells, and subsequently identified on uveal melanoma cells. In an early study, Van der Pol *et al.* [1] applied monoclonal antibodies directed against a range of antigens previously associated with cutaneous melanoma (cMAA). Van der Pol analysed the expression of seven different cMAA in a series of twenty-five uveal melanomas, and studied the degree of heterogeneity between uveal melanomas and potential correlations with known prognostic markers. One of the antigens that was often expressed on uveal melanoma was recognized by MoAb NKI-beteb, which was later identified as acting against gp100, a differentiation antigen [2]. M.2.2.4, which recognizes a differentiation antigen on skin melanoma and nevi, reacted with 50% of the tumors. Expression was lower after pre-operative radiotherapy with four Gray on the two days prior to enucleation. Two MoAbs that showed a large heterogeneity between tumors were MoAb AMF-1, which recognizes a cellular adhesion molecule, and PAL-M1, which is directed against an antigen that was mainly observed on skin melanoma metastases. MoAb R-24 which recognizes ganglioside GD3, was hardly expressed. It is of interest that several of these antigens are now being used as targets for immunotherapy in skin melanoma. No correlation with any of the known histopathological parameters in uveal melanoma was observed.

Melanoma antigens

The melanoma antigens that have been recognized so far can be divided into three general categories [3]. The first category can be characterized as melanocyte-differentiation antigens. This category includes antigens that are not only present in melanoma cells but also in normal skin and uveal melanocytes. Antigens belonging to this category are tyrosinase, gp100, MART-1/Melan A, and gp75. A second category can be characterized as tumor-associated antigens. This category includes the members of the MAGE gene family, antigens that were found to be expressed not only on melanomas, but in a number of tumors and in adult testis as well. A third group of antigens can be characterized as truly tumor-specific antigens, resulting from tumor-specific point mutations. Several investigators studied the presence of MAGE, gp100, and tyrosinase gene expression in uveal melanoma. Mulcahy *et al.* [4] performed a similar study on primary uveal melanoma and metastases. MAGE 1–4 were not found on primary tumors, while two out of 26 metastases expressed MAGE-1 and MAGE-4. When using more PCR cycles, a slight expression was found in more tumors. Tyrosinase, Melan-A/Mart-1, and gp100 were expressed on almost all primary uveal melanomas as well as on the metastases.

TABLE 1. *Expression of MAGE, tyrosinase and gp100 on uveal melanoma.*

	MAGE-1	MAGE-2	MAGE-3	tyrosinase	gp100
Mulcahy (1996)					
primary tumor $n = 27$	0	0	0	26	26
metastases $n = 26$	0	0	0	24	24
Luyten (1998)					
primary cell line $n = 5$	1	1	1	5	4
metastatic cell line $n = 3$	1	1	1	3	1
Chen (1997)					
skin melanocytes	neg	neg	neg		
choroidal melanocytes	neg	neg	neg		
retinal pigment epithelium	neg	neg	neg		
cultured uveal mel. $n = 17$	7	9	9		

Chen, Ksander and co-workers [5] used freshly cultured uveal melanomas and cell lines to determine MAGE expression. A total of 17 uveal melanomas were dissected and cultured (the number of times tumor cell cultures were passaged *in vitro* before testing varied from 3 to 33 times). A MAGE-1, -2, -3 positive and negative skin melanoma cell line were used as controls. A total of 10 out of 17 short-term cultures were positive for MAGE-1, 9 for MAGE-2, and 9 for MAGE-3, when assayed with reverse-transcription-polymerase chain reaction specific for either MAGE-1, -2, or -3. Fresh or cultured choroidal melanocytes or retinal pigment epithelium cells were negative with regard to all three antigens [6]. This may explain the phenomenon that patients do not develop ocular problems following immunotherapy with MAGE-specific peptides for skin melanoma. In another study, Chen *et al.* [5] compared material obtained from a freshly enucleated uveal melanoma with cells from the same tumor that were cultured *in vitro*, and with metastases from that uveal melanoma. A total of 17 tumor clones was obtained from the primary melanoma and all clones expressed MAGE-1, -2, and -3. Three out of four cultures obtained from metastases expressed MAGE-1, -2, and -3. One metastasis did not express MAGE antigens when tested after culture *in vitro*, but started to express the MAGE antigens after treatment with a demethylating agent.

Luyten *et al.* [7] evaluated expression of MAGE-1, -2, and -3, and of gp100 and tyrosinase on five primary and three metastatic uveal melanoma cell lines by reverse transcriptase PCR technique. All three MAGE antigens were expressed on two cell lines (OCM-1 and OMM-1), gp100 was expressed on all cell lines and tyrosinase on six. It is interesting that all five antigens were expressed on OCM-1, a cell line that had previously successfully been used by Kan-Mitchell *et al.* [8] to induce anti-uveal melanoma T cell clones. In conclusion, it is clear that the MAGE antigens have almost no expression on fresh tissue, but are expressed on around 50% of primary tumors after short-term culture. However, tyrosinase, Melan-A/Mart-1, and gp100 are expressed on most uveal melanomas and their metastases, and should therefore be appropriate targets for immunotherapy.

CTL-mediated lysis *in vitro*

The occurrence of tumor-specific lymphocytes inside the uveal melanoma was described by Ksander *et al.* [9,10]. Tumor-infiltrating lymphocytes (TIL) were obtained from a series of human choroidal melanomas and expanded *in vitro* with IL-2. TIL from four out of six tumors reacted only against autologous melanoma cells and not against allogeneic tumors. TIL from two patients were unable to lyse autologous melanoma cells, although these cells expressed backbone HLA-Class I molecules. It is possible that the tumor cells did not express the specific HLA Class I epitope necessary for CTL recognition (see Chapter 10). Histological analysis of most of the tumors that gave rise to TIL revealed no or few tumor-infiltrating lymphocytes. The specificity of these TIL has not yet been defined. One of the reasons is, that in contrast with T cells against skin melanoma, TIL obtained from uveal melanoma were very difficult to maintain and to stimulate *in vitro*.

We wondered whether cytotoxic T cells that had been generated against epitopes on skin melanoma would also be able to lyse uveal melanoma cells *in vitro*. *In vitro* grown cytotoxic T lymphocytes recognizing the melanocyte differentiation antigen Melan-A/MART-1 (clone 4/15) were used as effector cells. This anti-Melan-A/Mart-1 CTL clone had been induced by incubating peripheral blood leukocytes with peptide-pulsed dendritic cells [11]. A sensitive WEHI bioassay for Tumor Necrosis Factor release was utilized [12]. This CTL clone deed indeed recognize Melan-A/Mart-1 positive uveal melanoma cells with the right HLA type (Figure 1).

Membrane-bound regulators of complement

Tumor cells use many mechanisms that help the tumor cell escape from the immune system. Membrane-bound regulators of complement activation (mRCA) play an important role in the protection of host cells from the complement-mediated antibody-dependent lysis. They also play a role in the down-regulation of autologous anti-tumor antibody responses and may limit the therapeutic application of monoclonal antibodies. Some of the regulators of complement activation are membrane cofactor protein (MCP or CD46), decay-accelerating factor (DAF, CD55) and homologous restriction factor 20 (HRF20, CD59). The presence of these three RCAs was determined on sections of uveal melanoma and on uveal melanoma cell lines [13]. CD59 was intensely expressed on all tumors, while CD46 and CD55 showed a less intense staining, but showed staining on almost all sections. Three cell lines obtained from a primary uveal melanoma and one from a metastasis showed a high expression of CD59 and a lower expression of CD46. CD55 was quite low on two of the four cell lines. Exposure of cultured cells to phosphatidylinositol-specific phospholipase C decreased the expression of CD59 and CD55, and gave a moderate increase in the lysability of the tumor cells by complement-mediated antibody-dependent lysis. Since many patients

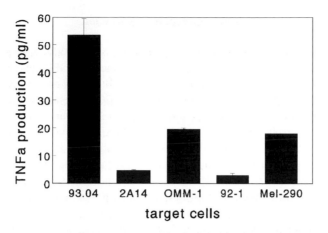

Cell lysis by Melan-A/Mart-1 specific CTLs. The release of Tumor Necrosis Factor was measured, following incubation of different tumor cell lines with Melan-A/Mart-1 specific CTLs. Cell lines 93.04 and 2A14 are the positive and negative control, respectively. Cell lines OMM1, 92-1, and Mel290 are uveal melanoma cell lines, of which 92-1 carries the HLA-A2.6 epitope, while the other two are HLA-A2.1 positive.

develop tumor-specific antibodies, it is possible that the RCA's play a role in the escape from the immune system in uveal melanoma.

Multidrug resistance proteins

The prognosis of patients with metastatic choroidal melanoma is extremely poor. Once the diagnosis of hepatic metastasis has been made, the median survival time is two to seven months. The resistance to chemotherapy is one of the major reasons for the lack of appropriate chemotherapeutic regimens for this disease. Tumor cells are resistant to specific drugs or groups of chemotherapeutic agents and several mechanisms can play a role in the resistance to these agents. A common mechanism in multidrug resistance involves overexpression of a 170-kDa plasma membrane protein, P-glycoprotein. This protein acts as an adenosine triphosphate-driven drug efflux pump and confers resistance to a wide range of agents, including anthracyclines and actinomycin. Other multidrug-resistance molecules are MDR-related protein (MRP) and Lung resistance protein (LRP). Van der Pol *et al.* [14] examined the expression of these molecules on sections of 12 uveal melanoma and on uveal melanoma cell lines. LRP was expressed on all uveal melanomas tested, MRP on 11 and P-glycoprotein on 5. A similar pattern was observed on cell lines. This expression plays a role in the resistance against chemotherapy that is clinically observed.

EGF-R receptor expression

The epidermal growth factor receptor (EGFR) is a 170 kDa transmembrane glycoprotein, that can bind epidermal growth factor (EGFR) and hepatocyte growth factor (HGF). Overexpression of EGFR occurs on a wide range of malignancies. Binding of HGF or EGF to the EGFR results in an increased cell proliferation, increased adhesion and motility. Ma and Niederkorn [15] observed a correlation between expression of EGFR on uveal melanoma cell lines and the development of liver metastases following injection of the cells in nude mice. Jager, Hurks and co-workers [16] analysed expression on sections of uveal melanoma by immunohistology and observed that the presence of EGFR was correlated with death due to melanoma metastases.

Future

Immunotherapeutic approaches are considered promising tools in future treatment or prevention of uveal melanoma metastases. Several epitopes like gangliosides and differentiation antigens are expressed on the primary tumor and its metastases, and future use as target for immunotherapy with cytotoxic T cells or specially created antibodies is not unthinkable. In addition, new approaches are necessary to circumvent the mechanisms that will make the tumor resistant to various treatments, such as loss of HLA Class I antigens, expression of regulators of complement activation and multidrug resistance molecules. Finally, once the mechanisms that lead to the development of metastases are elucidated, specific preventive measures, such as the application of EGFR-blocking antibodies, may be developed and used clinically.

References

1. Van Der Pol, J.P., Jager, M.J., De Wolff-Rouendaal, D., Ringens, P.J., Vennegoor, C., and Ruiter, D.J., *Curr. Eye Res.* 6: 757–765, 1987.
2. Bakker, A.B.H., Schreurs, M.W.J., Tafazzul, G., De Boer, A.J., Kawakami, Y., Adema, G.J., and Figdor, C.G., *Int. J. Cancer* 62: 97–102, 1995.
3. Ksander, B.R. in *Immunology of the Skin and the Eye*, Zierhut, M. and Thiel, H.-J. (eds.), pp. 269–288, Aeolus Press, Buren, The Netherlands, 1999.
4. Mulcahy, K.A., Rimoldi, D., Brasseur, F., Rodgers, S., Lienard, D., Marchand, M., Renniem I.G., Murraym A.K., McIntyre, C.A., Platts, K.E., Leyvraz, S., Boon, T., and Rees R.C., *Int. J. Cancer* 66: 738–742, 1996.
5. Chen, P.W., Murray, T.G., Uno, T., Salgallar, M., Reddy, R., and Ksander, B.R., *Clin. Exp. Metastasis* 15: 509–518, 1996.
6. Chen, P.W., Murray, T.G., Salgaller, M.L., and Ksander, B.R., *J. Immunother.* 20: 265–275, 1997.
7. Luyten, G.P.M., Van der Spek, C.W., Brand, I., Sintnicolaas, K., De Waard-Siebinga, I., Jager, M.J., De Jong, P.T.V.M., Schrier, P.I., and Luider, T.M., *Melanoma Res.* 8: 11–16, 1998.

M. J. Jager et al.

8. Kan-Mitchell, J., Liggett, P.E., Harel, W., Steinman, L., Nitta, T., Oksenberg, J.R., Posner, M.R., and Mitchell, M.S., *Cancer Imm. Immunother.* 33: 333–340, 1991.

9. Ksander, B.R., Rubsamen, P.E., Olsen, K.R., Cousins, S.W., and Streilein, J.W., *Invest. Ophthalmol. Vis. Sci.* 32: 3198–3208, 1991.

10. Ksander, B.R., Geer, D.C., Chen, P.W., Salgaller, M.L., Rubsamen, P., and Murray, T.G., *Curr. Eye Res.* 17: 165–173, 1998.

11. Van Elsas, A., Van der Burg, S.H., Van der Minne, C.C., Borghi, M., Mourer, J.S., Melief, C.J.M., and Schrier, P.I., *Eur. J. Imunol.* 26: 1683–1689, 1996.

12. Espevik, T., and Nissen-Meyer, J., *J. Immunol. Methods* 95: 99–105, 1986.

13. Goslings, W.R.O., Blom, D.J.R., De Waard-Siebinga, I., Van Beelen, E., Claas, F.H.J., Jager, M.J., and Gorter, A., *Invest. Ophthalmol. Vis. Sci.* 37: 1884–1891, 1996.

14. Van Der Pol, J.P., Blom, D.J.R., Flens, M.J., Luyten, G.P.M., De Waard-Siebinga, I., Koornneef, L., Scheper, R.J., and Jager, M.J., *Invest. Ophthalmol. Vis. Sci.* 38: 2523–2530, 1997.

15. Ma, D., and Niederkorn, J.Y., *Invest. Opthalmol. Vis. Sci.* 39: 1067–1075, 1998.

16. Jager, M.J., Hurks, M.H.M., Metzelaar-Blok, J.A., Schipper, R.F., and De Wolff-Rouendaal, D., *Invest. Opthalmol. Vis. Sci.* 40: S185, 1999.

RENÉ E.M. TOES, LINDA DIEHL, ANNEMIEKE TH. DEN
BOER, ELLEN I.H. VAN DER VOORT, CORNELIS J.M.
MELIEF AND RIENK OFFRINGA

CD40–CD40-ligand-interactions and their role in cytotoxic T lymphocyte priming and anti-tumor immunity

Abstract

Cytotoxic T lymphocytes (CTL) specific for cellular antigens are in general activated by professional antigen-presenting cells that indirectly present antigens derived from cells in the periphery. This "cross-priming" of $CD8^+$ T cells is dependent on the presence of help provided by $CD4^+$ T-helper cells. In the absence of helper-activity, antigen recognition by CTL can result in CTL tolerance. Thus, the outcome of antigen recognition by naïve $CD8^+$ CTL is orchestrated by $CD4^+$ T-helper cells. Although the dependency on "help" for efficient CTL priming has been well documented, it was only recently that more mechanistic insight into the nature of this help has been obtained. In the absence of $CD4^+$ T-helper cells, signalling of professional antigen-presenting cells through CD40 can replace "help" required for priming of $CD8^+$ T cells. Blockade of CD40Ligand expressed by T-helper cells severely inhibit priming of tumor-specific CTL. Moreover, triggering of CD40 *in vivo* can revert CTL tolerization induced by immunization with an tolerogenic peptide vaccine into strong CTL priming. These findings indicate that the CD40–CD40Ligand pair can act as a "switch" determining the activation state of professional antigen-presenting cells and thereby setting the balance between T cell tolerization and T cell activation.

Keywords: Cytotoxic T lymphocyte, priming, CD40, Th cell activity, dendritic cells

Department of Immunohematology and Blood Bank, University Hospital Leiden,
PO Box 9600, 2333 AZ Leiden, The Netherlands

Cross-presentation of antigen can lead both to priming and tolerization of CTL

Most solid tumors express MHC class I-molecules, but lack costimulatory molecules that are required for appropriate CTL activation [1,2]. Therefore, for optimal tumor-specific CTL induction, presentation of tumor-derived antigens by professional antigen presenting cells (APC) is routinely required. This re- or cross-presentation of antigens provides the immune system with a mechanism by which it can detect and respond to antigens expressed in non-lymphoid tissues, as well as with a means to survey neoantigens expressed by tumors. The first indications that cross-presentation of antigens to CTL is an important mechanism for the induction of CTL-responses came from studies in the late 1970s that showed that an antigen-specific T cell response can be induced independent of the haplotype of the immunising cell [3,4]. Since then, increasing evidence has been collected indicating that MHC class I-restricted tumor-specific immunity requires cross-presentation of antigens that have been captured by professional APC [5–8]. These studies describe the efficient priming of tumor-specific CTL in a situation in which the tumor cell used for immunisation is unable to directly prime or activate T cells because of the lack of relevant MHC-molecules. Cross-presentation of antigens by professional APC is important for efficient CTL-induction, but the same mechanism could also be important for tolerization of (autoreactive) CTL. Kurts and co-workers have shown in studies using transgenic mice expressing a membrane-bound form of ovalbumin (OVA) in pancreatic islets that OVA was represented to OVA-specific CTL in lymph nodes draining the site of antigen-expression [9]. However, after an initial phase of proliferation, OVA-specific CTL were ultimately deleted [10]. This deletion only required antigen recognition on an APC. Thus, cross-presentation of antigens can also lead to tolerization of CTL.

The balance between CTL-priming and tolerization is regulated by CD4$^+$ T-helper cells

The studies described above provide a mechanism by which potentially auto-reactive CTL can be deleted from the periphery when the antigen recognised by these CTL is expressed outside the recirculation pathway of naive T cells, but contrasts with the activation of OVA-specific CTL by cross-priming APC that occurs when OVA-expressing cells are used to immunize [11]. The discrepancy between these observations could be explained by the lack (in the case of tolerization) or presence (in the case of priming) of antigen-specific CD4$^+$ T-helper cells (Th cells). The presence or absence of CD4$^+$ T cell-mediated helper activity as important factor influencing the outcome of CTL responsiveness was first shown in a model using Qa-1 as antigen. Systemic presentation of Qa-1 in the absence of helper activity tolerized Qa-1-specific CTL, whereas Qa-1-specific CTL are primed in the presence of helper

René E. M. Toes et al.

activity [12]. Initial exposure to Qa-1 allodeterminants in the absence of T cell help leads to a state of Qa-1-specific transplantation tolerance, as animals "primed" in the absence of help are rendered tolerant to subsequent Qa-1-disparate skin allografts [13]. Furthermore, it has been shown in the OVA-transgenic mouse system, that injection of OVA-specific CD4$^+$ Th cells prevents the deletion of OVA-specific CTL and favours the induction of autoimmunity [14]. These observations indicate that provision of help by CD4$^+$ Th cells is an important factor in the prevention of peripheral CTL-tolerance as well as for the induction of CTL-immunity.

CD4$^+$ T cell help for CTL-priming is mediated through CD40–CD40Ligand interactions

The ability of Th cells to generate and augment the activity of CTL has been extensively characterised [15,16]. Although numerous studies have shown that priming of CD8$^+$ CTL *in vivo* requires the participation of CD4$^+$ Th cells, the nature of the "help" provided was until recently unknown. Previously, it has been suggested T help for CTL-priming is mediated by cytokines, such as interleukin-2 (IL-2), produced by Th cells activated in the proximity to the CTL precursor at the surface of the same APC [15,17]. Dissection of the cellular interactions involved in CTL-priming by cross-presentation of MHC class I-restricted epitopes has revealed that Th cells must recognise antigen on the same APC that presents the CTL-epitope [11]. These results could be explained by a proximity requirement for the efficient delivery by Th cells of soluble factors, such as IL-2. However, another possibility is that a cognate interaction between Th cell and APC is required to convert the APC to a "CTL-priming state", as first proposed by Guerder and Matzinger [12]. By interacting with the cross-presenting APC, a T-helper cell can assist in CTL priming without requiring the simultaneous interaction of a relatively rare antigen-specific CTL, the presence of which cannot be detected by the Th cell (murine CTL are class II-negative). Moreover, in this way the activity of only a few antigen-specific Th cells can in this way be amplified, since one Th cell can activate several APC which can then prime many antigen-specific CTL.

Interested in the mechanism by which T-helper activity for CTL-priming is mediated, we studied the role of CD40 CD40Ligand interaction in the delivery of help for CTL response induction. CD40Ligand is a member of the tumor necrosis factor gene family and is preferentially expressed on mast cells and (shortly following T cell receptor triggering) on CD4$^+$ T cells. CD40, the receptor for CD40Ligand is expressed on several cell types, including dendritic cells (DC), B cells, macrophages, endothelial cells and proximal tubular epithelial cells in the kidney (for review see [18]).

CD40–CD40Ligand interactions play an important role in the development of several effector functions. Studies in CD40- and CD40Ligand-deficient mice show that the generation of primary and secondary humoral immune responses and the formation of germinal centres to a variety of thymus-dependent antigens are dependent on this molecular interaction [19,20]. These observations indicate that CD40–CD40Ligand interactions play a crucial role in the delivery of T cell help to B cells. Furthermore, CD40–CD40 Ligand interactions are important for the generation of Th1 responses, the induction of T cell responses directed against viruses and bacteria [21,22], as well as for the induction of protective anti-tumor immunity after vaccination with a tumor cell vaccine [23].

CD40 signals are part of a critical pathway in T cell dependent macrophage and DC activation. Recombinant soluble CD40Ligand stimulates human monocytes to release proinflammatory cytokines [24], whereas triggering of CD40 on DC or interactions between DC and $CD4^+$ T cells leads to the production of interleukin-12. In the latter case, IL-12 production by DC is inhibited by blockade of CD40Ligand on the $CD4^+$ T cell [25]. Moreover, CD40 ligation is a potent stimulus to upregulate the expression of ICAM-1, CD80 and CD86 molecules [26,27]. Because CD40-induced activation of professional APC results in the expression of cytokines and costimulatory molecules important for CTL priming, this activation is likely to play an important role in the delivery of T help to CTL.

We have demonstrated that CD40-triggering can replace $CD4^+$ T cells in priming of helper-dependent $CD8^+$ CTL responses [28]. Vaccination of B6 mice (H-2D^b) with completely allogeneic tumor cells of BALB/c origin (H-2^d), transformed by the human adenovirus type 5 early region 1 (Ad5E1), leads to the induction of a potent H-2D^b-restricted CTL-response directed against an Ad5E1-encoded CTL-epitope [8,29]. Since these tumor cells themselves cannot present the Ad5E1-derived CTL epitope to E1-specific CTL directly (they lack H-2^b), the CTL must be primed by non-tumor cells that have processed and presented the Ad5E1-peptide to Ad5E1-specific CTL (cross-priming). Cross-priming of E1-specific CTL is strictly Th cell dependent, as mice depleted for $CD4^+$ Th cells prior to immunisation with BALB/c Ad5E1 cells no longer mount an E1-specific CTL response [28]. Administration of a CD40-activating monoclonal antibody (mAb) [30] to mice lacking functional MHC class II-restricted $CD4^+$ T cells in the periphery [31], resulted in efficient restoration of E1-specific CTL responses [28]. Moreover, blockade of CD40Ligand by *in vivo* administration of a mAb that blocks CD40Ligand on the $CD4^+$ T cells [32], resulted in a profound inhibition of CTL-priming. This inhibition is overcome by CD40 triggering. Similar observations were also made in another model. CD40- or CD40Ligand-deficient mice are unable generate OVA-specific CTL-responses after vaccination with OVA-expressing cells, showing that expression of both CD40 and CD40ligand is required for cross-priming of CTL. Moreover, mice devoid of $CD4^+$ Th cells, are not able to mount OVA-specific CTL after vaccination with OVA-expressing cells, unless immunisation is performed together with injection of a mAb that triggers CD40 [33]. Taken together, these results shown that CTL can be primed in the absence of Th-derived cytokines, and demonstrate the crucial importance of CD40–CD40Ligand interaction in delivery of T cell help for

René E. M. Toes et al.

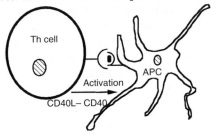

TH cell activates APC via CD40Ligand–CD40 interaction

Th cell

Activation

CD40L– CD40

APC

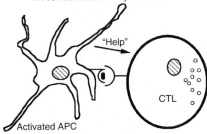

TH cell activated APC prime CTL

"Help"

CTL

Activated APC

FIGURE 1. *Model for delivery of T cell help for CTL-priming. An antigen-specific T-helper cells recognizes an APC that presents an peptide in the context of MHC class II. Upon antigen recognition, the Th cell activates the APC through trig-gering of CD40 expressed by the APC and CD40Ligand expressed by the Th cell. This CD40-triggered APC is now enabled to provide "help" for the priming of MHC class I-restricted CTL [12,28,33,34].*

CTL priming. These results also indicate that, rather than directly stimulating the CTL, the contribution of CD4$^+$ Th cells involves the activation of professional APC via CD40–CD40Ligand interactions (Fig. 1). It has been reported that help for priming of H-Y-specific CTL can be bypassed by acti-vation of DC through CD40. Female MHC class II knock-out mice are not able to mount an H-Y-response when injected with male DC, but do respond when CD40-modulated DC are used for vaccination [34]. Thus, Th cell and CTL do not need to meet simultaneously at the surface of the antigen-presenting DC to enable CTL-priming. Moreover, these results indicate that DC that have received an activation signal through CD40–CD40Ligand inter-actions can prime naive CTL, whereas unmodulated DC that have not been in contact with antigen-specific, CD40Ligand-expressing Th cells are not able to do so.

CD40 activation overcomes peptide-induced peripheral CTL tolerance

Since CD4$^+$ Th cells play a crucial role in orchestrating the outcome of the CTL-response to antigenic challenge, leading either to CTL immunity or

CTL tolerance, we sought to determine whether provision of help by triggering of CD40 *in vivo* is sufficient to prevent peripheral tolerization of CTL.

Vaccines consisting of minimal CTL epitopes emulsified in adjuvants can induce protective viral- and tumor-specific CTL immunity [35–37]. However, in certain cases such immunizations have adverse effects causing peripheral CTL tolerance [38]. For example, a minimal CTL epitope derived from the Ad5E1-region readily induces E1-specific CTL-tolerance that is associated with the inability of vaccinated animals to resist an, otherwise, non-lethal tumor [39,40]. Injection of syngeneic DC loaded with this peptide, however, induces strong protective anti-tumor CTL immunity [41], indicating that not the peptides themselves determines the outcome of vaccination. Moreover, these data indicate that when these peptide are presented by properly activated DC displaying their full co-stimulatory potential, they do induce a CTL-response. Since the peptide used for vaccination only represents a minimal CTL-epitope, but not a Th epitope, we studied whether provision of help through CD40-activation leading to activation of APC would now result in CTL-priming. Simultaneous injection of peptide and an agonistic anti-CD40 antibody overcame peripheral CTL tolerance that is normally induced when the peptide alone is used for vaccination [42]. Mice treated with both the peptide vaccine and the anti-CD40 mAb mounted a strong peptide- and tumor-specific CTL-response.

Not only the outcome of vaccination with a tolerogenic peptide is improved by *in vivo* CD40-triggering, but also the efficacy of an anti-tumor vaccine that leads to protective immunity (instead of tolerance). A peptide encompassing a CTL-eptiope derived from the human papillomavirus type 16 that normally induces protective anti-tumor immunity can be given tumor-eradicating potential when vaccination is combined with *in vivo* anti-CD40 triggering. In a model involving adoptive transfer of naïve tumor-specific CD4$^+$ T cells into tumor-bearing mice, CD40-triggering not only preserved tumor-specific CD4$^+$ T cell tolerance to T cell priming, but resulted also in their endogenous activation [43]. Moreover, established tumors regressed in vaccinated mice treated with antibody against CD40 at a time when no response was achieved with vaccination alone. Thus, manipulation of the immune system through CD40 can convert peripheral CTL tolerization induced by minimal CTL epitopes into efficient CTL priming and can augment the biological effects of a non-tolerizing peptide. This emphasizes the role of CD40–CD40L interactions in the control of T cell immunity and sheds light on the delicate balancing role of CD40–positive APC as essential guardians of CTL-activity.

Acknowledgements

The research of Dr. R.E.M. Toes has been made possible by a fellowship of the Royal Netherlands Academy of Arts and Sciences. Part of the work presented in this review was supported by the Dutch Cancer Foundation (Grants RUL 97-1449, RUL 97-1450 and RUL 99-2025).

René E. M. Toes et al.

References

1. Allison, J.P., *Curr. Opin. Immunol.* 6: 414–419, 1994.
2. Townsend, S.E., and Allison, J.P., *Science* 259: 368–370, 1993.
3. Bevan, M.J., *J. Exp. Med.* 143: 1283–1288, 1976.
4. Matzinger, P., and Bevan, M., *Cell. Immunol.* 33: 92–100, 1977.
5. Seung, S., Urban, J.L., and Schreiber, H., *J. Exp. Med.* 178: 933–940, 1993.
6. Huang, A.Y.C., Golumbek, P., Ahmadzadeh, M., Jaffee, E., Pardoll, D., and Levitsky, H., *Science* 264: 961–965, 1994.
7. Tzy-Choo Wu, Huang, A.Y.C., Jaffee, E.M., Levitsky, H.I., and Pardoll, D.M., *J. Exp. Med.* 182: 1415–1421, 1995.
8. Toes, R.E.M., Blom, R.J.J., van der Voort, E., Offringa, R., Melief, C.J.M., and Kast, W.M., *Cancer Res.* 56: 3782–3787, 1996.
9. Kurts, C., Heath, W.R., Carbone, F.R., Allison, J., Miller, J.F.A.P., and Kosaka, H., *J. Exp. Med.* 184: 923–930, 1996.
10. Kurts, C., Kosaka, H., Carbone, F.R., Miller, J.F.A.P., and Heath, W.R., *J. Exp. Med.* 186: 239–245, 1997.
11. Bennett, S.R.M., Carbone, F.R., Karamalis, F., Miller, J.F.A.P., and Heath, W.R., *J. Exp. Med.* 186: 65–70, 1997.
12. Guerder, S., and Matzinger, P., *J. Exp. Med.* 176: 553–564, 1992.
13. Rees, M., Rosenberg, A.S., Munitz, T.I., and Singer, A., *Proc. Natl. Acad. Sci. USA.* 87: 2765–2769, 1990.
14. Kurts, C., Carbone, F.R., Barnden, M., Blanas, E., Allison, J., Heath, W.R., and Miller, J.F.A.P., *J. Exp. Med.* 186: 2057–2062; 1997.
15. Keene, J., and Forman, J., *J. Exp. Med.* 155: 768–782, 1982.
16. Mitchison, N.A., and O'Malley, C., *Eur. J. Immunol.* 17: 1579–1583, 1987.
17. Cassel, D., and Forman, J., *Ann. N.Y. Acad. Sci.* 532: 51–60, 1988.
18. Grewal, I.S., and Flavell, R.A., *Immunol. Today* 17: 410–414, 1996.
19. Kawabe, T., Naka, T., Yoshida, K., Tanaka, T., Fujiwara, H., Suematsu, S., Yoshida, N., Kishimoto, T., and Kikutani, H., *Immunity* 1: 167–178, 1994.
20. Renshaw, B.R., Fanslow, W.C., Armitage, R.J., Campbell, K.A., Liggitt, D., Wright, B., Davison, B.L., and Maliszewski, C.R., *J. Exp. Med.* 180: 1889–1900, 1994.
21. Kamanaka, M., Yu, P., Yasui, T., Yoshida, K., Kawabe, T., Horii, T., Kishimoto, T., and Kikutani, H., *Immunity* 4: 275–281, 1996.
22. Yang, Y., and Wilson, J.M., *Science* 273: 1862–1864, 1996.
23. Mackey, M.F., Gunn, J.R., Ting, P.P., Kikutani, H., Dranoff, G., Noelle, R.J., and Barth Jr., R.J., *Cancer Res.* 57: 2569–2574, 1997.
24. Kiener, P.A., Moran, D.P., Rankin, B.M., Wahl, A.F., Aruffo, A., and Hollenbaugh, D., *J. Immunol.* 155: 4917–4925, 1995.
25. Koch, F., Stanzl, U., Jennewein, P., Janke, K., Heufler, C., Kampgen, E., Romani, N., and Schuler, G., *J. Exp. Med.* 184: 741–746, 1996.
26. Cella, M., Scheidegger, D., Palmer-Lehmann, K., Lane, P., Lanzavecchia, A., and Alber, G., *J. Exp. Med.* 184: 747–752, 1996.
27. Shinde, S.E.A., *J. Immunol.* 157: 2764–2768, 1996.
28. Schoenberger, S.P., Toes, R.E.M., van der Voort, E.I.H., Offringa, R., and Melief, C.J.M., *Nature* 393: 480–483, 1998.
29. Toes, R.E.M., Offringa, R., Blom, H.J.J., Brandt, R.M.P., Van der Eb, A.J., Melief, C.J.M., and Kast, W.M., *J. Immunol.* 154: 3396–3405, 1995.
30. Rolink, A., Melchers, F., and Andersson, J., *Immunity* 5: 319–330, 1996.

31. Grusby, M.J., Johnson, R.S., Papaioannou, V.E., and Glimcher, L.H., *Science* 253: 1417–1420, 1991.
32. Noelle, R.J., Roy, M., Shepherd, D.M., Stamenkovic, I., Ledbetter, J.A., and Aruffo, A., *Proc. Natl. Acad. Sci. USA.* 89: 6550, 1992.
33. Bennet, S.R.M., Carbone, F.R., Karamalis, F., Flavell, R.A., Miller, J.F.A.P., and Heath, W.R., *Nature* 393: 478–480, 1998.
34. Ridge, J.P., Di Rosa, F., and Matzinger, P., *Nature* 393: 474–478, 1998.
35. Kast, W.M., Roux, L., Curren, J., Blom, H.J.J., Voordouw, A.C., Meloen, R.H., Kolakofski, D., and Melief, C.J.M., *Proc. Natl. Acad. Sci. U.S.A.* 88: 2283–2287, 1991.
36. Aichele, P., Hengartner, H.P., Zinkernagel, R.M., and Schulz, M., *J. Exp. Med.* 171: 1815–1820, 1990.
37. Feltkamp, M.C.W., Smits, H.L., Vierboom, M.P.M., Minnaar, R.P., De Jongh, B.M., Drijfhout, J.W., Ter Schegget, J., Melief, C.J.M., and Kast, W.M., *Eur. J. Immunol.* 23: 2242–2249, 1993.
38. Aichele, P., Kyburz, D., Ohashi, P.S., Odermatt, B., Zinkernagel, R.M., Hengartner, H., and Pircher, H., *Proc. Natl. Acad. Sci. USA.* 91: 444–448, 1994.
39. Toes, R.E.M., Offringa, R., Blom, R.J.J., Melief, C.J.M., and Kast, W.M., *Proc. Natl. Acad. Sci. USA.* 93: 7855–7860, 1996.
40. Toes, R.E.M., Blom, R.J.J., Offringa, R., Kast, W.M., and Melief, C.J.M., *J. Immunol.* 156: 3911–3918, 1996.
41. Toes, R.E.M., van der Voort, E.I.H., Schoenberger, S.P., Drijfhout, J.W., van Blois, L., Storm, G., Kast, W.M., Offringa, R., and Melief, C.J.M., *J. Immunol.* 160: 4449–4456, 1998.
42. Diehl, L., den Boer, A.T., Schoenberger, S.P., van der Voort, E.I.H., Schumacher, T.N.M., Melief, C.J.M., Offringa, R., and Toes, R.E.M., *Nature Med.* 5: 774–779, 1999.
43. Sotomayor, E.M., Borrello, I., Tubb, E., Rattis, F., Bien, H., Lu, Z., Fein, S., Schoenberger, S., and Levitsky, H., *Nature Med.* 5: 780–787, 1999.

René E. M. Toes et al.

MICHAEL WELLER, WOLFGANG WICK, JOACHIM P.
STEINBACH, BETTINA WAGENKNECHT, ULRIKE NAUMANN
AND WILFRIED ROTH

The role of apoptosis in cancerogenesis and resistance to therapy: Lessons from malignant glioma

———

Abstract

The concepts of apoptosis and programmed, physiological or active cell death have had a great impact on our understanding of cancerogenesis and of tumor cell resistance to cytotoxic therapies. First, the p53 tumor suppressor gene, which is a mutational target in a large proportion of human cancers, is also a potent mediator of apoptosis in response to genotoxic stress. A number of different p53-responsive genes are involved in modulating apoptotic responses. Despite the plethora of experimental and clinical studies on the role of p53 in cancerogenesis and response to therapy, many questions regarding p53 have remained unanswered. Second, genetic analyses of the nematode, *C. elegans*, have been instrumental in characterizing two principal families of genes, the Bcl-2 and caspase families, which are critical in the control and in the execution of apoptotic cell death. Imbalances in the biological activity of these genes contribute to tumor formation, malignant progression, and resistance to therapy. Third, specific induction of apoptosis by death ligands (tumor necrosis factor-alpha, TNF-α; CD95 ligand, CD95L; Apo2 ligand/tumor necrosis factor-related apoptosis-inducing ligand, Apo2L/TRAIL) acting on their corresponding death receptors emerges as a novel therapeutic approach to cancers which resist current strategies of surgery and adjuvant radiochemotherapy. In contrast, death ligand/receptor interactions are probably not the critical mediators of radiotherapy- or cancer chemotherapy-induced cell death in most types of human cancer.

Keywords: Apoptosis, glioma, Bcl-2, CD95, p53

Laboratory of Molecular Neuro-Oncology, Department of Neurology,
University of Tübingen, Tübingen, Germany

131

Apoptosis, programmed and physiological cell death, and active cell death: an introduction

It has long been known that the development of mammals involves the loss of numerous cells in various organs at predetermined phases of ontogenesis. This type of cell death, which plays a major role, e.g., in shaping the immune and central nervous systems, is a physiological process and may therefore be aptly termed *developmental* or *programmed cell death*. This concept of programmed cell death has been developed in contradistinction to various other instances of cell death which are unscheduled and which are caused, e.g., by mechanical trauma, inflammation, or ischemia.

Many types of programmed cell death are characterized by typical morphological changes collectively referred to as apoptosis [1]. These include condensation and fragmentation of chromatin and nuclear remnants as well as cytoplasmic compartmentalization, resulting in membrane blebbing and the formation of apoptotic bodies. The latter are efficiently cleared from the tissue by nonprofessional phagocytes which recognize signals on display on the surface of apoptotic cells and cell fragments. This may account for the lack of inflammatory responses and of macrophage activation in response to cell death during ontogeny. Apoptotic cell death tends to eliminate solitary cells within a given target tissue. In contrast, tissue loss by necrosis, a process aptly considered an *accidental* cell death, mostly affects continuous parts of a tissue.

The latter type of death features disturbances of energy metabolism, cell swelling, osmotic lysis, degeneration of organelles, activation of catabolic enzymes such as proteases and endonucleases, and the release of proinflammatory mediators.

Most, but not all, types of apoptotic cell death share the biochemical features of caspase activation and DNA fragmentation. The caspases are a growing family of proteases which degrade specific proteins during the apoptotic process and which are considered the execution machinery of apoptosis. The DNA lesions may be restricted to the formation of large DNA fragments of up to 300 kilobase pairs. The classical nucleosomal size, ladder-like pattern of DNA fragmentation that is almost always observed in lymphoid cells undergoing apoptosis may be lacking in apoptosis of nonlymphoid cells. The typical ladder pattern of apoptotic cell death derives from the preferential cleavage of DNA in nucleosomal linker regions which results in the release of 180 base pair fragments and multiples thereof.

Programmed cell death is often considered in a somewhat anthropomorphous way as a suicidal cell death since there is evidence for an active participation of the dying cell during most instances of programmed cell death, e.g., the morphological process of apoptosis is energy-consuming. Further, inhibition of RNA and protein synthesis prevents cell death in many paradigms of apoptosis, notably in nontransformed cells, e.g., neurons. This suggests that cells induced to undergo apoptosis may synthesize mRNA encoded by *killer genes* which is translated into *killer proteins* which execute cellular suicide from within. However, it is important to note that inhibitors of RNA and protein synthesis are themselves potent inducers of death in many tumor cell types, presumably because such drugs interfere with the synthesis of proteins essential for survival.

The present article will highlight recent advances in the fields of apoptosis, cancerogenesis and cancer therapy with special emphasis on malignant glial brain tumors.

p53, apoptosis, cancer, and chemotherapy

Loss of wild-type p53 function is the most common molecular event in the pathogenesis of cancer that has been identified so far. p53 is a stress-responsive regulator of gene transcription that controls cellular responses to DNA damage in particular. The most important genes induced by p53 include the cyclin-dependent kinase (CDK) inhibitor, p21$^{WAF/Cip1}$, which mediates growth arrest, and members of the Bcl-2 gene family, notably the proapoptotic bax gene. Loss of p53 promotes the accumulation of genetic changes which provide a cell with altered properties regarding, e.g., responses to external stimuli, growth control, migration, and adhesion. p53 alterations have also been suggested to account for the failure of most cancers to respond to radiotherapy and chemotherapy (for review, see [2]). However, despite the plethora of studies on p53 in various human cancers, no clear-cut picture on the prognostic value of assessing p53 status in human cancers has emerged. In fact, several lines of evidence indicate that loss of p53 enhances rather than decreases vulnerability to apoptosis in untransformed cells. Further, naturally occurring or targeted alterations of the p53 status in human cancer cells often result in unpredictable biological effects which commonly include gain-of-function type effects and which are unlikely to be applicable for cancer therapy. We have carried out a series of such experiments in human glioma cells [3,4] but our literature review on p53 and response to cancer chemotherapy indicates that systematic studies in other types of cancer would also arrive at these conclusions [2]. Of note, even in the simplified paradigm of a panel of long-term glioma cell lines, each of which has a stable genotype, no correlation between sensitivity to cytotoxic therapy and genetic or functional p53 status or expression of p53 response genes became apparent [2].

Control of apoptosis by Bcl-2 and caspase family proteins

The analysis of developmental cell death in the nematode, *C. elegans*, has led to the detection and extensive study of two major protein familes which exert opposite functions in the regulation of apoptotic cell death (Fig. 1). The homologs of the antiapoptotic *C. elegans* gene, ced-9, constitute the Bcl-2 protein family which consists of multiple antiapoptotic and proapoptotic family members [5]. The homologs of the ced-3 gene form the growing caspase family which consists of at least 14 different enzymes [6]. Antiapoptotic Bcl-2

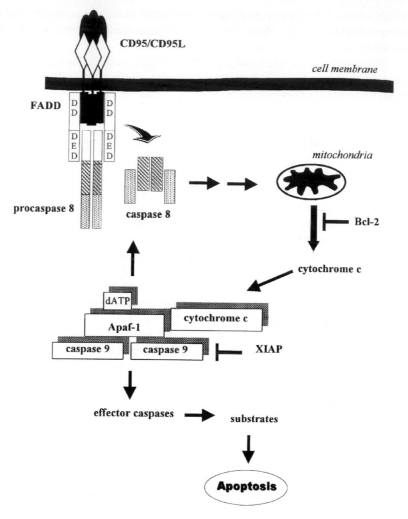

FIGURE 1. *Current model of the death ligand/receptor-dependent apoptotic pathway and its modulation by antiapoptotic proteins of the Bcl-2 and XIAP protein families (for details, see text).*

family proteins appear to act by multiple mechanisms although a principal action seems to maintain mitochondrial integrity and prevention of cytochrome c release from mitochondria [7]. The caspases are proteases which cleave multiple protein substrates in a site-specific manner and which are the principal executioners of apoptosis. Interestingly, a novel family of antiapoptotic proteins, the inhibitor-of-apoptosis protein (IAP) family has recently been characterized as a class of proteins that specifically bind and inactivate caspases [8]. These IAP proteins are highly expressed in human glioma cell lines [9].

Various members of the Bcl-2 protein family are known to be expressed in malignant gliomas. Some studies reported increased expression of

Michael Weller et al.

antiapoptotic Bcl-2 family proteins or reduced expression of proapoptotic proteins such as Bax in gliomas with higher grades of malignancy [10,11] whereas other authors failed to note such a correlation [12–15]. More recently, several studies have addressed the possible prognostic significance of Bcl-2 family protein expression in human gliomas. No clear-cut pattern for a predictive role of Bcl-2 for patient outcome has been delineated so far [16,17]. We observed that high expression of the MCL-1 protein was associated with shortened progression-free survival in glioma patients receiving adjuvant radiochemotherapy [17]. Further, a comparison of first versus recurrent resections showed a changing pattern of Bcl-2 family protein expression toward a more apoptosis-resistant phenotype [18]. Detailed studies on changes in the patterns of caspase expression or expression of IAP in glial tumors of different malignancy grades have not been performed to date.

Therapeutic induction of apoptosis by death ligands

The characterization of the apoptosis-inducing antibodies CH-11 and APO-1 in 1989 and the independent identification of a common target antigen for these antibodies, the cytokine receptor CD95 (Fas/APO-1), by S. Nagata and P. Krammer led to the development of a key field of apoptosis research, the study of death receptors and death ligands [19]. It is now apparent that there is a growing family of death ligands such as TNF-α, CD95L and Apo2L/TRAIL which interact with one or more receptors [20]. The presence of both agonistic, that is, death signal-tranducing, and antagonistic, that is, death-inhibitory, receptors, e.g., for Apo2L/TRAIL, has added significantly to the complexity of the death ligand/receptor system.

The expression of death receptors in human gliomas has not been studied in detail. Adequate analyses have only been performed for CD95 [21–23]. These studies showed that the expression of CD95 mRNA increases with grade of malignancy and that CD95 protein is preferentially expressed in perinecrotic areas of human glioblastomas. An attractive hypothesis predicts that hypoxia will eliminate p53 wild-type-retaining cells and thus promote the emergence of p53 mutant clones upon malignant progression. Although controversial data regarding the control of CD95 expression by p53 have been published [24,25], we have observed that the wild-type p53-dependent increase in CD95 expression in glioma cells does not result in enhanced susceptibility to CD95-mediated apoptosis [25], questioning the relevance of p53-mediated changes of CD95 expression in glioma progression.

Surprisingly, several studies have confirmed that glioma cells co-express CD95 and CD95L, yet do not undergo suicidal or fratricidal CD95-mediated cell death [26–29]. Further, CD95L expressed on some glioma cell lines is biologically active and kills target T cells, and the same glioma cells are susceptible to cell death induced by exogenous CD95L (see below). These diverging observations have not been incorporated into a unifying hypothesis as to the regulation of CD95/CD95L function in glioma cells. Moreover, similar data on complex patterns of CD95 and CD95L expression and function have recently been reported for various nonglial cell lines, suggesting that these issues will receive increasing attention in the coming years of apoptosis research.

The majority of human glioma cell lines are sensitive to apoptosis induced by agonistic CD95 antibodies [23] or soluble CD95L [30] or viral vectors encoding CD95L [31]. CD95-mediated apoptosis is greatly facilitated when RNA or protein synthesis are inhibited, suggesting that glioma cells express cytoprotective proteins, which block the killing pathway, constitutively or in response to CD95 triggering [23]. Interestingly, human fetal astrocytes may be more resistant to CD95L than neoplastic astrocytes [32], suggesting a link between transformation and sensitivity to CD95-mediated apoptosis.

In vivo, the therapeutic application of TNF-α has not gained a relevant role in clinical oncology, both because of systemic side effects (shock, cachexia) and because of low antitumor activity at tolerable doses. The CD95L has been considered too toxic since the systemic activation of the CD95 system results in fulminant liver failure within few hours [33]. The local application of adeno-viral vectors expressing CD95L may be a strategy to circumvent systemic side effects in the case of gliomas [34]. Transferring a therapeutic gene encoding a cytoplasmic component of the CD95-dependent killing cascade, *Fas-associated protein with death domain* (FADD), into glioma cells was also effective in controlling tumor cell growth *in vitro* and *in vivo* [35]. Finally, even more down-stream effectors of death receptor-mediated apoptosis, the caspases, have been successfully employed to promote glioma cell death *in vitro* and *in vivo* [36,37]. Clearly, targeting potent intracellular mediators of apoptosis is only feasible clinically if major problems of therapeutic gene delivery will be solved, involving both efficacy and specificity. For instance, caspase 3 gene transfer will only kill cancer cells that are transduced, and caspase 3 is also a potent inducer of apoptosis in neurons, suggesting that neurotoxicity might become a problem *in vivo*. Therefore, activating signalling pathways that are selectively available in tumor cells is still most attractive. At present, we believe that inducing cancer cell apoptosis via local or systemic application of Apo2L/TRAIL is probably one of the most attractive strategies of cancer therapy that is based on recent insights into the molecular regulation of apoptotic cell death [38,39].

Endogenous death ligand/receptor interactions and radiochemotherapy for cancer

An attractive hypothesis has recently proposed that cytotoxic cancer therapy, including chemotherapy and radiotherapy, may rely on the endogenous triggering of apoptosis *via* death ligands and death receptors. In fact, both chemotherapy and radiotherapy have been shown to enhance, e.g., CD95 and CD95L expression at the cell surface of cancer cells of various histogenetic origins. Yet, the precise role of CD95 and CD95L in cancer chemotherapy is currently a field of much controversy. In the case of malignant glioma, a causal role for death receptor/ligand interactions in mediating cell death induced by radiochemotherapy was excluded [40]. Further studies will have to clarify the role of death receptors in the response to cancer therapy in other cancer cell types. On the other hand, caspase activation, proceeding in a death receptor-independent manner, plays a role in drug-induced apoptosis of cancer cells, including glioma cells [36,40], although the specific caspases essential for drug-induced apoptosis remain to be identified.

Conclusions

Research into the basic biochemical mechanisms of programmed cell death and apoptosis has influenced current concepts of cancerogenesis and experimental cancer therapy more than any other field of research in the recent decade. The present summary focused on the field of malignant glial brain tumors. Similar investigations have been performed in most other types of cancer as well, yielding mostly similar findings, but also some tumor type-specific pathways of how susceptibility to apoptotic cell death is regulated. Overcoming Bcl-2-mediated cytoprotection, facilitating caspase activation in response to cytotoxic cancer therapy, and exploiting the great therapeutic potential of death ligands, notably Apo2 ligand, will be the key issues of apoptosis research in oncology for the coming decade.

References

1. Kerr, J.F.R., Wyllie, A.H., and Currie, A.R., *Br. J. Cancer* 26: 239–257, 1972.
2. Weller, M., *Cell Tissue Res.* 292: 435–445, 1998.
3. Bartussek, C., Naumann, U., and Weller, M., *Exp. Cell Res.* 253: 432–439, 1999.
4. Trepel, M., Groscurth P., Malipiero, U., Gulbins, E., Dichgans, J., and Weller, M., *J. Neuro-Oncol.* 39: 19–32, 1998.
5. Strasser, A., Huang, D.C.S., and Vaux, D.L., *Biochim. Biophys. Acta* 1333: F151–F178, 1997.
6. Villa, P., Kaufmann, S.H., and Earnshaw, W.C., *Trends Biochem. Sci.* 22: 388–393, 1997.
7. Green, D.R., and Reed, J.C., *Science* 281: 11309–11316, 1998.
8. LaCasse, E.C., Baird, S., Korneluk, R.G., and MacKenzie, A.E., *Oncogene* 17: 3247–3259, 1998.
9. Wagenknecht, B., Glaser, T., Naumann, U., Kügler, S., Isenmann, S., Bähr, M., Korneluk, R., Liston, P., and Weller, M., *Cell Death Differ.* 6: 370–376, 1999.
10. Hara, A., Hirose, Y., Yoshimi, N., Tanaka, T., and Mori, H., *Neurol. Res.* 19: 623–628, 1997.
11. Weller, M., Malipiero, U.V., Aguzzi, A., Reed, J.C., and Fontana, A., *J. Clin. Invest.* 95: 2633–2643, 1995.
12. Ellison, D.W., Steart, P.V., Gatter, K.C., and Weller, R.O., *Neuropathol. Appl. Neurobiol.* 21: 352–361, 1995.
13. Krajewski, S., Krajewska, M., Ehrmann, J., Sikorska, M., Lach, B., Chatten, J., and Reed, J.C., *Am. J. Pathol.* 150: 805–814, 1997.

14. Krishna, M., Smith, T.W., and Recht, L.D., *J. Neurosurg.* 83: 1017–1022, 1995.
15. Nakasu, S., Nakasa, Y., Nioka, H., Nakajima, M., and Handa, J., *Acta Neuropathol.* 88: 520–526, 1994.
16. Newcomb, E.W., Bhalla. S.K., Parrish, C.L., Hayes, R.L., Cohen, H., and Miller, D.C., *Acta Neuropathol.* 94: 369–375, 1997.
17. Rieger, L., Weller, M., Bornemann, A., Schabet, M., Dichgans, J., and Meyermann, R., *J. Neurol. Sci.* 155: 68–75, 1998.
18. Strik, H., Deininger, M., Streffer, J., Grote, E., Wickboldt, J., Dichgans, J., Weller, M., and Meyermann, R., *J. Neurol. Neurosur. Ps.* 67: 763–768, 1999.
19. Peter, M.E., and Krammer, P.H., *Curr. Opin. Immunol.* 10: 545–551, 1998.
20. Ashkenazi, A., and Dixit, V.M., *Science* 281: 1305–1309, 1998.
21. Tachibana, O., Nakazawa, H., Lampe, J., Watanabe, K., Kleihues, P., and Ohgaki, H., *Cancer Res.* 55: 5528–5530, 1995.
22. Tachibana, O., Lampe, J., Kleihues, P., and Ohgaki, H., *Acta Neuropathol.* 92: 431–434, 1996.
23. Weller, M., Frei, K., Groscurth, P., Krammer, P.H., Yonekawa, Y., and Fontana, A., *J. Clin. Invest.* 94: 954–964, 1994.
24. Pohl, U., Wagenknecht, B., Naumann, U., and Weller, M., *Cell Physiol. Biochem.* 9: 29–37, 1999.
25. Tohma, Y., Gratas C., Van Meir, E.G., Desbaillets, I., Tenan, M., Tachibana, O., Kleihues, P., and Ohgaki, H., *J. Neuropathol. Exp. Neurol.* 57: 239–245, 1998.
26. Gratas, C., Tohma, Y., Van Meir, E.G., Klein, M., Tenan, M., Ishii, N., Tachibana, O., Kleihues, P., and Ohgaki, H., *Brain Pathol.* 7: 863–869, 1997.
27. Husain, N., Chiocca, E.A., Rainov, N., Louis, D.N., and Zervas, N.T., *Acta Neuropathol.* 95: 287–290, 1998.
28. Saas, P., Walker, P.R., Hahne, M., Quiquerez, A.L., Schnuriger, V., and Perrin, G., *J. Clin. Invest.* 99: 1173–1178, 1997.
29. Weller, M., Weinstock, C., Will, C., Wagenknecht, B., Dichgans, J., Lang, F., and Gulbins, E., *Cell. Physiol. Biochem.* 7: 282–288, 1997.
30. Roth, W., Fontana, A., Trepel, M., Dichgans, J., Reed, J.C., and Weller, M., *Cancer Immunol. Immunother.* 44: 55–63, 1997.
31. Shinoura, N., Yoshida, Y., Sadata, A., Hanada, K.I., Yamamoto, S., Kirino, T., Asai, A., and Hamada, H., *Human Gene Ther.* 9: 1983–1989, 1998.
32. Becher, B., D'Souza, D., Troutt, A.B., and Antel, J.P., *Neuroscience* 84: 627–634, 1998.
33. Ogasawara, J., Watanabe-Fukunaga, R., Adachi M., Matsuzawa, A., Kasugai, T., Kitamura,Y., Itoh, N., Suda, T., and Nagata, S., *Nature* 364: 806–809, 1993.
34. Ambar, B.B., Frei, K., Malipiero, U., Morelli, A.E., Castro, M.G., Lowenstein, P.R., and Fontana A., *Human Gene Ther.* 10: 1641–1648, 1999.
35. Kondo, S., Ishizaka, Y., Okada, T., Kondo, Y., Hitomi, M., Tanaka, Y., Haqqi, T., Barnett, G.H., and Barna, B.P., *Human Gene Ther.* 9: 1599–1608, 1998.
36. Kondo, S., Barna, B.P., Morimura, T., Takeuchi, J., Yuan, J., Akbasak, A., and Barnett, G.H., *Cancer Res.* 55: 6166–6171, 1996.
37. Yu, J.S., Sena-Esteves, M., Paulus W., Breakefield, X.O., and Reeves, S.A., *Cancer Res.* 56: 5423–5427, 1998.
38. Ashkenazi, A., Pai, R.C., Fong, S., Leung, S., Lawrence, D.A., Marsters, S.A., Blackie, Chang, L., McMurtrey, A.E., Hebert, A., DeForge, L., Koumenis, I.L., Lewis, D., Harris, L., Bussiere, J., Koeppen, H., Shahrokh, Z., and Schwall, R.H., *J. Clin. Invest.* 104: 155–162, 1999.

39. Roth, W., Isenmann, S., Naumann, U., Kügler, S., Bähr, M., Dichgans, J., Ashkenazi, A., and Weller, M., *Biochem. Biophys. Res. Commun.* 265: 479–483, 1999.
40. Glaser, T., Wagenknecht, B., Groscurth, P., Krammer, P.H., and Weller, M., *Oncogene* 18: 5044–5053, 1999.
41. Weller, M., Rieger, J., Grimmel, C., Van Meir, E.G., De Tribolet, N., Krajewski, S., Reed, J.C., Von Deimling, A., and Dichgans, J., *Int. J. Cancer* 79: 640–644, 1998.

JÜRGEN C. BECKER, PATRICK TERHEYDEN AND
EVA-B. BRÖCKER

Treatment of disseminated uveal melanoma: A continuing dilemma?

Abstract

At the time of initial diagnosis of uveal melanoma, most patients have no evidence of metastatic disease. Within 10 years, however, metastases appear in at least 30% of patients. Unlike cutaneous melanoma, uveal melanoma is remarkable for its tendency to metastasize to the liver, which is involved in up to 95% of patients even though 50% of the patients also suffer from extrahepatic metastases. Treatment options for metastatic uveal melanoma include surgery, chemoembolization, intra-arterial chemotherapy, and systemic chemoimmunotherapy. Recently, treatment strategies shifted from an emphasis on palliative therapy given on an individual basis to controlled clinical trials. Although initial results from these studies provide encouraging evidence that the course of the disease can be influenced, it is also evident that new drug combinations are required to improve efficacy and feasibility of therapeutic approaches.

Keywords: Metastatic uveal melanoma, screening protocol, surgery, regional therapy, systemic therapy

Introduction

Although primary melanoma either originating from the skin or the uveal tract can almost always be controlled locally, management of distant metastases from melanoma in general and from uveal melanoma in particular remains extremely disappointing [1,2]. Thus, it is not surprising that although the diagnosis and treatment of primary uveal melanoma has been well covered by the ophthalmalogic literature, the therapy of disseminated uveal melanoma has received less attention. However, it should be kept in mind that, regardless of the method of management, at least 30% of affected patients will develop metastatic disease within 10 years of successful local control of the

Department of Dermatology, University of Würzburg,
Josef-Schneider-Str. 2, D-97080 Würzburg, Germany

primary tumor [3]. Factors reported to influence the prognosis include tumor size and location, scleral invasion, cell type, number of mitoses, expression of MHC class I molecules, or the presence of anti-ganglioside antibodies in the serum [4–8].

Uveal melanoma is remarkable for purely hematogenous dissemination and its tendency to metastasize to the liver. The latter is involved in up to 95% of patients even though 50% of the patients also suffer from extrahepatic metastases, most often the lungs, bone, skin and the brain [9]. Despite this knowledge it is still unclear what constitutes an adequate screening program for early detection of metastasis. The lack of information on the clinical and laboratory findings of patients with metastatic disease are reflected in the differences in current screening programs. In a recent report, based on the experience of more than 10 years in which 390 patients with uveal melanoma were followed and 62 of these subsequently developed metastasis, it was concluded that semiannual screening with liver function tests and abdominal ultrasound will detect more than 95% of patients with disseminated melanoma in an asymptomatic state [10]. Detection of such patients is of particular importance since treatment strategies shifted from an emphasis on palliative chemotherapy given on an individual basis to controlled clinical trials. This shift is mandatory for the development of an effective treatment for metastatic uveal melanoma. This paper reviews some of the studies that evaluated different treatment options including regional and systemic chemo/chemoimmunotherapy.

Regional therapy

The recognition that most patients with disseminated uveal melanoma have liver involvement and, notably, that in more than half of these patients the liver is the sole site of disease, has led to the evaluation of regional therapies such as hepatic intra-arterial chemotherapy or chemoembolization. In a retrospective study Bedikian et al. reviewed the M.D. Anderson Cancer Center experience on several treatment modalities [11]. From their data it became evident that chemoembolization with cisplatin was the most effective treatment inducing objective responses in up to 36% of patients. The overall survival, however, was not influenced by any of the applied therapies including the latter. These results should be interpreted in the context that this was a retrospective study with a heterogeneous patient population ranging from asymptomatic, chemo-naive to symptomatic, heavily pretreated patients. In this respect, two recently published prospective studies in defined patient populations demonstrated a more favorable response to regional therapy [12,13].

The first study was based on anecdotal results demonstrating a prolonged survival after surgical resection and hepatic intra-arterial chemotherapy for liver metastases from uveal melanoma [12]. Over a period of 5 years 75 patients were treated by surgical removal of as much liver disease as possible, implantation of an intra-arterial catheter which was used for inter-arterial

Jürgen C. Becker, Patrick Terheyden and Eva-B. Bröcker

chemotherapy with either fotemustine or DTIC/cisplatin. Macroscopically curative surgery was possible in one fourth of the patients, with an additional two fourth of patients receiving a significant tumor reduction. Sixty-one patients received the complete course of intra-arterial chemotherapy. The median overall survival of these patients was 10 months, which was only a slight improvement to that of historical controls. However, when curative resection was possible, survival increased to 22 months [12].

The objective of the second study was to establish the efficacy and toxicity of hepatic intra-arterial fotemustine in asymptomatic patients with liver metastases as sole disease manifestation [13]. Fotemustine is a third-generation nitrosourea which contains an aminophosphoic acid group that facilitates the passage across membranes. It has a high plasma clearance which approximates the hepatic blood flow and the first-pass liver extraction ratio ranges between 0.4 and 0.9. These characteristics make fotemustine an ideal drug for hepatic intra-arterial chemotherapy. The concentration in the liver can be expected to be 7.9 to 47 times higher than in other tissues if administered via this route. Thirty-one patients were enrolled into this study, of 30 assessable patients four achieved a complete and eight a partial response, for an overall response rate of 40% [13]. The median overall survival of this patient cohort was 14 months. Furthermore, the response to treatment selected for a better survival, with a median of 20 months as compared with 11 months for non-responders. These promising results, however, should be seen in the context of a well-defined and selected patient population. Metastatic disease of most of the patients were discovered in the course of semiannual abdominal ultra-sound screening; thus, all patients were asymptomatic with a good perform-ance status. As stated by Eskelin *et al.* it is important to realize that, even in the absence of any therapy, the apparent survival of patients who are screened with liver imaging will be a few months longer than that of patients who are screened only by liver function tests or not at all [10]. Notably, in this study pathological liver function tests, i.e., serum LDH or alkaline phosphatase, were associated with a reduced survival time even in responding patients [13]. These comments are not intended to dwarf the findings reported by Leyvraz *et al.* but to stress the importance of standardized screening pro-grams for patients with uveal melanoma.

Our own experience with 20 patients receiving hepatic intra-arterial chemotherapy with fotemustine in combination with immunotherapy as part of a multi-institutional trial which was initiated to substantiate the sporadic observation that patients with disseminated uveal melanoma benefited from such a combination even if the fotemustine was administered intravenously, did not result in an objective response rate as favourable as reported by Leyvraz (unpublished results). To date only two objective responses among 13 assessable patients were observed. However, these patients were not selected and the majority were suffering from symptomatic liver involvement. Nevertheless, for six additional patients the disease progression could be stabilized and the median survival of the cohort was 9 months with four of the patients being still alive. The eligible criteria for this study did not exclude extra-hepatic disease, but patients were stratified according to the metastatic sites to either receive fotemustine intra-arterial or intravenously. Hence, an additional 26 patients received fotemustine systemically and 18 of these were assessable until September 1999; four patients of this cohort achieved an objective response. The results of this group will be discussed in more detail in the following paragraph.

Systemic therapy

Until recently systemic chemotherapy for disseminated uveal melanoma has been regarded as largely unsuccessful with response rates of less than 1% [1–4]. This was likely due to the fact that treatment strategies have relied on the experience with cutaneous melanoma based on the premise that because both cutaneous and uveal melanoma are derived from melanocytes, they may respond similarly, despite the many genetic and phenotypic differences between them. While occasional responses have been reported, there are only few trial-based data on systemic therapy for uveal melanoma from which response rates can be obtained.

Recently it has been reported that chemoimmunotherapy with a four-drug chemotherapy regimen and interferon α is able to induce considerable objective responses and may contribute to prolonged survival [14]. Specifically, bleomycin, vincristine, lomustine and DTIC (BOLD) were administered every 28 days together with low dose intercycle interferon α. Twenty-three patients were enrolled into this study and among 20 evaluable patients, four objective responses were observed. However, the anti-tumor activity of this treatment was associated with severe toxicity. While hematologic and neurologic side effects were manageable, an unexpected and severe pulmonary toxicity was observed in three patients. The latter is likely to be due to an acquired hypersensitivity reaction or a cumulative toxic effect of two or more of the agents; the pattern of occurrence and clinical course of these pulmonary events were similar to those induced by the combination of fotemustine and DTIC [15]. The feasibility of this regimen was recently tested in a multi-center trial (EORTC 88941); unfortunately this trial was prematurely stopped due to the pulmonary toxicity.

By making the usual mistake to enroll patients with disseminated uveal melanoma into a protocol designed for metastatic cutaneous melanoma we observed a rather favorable outcome for these patients [16]. The therapy regimen consisted of intravenously applied fotemustine together with intermediate dose interleukin 2 and interferon α. As a matter of fact, this therapy induced a partial response of more than 49 months duration in one out of three patients, whereas for the remaining patients the disease progression could be stabilized for eight and 16 months, respectively. This therapeutic success was reflected by a prolonged survival, i.e., 14, 46 and 63 months. Thus, we felt encouraged to initiate a multi-center trial to determine the activity and feasibility of this regimen. To date, 26 patients were enrolled and 18 of these were assessable for response; four patients of this cohort achieved an objective response, while for three patients the disease progression could be stabilized. The duration of the objective responses are 4, 4+, 11, 12+ months (unpublished results). As mentioned above, within this trial the administration route of fotemustine was stratified according to the presence or absence of extra-hepatic metastasis; hence, the final analysis may provide information on the differential activity of this drug combination with respect to the administration route even if the trial design was not prospectively randomized to answer this question and differential prognostic parameters may be present in the two cohorts.

Perspectives

Therapeutic trials are mandatory for the development of an effective treatment for metastatic uveal melanoma. Since chances for therapy are generally highest when the metastatic burden is small, patients should be enrolled in screening programs after diagnosis and therapy of the primary tumor. These screening programs should include liver function tests and liver imaging on a semiannual basis [10]. The availability of ATP-based tumor chemosensitivity assays may allow to predict new drug combinations suitable for therapy of this tumor [17]; recent reports on the *in vitro* activity of the combination of treosulfan with gemcitabine already stimulated several phase II trials to test this combination *in vivo*.

References

1. Pyrhonen, S., *Eur. J. Cancer* 34 (Suppl. 3) S27–S30, 1998.
2. Kath, R., Hayungs, J., Bornfeld, N., Sauerwein, W., Hoffken, K., and Seeber, S., *Cancer* 72: 2219–2223, 1993.
3. Sato, T., Babazono, A., Shields, J.A., Shields, C.L., De Potter, P., and Mastrangelo, M.J., *Cancer Invest.* 15: 98–105, 1997.
4. Mooy, C.M., de J.P., *Surv. Ophthalmol.* 41: 215–228, 1996.
5. Luyten, G.P., Mooy, C.M., Post, J., Jensen, O.A., Luider, T.M., and de J.P., *Cancer* 78: 1967–1971, 1996.
6. Niederkorn, J.Y., Mellon, J., Pidherney, M., Mayhew, E., and Anand, R., *Curr. Eye Res.* 12: 347–358, 1993.
7. White, V.A., Chambers, J.D., Courtright, P.D., Chang, W.Y., and Horsman, D.E., *Cancer* 83: 354–359, 1998.
8. Blom, D.J., Mooy, C.M., Luyten, G.P., Kerkvliet, S,, Onwerkerk, I., Zwinderman, A H., Schrier, P.I., and Jager, M.J., *J. Pathol.* 181: 75–79, 1997.
9. Gragoudas, E.S., Egan, K.M., Seddon, J.M., Glynn, R.J., Walsh, S.M., Finn, S.M., Munzenrider, J.E., and Spar, M.D., *Ophthalmology* 98: 383–389, 1991.
10. Eskelin, S., Pyrhonen, S., Summanen, P., Prause, J.U., and Kivela, T., *Cancer* 85: 1151–1159, 1999.
11. Bedikian, A.Y., Legha, S.S., Mavligit, G., Carrasco, C.H., Khorana, S., Plager, C., Papadopoulos, N., and Benjamin, R.S., *Cancer* 76: 1665–1670, 1995.

12. Salmon, R.J., Levy, C., Plancher, C., Dorval, T., Desjardins, L., Leyvraz, S., Pouillart, P., Schlienger, P., Servois, V., and Asselain, B., *Eur. J. Surg. Oncol.* 24: 127–130, 1998.
13. Leyvraz, S., Spataro, V., Bauer, J., Pampallona, S., Salmon, R., Dorval, T., Meuli, R., Gillet, M., Lejeune, F., and Zografos, L., *J. Clin. Oncol.* 15: 2589–2595, 1997.
14. Nathan, F.E., Berd, D., Sato, T., Shield, J.A., Shields, C.L., De Potter, P., and Mastrangelo, M.J., *J. Exp. Clin. Cancer Res.* 16: 201–208, 1997.
15. Gerard, B., Aamdal, S., Lee, S.M., Leyvraz, S., Lucas, C., D'Incalci, M., and Bizzari, J.P., *Eur. J. Cancer* 29A: 711–719, 1993.
16. Terheyden, P., Kampgen, E., Runger, T.M., Brocker, E.B., and Becker, J.C., *Hautarzt* 49: 770–773, 1998.
17. Neale, M.H., Myatt, N., Cree, I.A., Kurbacher, C.M., Foss, A.J., Hungerford, J.L., and Plowman, P.N., *Br. J. Cancer* 79: 1487–1493, 1999.

IAN A. CREE

Cytokine therapy and ocular melanoma

Abstract

Cytokines are widely used to treat melanoma both alone, often in the adjuvant setting, and combined with chemotherapy for more advanced disease. The rationale for their use is often an attempt to enhance anti-tumor immunity, although the type of immunity desired is not always clear. There is little clinical evidence that cytokine therapy can benefit patients with uveal melanoma, but there is an increasingly large body of experimental data suggesting that these agents may be useful. HLA antigen expression on uveal melanoma cells can be modulated by interferons and direct anti-proliferative effects of interferons on tumor derived cells have been observed. There is evidence for differences in HLA antigen expression between the primary intra-ocular tumor and liver metastases in at least some patients. However, therapeutic cytokines do not act within a vacuum: cytokines are produced by melanoma cells and the stromal cells within the tumor, both lymphoid and non-lymphoid. There is already evidence of heterogeneity of responsiveness of melanoma cells to interferon and other cytokines. The complex balance of cytokines can be altered by cytokine administration, but as yet prediction of an individual patient's response to such treatment is beyond our capability.

Keywords: Cytokines, melanoma, chemotherapy, interferons, eye

Introduction

Melanoma, even uveal melanoma, can undergo very occasional spontaneous remission. This fact more than any other has kept the hope of effective immunotherapy for cancer alive when many would otherwise have written off the idea of using the immune system to defeat cancer as science fiction. The explosion of knowledge about the immune system during the 1980s has not yet produced many effective therapies. Nevertheless, we are now at the point where we realise the full complexity of the immune system and the difficulty of directing it therapeutically.

Department of Pathology, Institute of Ophthalmology, University College London, Bath Street, London EC1V 9EL, Great Britain

Communication between cells that are not in direct contact is mediated by hormone-like peptides known as cytokines and by smaller chemical molecules such as arachidonic acid metabolites (prostaglandins and leukotrienes), histamine and nitric oxide. Cytokines are relatively easily studied and manufactured. As a result their potential as immunomodulatory agents has been extensively explored. There have been several successes, most notably in the use of colony-stimulating factors (CSFs) to regenerate bone marrow function during chemotherapy or following bone marrow transplantation. These allow the haematologist or oncologist to manipulate the white cell count, but not to alter specific immune reactions.

The pattern of an immune response can be altered by cytokine administration to patients to augment or reduce either cellular (Th1) or humoral (Th2) immunity via a number of different mechanisms. Co-administration of certain cytokines with antigen in particulate, soluble or cellular form can produce desired effects, at least in inbred strains of animals. Reproducible results are more difficult to achieve clinically although progress is being made and anti-cancer immune responses can be measured in patients following vaccine administration.

There is little published information about the effect of cytokines on uveal melanoma, and most of the information described hereafter relates to skin melanoma, which differs from uveal melanoma at genetic, molecular, cellular and clinical levels.

Regression in skin melanoma

Measurement of cytokine production in regressing skin melanoma is instructive [1]. Larger numbers of $CD4^+$ T lymphocytes within the tumor are associated with increased mRNA for IL2 and lymphotoxin (TNFβ), together with non-statistically significant increases in IFNα. There is no difference in Th2 or inflammatory cytokines [1]. The hypothesis is therefore that activated $CD4^+$ T cells may mediate melanoma regression by secretion of Th1 cytokines. Some (but not all) current strategies for the treatment of melanoma by exogenous cytokines are based on this hypothesis.

Cytokines produced by melanoma cells

Melanoma cells produce a number of different cytokines *in vitro*, notably basic fibroblast growth factor (bFGF), transforming growth factor alpha (TGFα), transforming growth factor beta (TGFβ), platelet-derived growth factor (PDGF) and melanoma growth stimulatory activity (MGSA), cytokines which are not expressed by normal human melanocytes [2]. Autocrine stimulation by simultaneous synthesis of growth factors and expression of their receptors by melanoma cells has been shown for bFGF and MGSA [2].

TGFβ can actually stimulate growth in some melanomas in contrast to the inhibition reported for melanocytes [2,3]. Part of the importance of cytokines produced by melanoma cells may be their effect on the immune system. Immunosuppression occurs in many types of cancer [4] and may be mediated by TGFβ or IL-10, both of which may be produced by melanoma cells. IL-10 is a Th2 cytokine which inhibits Th1 responses and downregulates HLA class I and II expression. It is produced by cutaneous melanoma cells and can act as an autocrine factor [5,6]. The role of IL-10 in uveal melanoma has not been reported.

Effects on melanoma cells

Many cytokines can show inhibitory effects on melanoma cells *in vitro*, but the relevance of these results to the situation *in vivo* is hard to judge, and there is certainly heterogeneity of responsiveness between tumors. Interferons (α, β and γ) have all been shown to inhibit melanoma cell proliferation and are of particular interest for immunotherapy.

Other cytokines can produce melanoma cell growth, including TGFα, epidermal growth factor (EGF), TGFβ, hepatocyte growth factor (HGF), stem cell growth factor (SCF), and the insulin-like growth factors (IGF1 and IGF2) [2,3] Again, the effects on both uveal and skin melanoma are erratic and there is heterogeneity between tumors of the same type [3].

Therapeutic effects on melanoma

There is a rapidly growing body of literature on the use of cytokines to treat melanoma. Given the pleotropic effects of these molecules, it is quite possible to formulate a rationale for many cytokines, particularly the interleukins and interferons, and this has produced a plethora of studies which it is almost impossible to interpret. This section therefore concentrates on the effects of cytokines in patients, classified by whether they are in use, or experimental, with a brief overview of the experimental approaches now current.

Cytokines in use

IFNα2b/IFNβ: The most recent major advance in cytokine therapy of skin melanoma has been the use of high dose IFNα2b for the adjuvant therapy of high risk skin melanoma [7–10]. However, a follow-up study failed to confirm the apparent improved cure rate and further trials will be needed to clarify the situation. In the Barts/Moorfields trial of high dose IFNα2b in high risk uveal melanoma patients, we set out to use the Kirkwood regimen (Plowman *et al.*, unpublished). However, the costs involved in providing this treatment mean that only the induction phase is being given. To date 30 patients have been randomised. This is too small a number to allow any useful data to be developed, but the treatment has been well-tolerated.

IFNβ has also been used for immunotherapy of malignant melanoma [11]. Systemic effects (e.g. increased neopterin levels) were only observed during the first four weeks of subcutaneous treatment. Immunostimulation may therefore be short-term with tachyphylaxis developing after a relatively short period. If a similar phenomenon is occurring with IFNα, this argues in favour of shortening the high dose regimen to one month, as is happening by default in the Barts/Moorfields trial in uveal melanoma. The one month induction phase for IFNα is also being tested by several groups for skin melanoma on the basis that the ECOG studies have shown early impact of IFNα on survival.

The reasons underlying the apparent effects of type I interferons on melanoma are unknown. Intracellular pathways are apparently intact [12]. De Waard-Siebinga et al. [13] reported the effects of IFNα and IFNγ on uveal melanoma cell lines, showing that they had effects on proliferation and HLA expression. IFNα enhanced HLA class I while IFNγ upregulated both HLA class I and II molecules. We have recently reported variable effects of IFNα2b on melanoma cells ex vivo in an ATP-based chemosensitivity assay [14].

IFNγ has been used in vivo at the time of surgery for uveal melanoma (Rennie personal communication), but the results are only now becoming mature and ready for analysis. Transduction of skin melanoma cells with IFNγ has been performed and irradiated transduced cells used as a vaccine. Paradoxically, one major study reported responses associated with humoral responses rather than the expected cellular responses following this treatment [15].

IL-2 has been used as a single agent or as part of combined chemoimmunotherapy regimens for nearly a decade [16]. Yet there is little trial-based evidence that these combinations have any great advantage over the single cytokine [17]. However it is also true that those who benefit from IL-2 may not be the same patients who benefit from IFNα2b or other cytokines. The mechanism of action is probably expansion of lymphocytes reacting to the melanoma—hopefully those which will attack the tumor cells rather than protect it. There is also evidence of more general pro-inflammatory effects [18]. IL-2 has also been targeted to melanoma by antibodies, with some apparent success, but this therapy is at any early stage of development [19,20]. One possible explanation for the effects of IL-2 and IFNα is the observed effect of this combination on DNA repair [21], although there are of course easier and less toxic ways of interrupting this aspect of melanoma biology using gemcitabine [22]. IL-2 has rarely been used with uveal melanoma and there are few reports of its efficacy [23].

GM-CSF has been used in one non-randomised phase II study of adjuvant therapy for cutaneous melanoma with apparently spectacular results (Spitler et al., unpublished). The ECOG group is considering a phase III randomised trial based on this data and the wealth of biologic information indicating the importance of this cytokine in dendritic cell differentiation.

Cytokines in combination

Most experience of combined cytokines in melanoma is with IL-2 and IFNα, usually in combination with cytotoxic drugs [24–26]. A recent study reported by Mainwaring *et al.* [25] had an 18% response rate with short duration. These regimens are extremely toxic and require frequent hospital attendance. The immunological rationale for combination of these two agents is debatable and sequence-mediated effects are likely to be important. The degree of heterogeneity of both tumor and host response are likely to make such regimens unpredictable at best and some tissue heterogeneity has been noted [25]. Such trials are probably not warranted at present in patients with uveal melanoma.

Experimental approaches

A surprisingly large number of cytokine genes have been transduced into lymphoid cells or tumor cells as potential vaccines [27]. This technology often shows some activity, but many studies fail to show convincing evidence that it is the gene transduction which is responsible for the effects observed. For instance, IL-7 can be transfected into melanoma cells as a potential way of producing a vaccine [28]. However, only 31% of melanomas established the cell lines necessary for this approach in one study [28] and there is no guarantee that such lines are representative of the original tumor.

IL-4 has been used with IL-2 for combined cytokine therapy. One study showed that IL-4 could modulate IL-2 effects by reducing LAK cell effects, but the effects on antibody production were not reported [29].

One of the latest candidates for cytokine therapy of melanoma is IL-12 [30]. This cytokine switches immune responses towards a Th1 phenotype, inducing IFNγ production, and is therefore of considerable interest for systemic therapy or for gene therapy approaches [31]. In early clinical trials, IL-12 produces 'flu-like symptoms with increased NK cell activity' [32]. IL-15 is an IL-12 like molecule which also looks promising [33,34].

Effects on melanoma-associated angiogenesis

The work of Folkman and others has resulted in a considerably enhanced profile for angiogenesis within tumors, since their growth to clinically detectable size depends upon the ability of the neoplastic cells to induce new blood vessel formation [35]. The main cytokines involved are VEGF/VPF and bFGF. The latter is involved in uveal melanoma progression and can be found in the tumors, but the evidence that VEGF is present is debatable. We have been unable to find either peptide or mRNA for VEGF in uveal melanomas fixed immediately following surgery, although there is VEGF in both aqueous and vitreous. In contrast, bFGF is present by immunocytochemistry in uveal melanomas in the absence of appreciable levels within vitreous or aqueous [36].

Cytokines and uveal melanoma treatment

Treatment of metastatic uveal melanoma has previously been disappointing [37,38], but IFNα has shown some effect in combination with systemic fotemustine and IL-2 [39], with intra-arterial fotemustine for liver metastases, or systemically in combination with the BOLD combination which induced a 20% (4/23) response rate [40]. However, multicentre studies have failed to confirm the efficacy of the BOLD + IFNα2b regimen and no further use of this toxic combination is warranted in metastatic uveal melanoma (EORTC-OOG, unpublished).

IFNα has recently been used to treat conjunctival and corneal intraepithelial neoplasia, with apparent success, using drops (1MIU/ml) and a perilesional injection (3MIU) [41].

Intra-ocular melanomas inhibit lymphocyte proliferation, probably as a result of FasL expression rather than alterations in HLA expression [42]. However, circulating lymphocytes do recognise and kill uveal melanoma cells [43] Creyghton et al. [44] examined the modulation of cell surface adhesion molecules on uveal melanoma cell lines by interferon alpha, interferon gamma and tumor necrosis factor alpha. There was heterogeneity of response between cell lines, and in terms of the integrins affected.

Most of the lymphocytes present in primary uveal melanomas are of the CD8$^+$ cytotoxic type [45] and require expression of HLA class I antigens to cause cytolysis. Ma and Niederkorn [46] reported that TGFβ downregulated HLA class I antigens on uveal melanoma cell lines, increasing their suscepibitility to attack by NK cells (which are also present), but potentially protecting them from CD8$^+$ cytotoxic T lymphocytes. IFNα upregulated HLA class I expression [46]. It has further been suggested that regulation of HLA [13] and the Fas/FasL system might be responsible for the differences observed between uveal primary and metastatic tumors, and that this could be modulated by cytokines to produce therapeutic advantages. At present most of this interesting data is based on cell line information, the relevance of which to the *in vivo* situation is questionable. Nevertheless, there is a clear biological argument in favour of interferon treatment of uveal melanoma and clinical trials are justified.

Conclusions

Uveal melanoma is a rare tumor. There is no place for "add it and see" trials of the type common to other types of tumor. Both resources and numbers of patients are limited. There is a need to establish a clear rationale for cytokine treatment in uveal melanoma based on experimental evidence of successful immune responses.

The gains produced by cytokine therapy of skin melanoma have been modest with single agents inducing 15–25% response rates similar to those achieved by cytotoxic chemotherapy. Combined chemo-immunotherapy has produced higher response rates, sometimes over 50%, but survival is rarely influenced [47]. Individualised therapy may be necessary, as shown by the growth stimulatory effect of IL-2 on occasional cell lines and apparently in patients [48], in addition to differences in HLA expression between tumors. Certainly, melanoma cells can become resistant to the effect of cytokines, just as they do to cytotoxic drugs [49]. Despite these caveats, there is likely to be a future for cytokine treatment of uveal melanoma and these agents may have considerable potential, particulary in the adjuvant setting.

References

1. Lowes, M.A., Bishop, G.A., Crotty, K., Barnetson, R.S., and Halliday, G.M., *J. Invest. Dermatol.* 108: 914–919, 1997.
2. Krasagakis, K., Garbe, C., and Orfanos, C.E., *Melanoma Res.* 3: 425–433, 1993.
3. Myatt, N., Cree, I.A., Neale, M.H., Foss, A.J.E., Hungerford, J.L., and Bhattacharya, S., *Ann. Oncol.* 2 (Suppl 2): 83, 1998.
4. Wojtowicz-Praga, S., *J. Immunother.*, 20: 165–177, 1997.
5. Fortis, C., Foppoli, M., Gianotti, L., Galli, L., Citterio, G., Consogno, G., Gentilini, O., and Braga, M., *Cancer Lett.* 104: 1–5, 1996.
6. Yue, F.Y., Dummer, R., Geertsen, R., Hofbauer, G., Laine, E., Manolio, S., and Burg, G., *Int. J. Cancer* 71: 630–637, 1997.
7. Kirkwood, J.M., Strawderman, M.H., Ernstoff, M.S., Smith, T.J., Borden, E.C., and Blum, R.H., *J. Clin. Oncol.* 14: 7–17, 1996.
8. Sondak, V.K., and Wolfe, J.A., *Curr. Opin. Oncol.* 9: 189–204, 1997.
9. Eggermont, A.M., *Eur. J. Cancer* 34 (Suppl 3): S22–S26, 1998.
10. Kirkwood, J.M., *Eur. J. Cancer* 34 (Suppl 3): S12–S17, 1998.
11. Fierlbeck, G., Ulmer, A., Schreiner, T., Stroebel, W., Schiebel, U., and Brzoska, J., *J. Interferon Cytokine Res.* 16: 777–781, 1996.
12. Grandér, D., Sangfelt, O., Skoog, L., and Hansson, J., *J. Interferon Cytokine Res.* 18: 691–695, 1998.
13. De Waard-Siebinga, I., Creyghton, W.M., Kool, J., and Jager, M.J., *Br. J. Ophthalmol.* 79: 847–855, 1995.
14. Neale, M., Myatt, N., Hungerford, J.L., Plowman, P.N., and Cree, I.A., *Ann. Oncol.* 9 (Suppl 2): 88, 1998.
15. Abdel-Wahab, Z., Weltz, C., Hester, D., Pickett, N., Vervaert, C., Barber, J.R., Jolly, D., and Seigler, H.F., *Cancer* 80: 401–412, 1997.
16. Whittington, R., and Faulds, D., *Drugs* 46: 446–514, 1993.
17. Dillman, R.O., *Cancer Biother.* 9: 183–209, 1994.
18. Fortis, C., Galli, L., Consogno, G., Citterio, G., Matteucci, P., Scaglietti, U., and Bucci, E., *Clin. Immunol. Immunopathol.* 76: 142–147, 1995.
19. Becker, J.C., Varki, N., Gillies, S.D., Furukawa, K., and Reisfeld, R.A., *Proc. Natl. Acad. Sci. U.S.A.* 93: 7826–7831, 1996.
20. Reisfeld, R.A., Becker, J.C., and Gillies, S.D., *Melanoma Res.* 7 (Suppl 2): S99–S106, 1997.
21. Buzaid, A.C., Ali-Osman, F., Akande, N., Grimm, E.A., Lee, J.J., Bedikian, A., Eton, O., Papadopoulos, N., Plager, C., Legha, S.S., and Benjamin, R.S., *Melanoma Res.* 8: 145–148, 1998.

22. Neale, M.H., Myatt, N., Cree, I.A., Kurbacher, C.M., Foss, A.J.E., Hungerford, J.L., and Plowman, P.N., *Br. J. Cancer* 79: 1487–1493, 1999.

23. Dorval, T., Fridman, W.H., Mathiot, C., and Pouillart, P., *Eur. J. Cancer* 28A: 2087, 1992.

24. Gause, B.L., Sznol, M., Kopp, W.C., Janik, J.E., Smith, J.W. 2nd, Steis, R.G., Urba, W.J., Sharfman, W., Fenton, R.G., Creekmore, S.P., Holmlund, J., Conlon, K.C., VanderMolen, L.A., and Longo, D.L., *J. Clin. Oncol.* 14: 2234–2241, 1996.

25. Mainwaring, P.N., Atkinson, H., Chang, J., Moore, J., Hancock, B.W., Guillou, P.J., Oskam, R., and Gore, M.E., *Eur. J. Cancer* 33: 1388–1392, 1997.

26. Andrès, P., Cupissol, D., Guillot, B., Avril, M.F., and Drèno, B., *Eur. J. Dermatol.* 8: 235–239, 1998.

27. Simons, J.W., and Mikhak, B., *Semin. Oncol.* 25: 661–676, 1998.

28. Finke, S., Trojaneck, B., Möller, P., Schadendorf, D., Neubauer, A., Huhn, D., and Schmidt-Wolf, I.G., *Cancer Gene Ther.* 4: 260–268, 1997.

29. Olencki, T., Finke, J., Tubbs, R., Tuason, L., Greene, T., McLain, D., Swanson, S.J., Herzog, P., Stanley, J., Edinger, M., Budd, G.T., and Bukowski, R.M., *J. Immunother. Emphasis Tumor Immunol.* 19: 69–80, 1996.

30. Nishimura, T., Watanabe, K., Yahata, T., Ushaku, L., Ando, K., Kimura, M., Saiki, I., Uede, T., and Habu, S., *Cancer Chemother. Pharmacol.* 38 (Suppl): S27–S34, 1996.

31. Nanni, P., Rossi, I., De Giovanni, C., Landuzzi, L., Nicoletti, G., Stoppacciaro, A., Parenza, M., Colombo, M.P., and Lollini, P.L., *Cancer Res.* 58: 1225–1230, 1998.

32. Ohe, Y., Kasai, T., Heike, Y., and Saijo, N., *Gan To Kagaku Ryoho* 25: 177–184 (abstract only), 1998.

33. De Jong, J.L., Farner, N.L., Javorsky, B.R., Lindstrom, M.J., Hank, J.A., and Sondel, P.M., *Clin. Cancer Res.* 4: 1287–1296, 1998.

34. Seidel, M.G., Freissmuth, M., Pehamberger, H., and Micksche, M., *Arch. Pharmacol.* 358: 382–389 (abstract only), 1998.

35. Rak, J.W., St Croix, B.D., and Kerbel, R.S., *Anticancer Drugs* 6: 3–18, 1995.

36. Cree, I.A., Boyd, S.R., Tan, D., Charnock-Jones, D.S., da Souza, L., and Hungerford, J.L., *ARVO 1999*, abstract # 3037.

37. Albert, D.M., Niffenegger, A.S., and Willson, J.K., *Surv. Ophthalmol.* 36: 429–438, 1992.

38. Pyrhönen, S., *Eur. J. Cancer* 34 (Suppl 3): S27–S30, 1998.

39. Terheyden, P., Kämpgen, E., Rünger, T.M., Bröcker, E.B., and Becker, J.C., *Hautarzt* 49: 770–773 (abstract only), 1998.

40. Nathan, F.E., Berd, D., Sato, T., Shield, J.A., Shields, C.L., De Potter, P., and Mastrangelo, M.J., *J. Exp. Clin. Cancer Res.* 16: 201–208, 1997.

41. Vann, R.R., and Karp, C.L., *Ophthalmology* 106: 91–97, 1999.

42. Verbik, D.J., Murray, T.G., Tran, J.M., and Ksander, B.R., *Int. J. Cancer* 73: 470–478, 1997.

43. Kan-Mitchell, J., Liggett, P.E., Harel, W., Steinman, L., Nitta, T., Oksenberg, J.R., Posner, M.R., and Mitchell, M.S., *Cancer Immunol. Immunother.* 33: 333–340, 1991.

44. Creyghton, W.M., de Waard-Siebinga, I., Danen E.H., Luyten, G.P., van Muijen, G.N., and Jager, M.J., *Melanoma Res.* 5: 235–242, 1995.

45. Durie, F.H., Campbell, A.M., Lee, W.R., and Damato, B.E., *Invest. Ophthalmol. Vis. Sci.* 31: 2106–2110, 1990.

Ian A. Cree

46. Ma, D., and Niederkorn, J.Y., *Immunology* 86: 263–269, 1995.
47. Villikka, K., and Pyrhönen, S., *Ann. Med.* 28: 227–233, 1996.
48. Han, D., Pottin-Clemenceau, C., Imro, M.A., Scudeletti, M., Doucet, C., Puppo, F., Brouty-Boye, D., Vedrenne, J., Sahraoui, Y., Brailly, H., Poggi, A., Jasmin, C., Azzarone, B., and Indiveri, F., *Oncogene* 12: 1015–1023, 1996.
49. Restifo, N.P., Marincola, F.M., Kawakami, Y., Taubenberger, J., Yannelli, J.R., and Rosenberg, S.A., *J. Natl. Cancer Inst.* 88: 100–108, 1996.

LISA S. KIERSTEAD[a], ELENA RANIERI[a],
JOHN M. KIRKWOOD[b], MICHAEL T. LOTZE[a],
THERESA WHITESIDE[c] AND
WALTER J. STORKUS[a]

Dendritic cell-based melanoma vaccines

Abstract

Dendritic cell (DC)-based vaccines have now been implemented in the treatment of a number of cancer histologies, including melanoma. The clinical efficacy of DCs is believed to be due to their potent ability to activate tumor-specific T cells that are capable of regulating the growth of, or causing the regression of, active disease. Based on the initial findings of our DC/melanoma peptide-based vaccine trial, we believe that DCs drive the early expansion of vaccine-specific CD8+ T cells *in situ* that may result in an expansion in the anti-tumor T cell repertoire over time. This "spreading" in the tumor-reactive T cell repertoire was most evident and durable in patients exhibiting objective clinical responses. This suggests that vaccines based on a restricted number of tumor epitopes may evolve highly-diversified immunity in clinical responders.

Keywords: Melanoma, vaccine, dendritic cells, peptide, epitope spreading

Melanoma vaccines: dendritic cell biology and clinical implications

An effective melanoma vaccine designed to elicit cellular anti-tumor immunity must select an optimal form of antigen, type of adjuvant, and mode of delivery (i.e. dose, route of administration, schedule) that favors the uptake and processing of the vaccine by "antigen presenting cells" (APC) in tissue [1,2]. The requirement for host APC (such as dendritic cells, DC) processing and presentation of tumor antigens in the effective induction of tumor-reactive T cells has been clearly delineated in murine models [3]. To involve a large number of DC *in situ*, either by recruiting these APC to cutaneous vaccine sites or by *ex vivo* manipulation and subsequent injection (subcutaneous, intravenous, or intratumoral) of antigen-laden DC in vaccines, appears a major goal of efficacious cancer vaccines [4,5]. Vaccine access to the potent

Departments of [a]Surgery, [b]Medicine, and [c]Pathology, University of
Pittsburgh School of Medicine and the University of Pittsburgh
Cancer Institute, Pittsburgh, PA 15261, USA

immunostimulatory DC may prove critical in the melanoma setting, since clinical success may require the "breaking of functional tolerance" and a resultant limited autoimmunity directed against "normal, self" melanocytic lineage antigens (such as Melan-A/MART-1, gp100/pmel17, tyrosinase, TRP-1/-2).

Mechanistically, the vaccine-activated or -administered DC serve as antigen transporting cells that traffic to draining lymphoid tissue via the afferent lymphatics (dermal injections) or peripheral blood (intravenous injection), where these APC form clusters with antigen-specific T-cells [6]. After appropriate activation, proliferation, and maturation has occurred, tumor-reactive CD4+ and CD8+ T-cells may leave the "priming" lymphoid organs. They recirculate throughout the body and into distal lesions, where they may directly mediate the regression of established disease or recruit additional immune cell infiltration as a result of the paracrine elaboration of cytokines/chemokines in DTH-like reactions [7].

Melanoma peptide/DC-based vaccines

Well-characterized melanoma antigens for implementation in vaccines may take the form of synthetic peptides derived from melanoma-associated antigens [8]. Tumor-associated peptides have demonstrated the capacity to promote antitumor CTL from the peripheral blood of normal donors and patients with melanoma both *in vitro* and *in vivo* [9,10]. In addition, they are inexpensive to produce, biochemically well-defined and generally quite stable, which are preferred parameters for an "off-the-shelf" clinical vaccine. The noted disadvantage of peptide-based vaccines is that a given melanoma peptide sequence may only be presented by a single or restricted set of MHC alleles, making only certain patients appropriate for protocol accrual. While tumor lesions are expected to exhibit phenotypic heterogeneity [11], for accrual purpose, at least some of the patient's tumor cells should express the vaccine-targeted antigen(s). This restriction may further diminish the pool of applicable patients. Some have argued that single epitope vaccines may prove therapeutically ineffective since epitope- and/or antigen-loss tumor variants may be immunoselected *in vivo*, however, the process of "epitope spreading" (see below) may alleviate some of these concerns, if *at least some* of the patient's tumor lesion(s) contain cells that express the vaccine-targeted antigen.

Despite such theoretical concerns, synthetic peptide-based vaccines have shown initial promise in melanoma vaccines. Notably, a synthetic MAGE-3 peptide injected subcutaneously in the absence of overt adjuvant, yielded objective clinical responses in three HLA-A1+ patients with melanoma [12]. In an independent clinical study, cultured autologous human peripheral blood APC (i.e. monocytes) pulsed with the MAGE-$1_{161-169}$ peptide epitope have been shown to elicit melanoma-specific CTL within the intradermal vaccine site and in the peripheral blood of HLA-A1 patients with metastatic melanoma [13]. Since DC are the prototype APC involved in the priming of "naive" T cells and melanoma antigen-specific CD8+ T cells in the majority of patients with melanoma exhibit a qualitatively CD45RA+ "naive" phenotype [14], the application of melanoma peptide epitopes in the context of autologous DC should have the greatest potential of promoting clinically-relevant immunity in the greatest number of patients.

Interim results of a melanoma peptide-DC vaccine trial

We have recently completed a phase I clinical trial (UPCI 95-060) of vaccines consisting of synthetic melanoma peptide-pulsed DC that was initiated in June 1995. Peripheral blood mononuclear cells were harvested from HLA-A2+ melanoma patients and DC generated by seven day culture of the derivative monocytes in serum-free media containing rhIL-4+ rhGM-CSF. DC were then harvested, washed and pulsed with AIM-V medium containing 10 μg/ml of each of the following peptides: MART-1 27–35 (AAGIGILTV), gp100 280–288 (YLEPGPVTA), tyrosinase 368–376D (YMDGTMSQV), and influenza matrix 58–66 (GILGFVFTL) (Fig. 1). Each week, DC were prepared from 60–100 cc of blood, pulsed with bulk peptides and injected into the autologous patient. Typically $0.5-1.5 \times 10^6$ DC (HLA-DR+, CD86+) were applied as a vaccine, with 10% of the yield injected s.c. (as a test of acute hypersensitivity) one hour prior to the remaining peptide-pulsed DC being injected i.v. No adverse reactions were observed.

Of note, of 23 patients evaluated, two displayed complete responses (CR; regression of all measurable disease) and one patient displayed a partial response (PR; greater than 50% reduction in total measurable disease). Peripheral blood was harvested one week prior to DC vaccination and one week after the fourth weekly injection of DCs for the immune monitoring of peripheral CD8+ T cell responses directed against the HLA-A2 presented peptides used in the vaccine. The IFN-γ ELISPOT assay was used in conjunction with the Zeiss AutoImaging system to quantitate the frequency of CD8+ T cells capable of secreting IFN-γ during the course of a 20h co-culture with T2 (HLA-A2+) cells pulsed with the individual synthetic peptides [15,16].

Grow DC	Pulse with Ag	Treat
Weeks 0–3 Draw 100 cc blood for DC expansion for 7d, IL–4 + GM-CSF	DC + MART-1 + gp100 + Tyrosinase + Flu matrix $0.5-2 \times 10^6$ DC Total	10% DC s.c. (1h pre-test) 90% DC i.v. Weeks 1–4

Clinical screen	Laboratory screen (pre-/post-)
Lesion shrinkage Depigmentation: Halo Nevi/Vitiligo DTH	Cytotoxicity Proliferation Cytokine production (ELISPOT)

FIGURE 1. *Schema for melanoma peptide/DC vaccine protocol.*

Dendritic cell-based melanoma vaccines

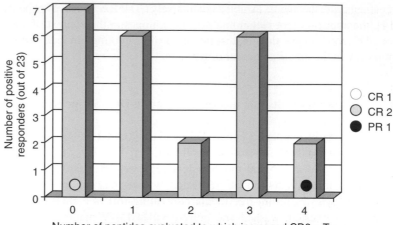

FIGURE 2. *Summary of patient peripheral blood T cell reactivity to vaccinated peptides. Peripheral blood CD8+ T cells were purified from patients prior to and one week after the last of four weekly vaccines (as outlined in Fig. 1). ELISPOT analyses (21, 22) for IFN-γ production were performed using these T cell responders and the HLA-A2+ T2 cell line ± the individual vaccine peptides as stimulators. A ratio of the frequency of peptide-specific CD8+ T cell responses post- vs. pre-vaccination was calculated for each patient. Patients were categorized based on the number of peptides against which their T cells yielded values >1 (i.e. increased response postvaccination) and the categories in which the two complete responders (CR) and the partial responder (PR) are indicated.*

A summary of the T cell response data is depicted in Figs 2 and 3. Of note, 16 out of 23 patients displayed an increase in the frequency of peripheral CD8+ T cells reactive against at least one of the vaccine-associated peptides, with 10 out of 23 patients' CD8+ T cell populations displaying elevated reactivity against at least two of these epitopes (Fig. 3).

While one patient exhibiting a CR and one patient with a PR reacted at an elevated frequency post-vaccination against three and four of the peptides, respectively, one patient with a CR displayed a reduction in response frequencies against the vaccine-associated epitopes (i.e. 0 peptide group). We hypothesize that this latter result may reflect the disseminated immune response occurring in this patient in which more than 100 lesions were simultaneously regressing during the four week course of vaccination, resulting in the largely tissue (and not blood)-associated localization of antigen-specific T cells at the time of the "post-vaccine" blood donation. If this hypothesis is true, it will clearly be important to extend the temporal range during which blood samples are acquired from the patients post-vaccination in order to establish a "baseline" of the impact of peptide vaccinations on the peripheral T cell repertoire of these patients. Bearing this caveat in mind, we observed significant variation of the range of increases in peptide-specific T cell frequencies

Lisa S. Kierstead et al.

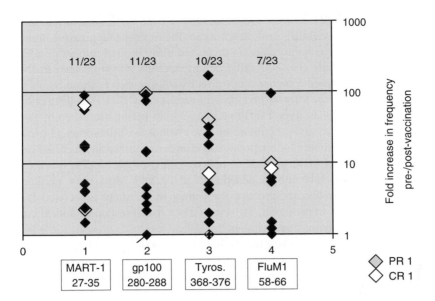

FIGURE 3. *Fold increases in the frequencies of vaccine-augmented, peptide-specific CD8+ T cells. The ratio of post- vs. pre-vaccine frequencies of CD8+ T cells reactive against the indicated peptides are reported. The total number of 23 patients that displayed ratios >1 for a given peptide are also reported. The data for one of the two complete responders (CR) and the partial responder are indicated.*

observed in the patients evaluated (Fig. 3). Approximately half of the patients displayed an increase in CD8+ T cell frequency responsive (i.e. > one-fold increase in frequency pre-/post-vaccination) against a given melanoma-associated peptide epitope (with either 10 or 11 out of 23 patients reacting better against the MART-1, gp100, or tyrosinase peptide epitopes post-vaccination). Interestingly, only 7 out of 23 patients displayed an elevated CD8+ T cell response against the influenza matrix 58–66 peptide (FluM1 58–66), despite the belief that this "immunodominant" epitope should serve as the prototype "positive control" peptide in vaccination of HLA-A2+ individuals. Overall, the range of increased responses was approximately 1–250 fold and a significant number of patients displayed increases in the 10–100 fold range for a given peptide, including one of the patients with a clinical CR and the patient with a clinical PR. We are currently performing long-term follow-up of the two CR patients who remain disease-free at more the 24 months post-vaccination in order to determine the durability of these antigen-specific T cell reactivities.

The clinical importance of CD4+ T cell-mediated anti-tumor immunity

It is clear that many issues must be addressed in order to foster optimal clinical efficacy of melanoma vaccines, including, identifying means to increase antigen-specific CTL numbers, to target these T cells to the sites of tumor, to maintain T cell viability and function in the immunosuppressive tumor micro-environment, and to promote increased infiltration of tumors by additional immune cells (i.e. NK cells, dendritic cells, macrophages, PMN). Clearly, CD4+ T cell responses may directly impact each of these issues by potentiating both the afferent and efferent aspects of CD8+ T cell function, and by mediating Th1-type DTH reactions within tumor sites, thereby promoting pro-inflammatory cytokine and/or chemokine production [17–20]. Cytokines may enhance locoregional vascular permeability and increase cellular expression of MHC-peptide complexes, thus, enhancing T cell reactivity. Chemokines (i.e. IFN-γ dependent IP-10 and Mig) may facilitate lymphocyte infiltration and promote the demise of the tumor-associated neovascular bed [21]. In particular, Th1-type CD4+ T cell responses appear crucial to such anti-tumor immune responses [22].

Despite the understanding that CD4+ T cells will play an important role in this complex biologic equation, few tumor antigen-derived peptides that serve as CD4+ T cell epitopes have been well-described to date. A limited series of CD4+ T cell melanoma epitopes have been identified (Table 1). We fully anticipate that CD4+ T cell responses against such epitopes *in situ* may be increased upon vaccination with defined melanoma peptides or proteins, and that these T cell responses will facilitate immune-mediated tumor regression or preclude disease recurrence. To that end, we have recently identified a series of HLA-DR4-presented peptide epitopes that are derived from the Melan-A/MART-1 [25], gp100, tyrosinase, and MAGE-3/-6 proteins and which are recognized by anti-melanoma CD4+ T cells. These peptides are currently being integrated into phase I clinical vaccine trials for the treatment of HLA-DR4+ patients with melanoma.

TABLE 1.   *Defined CD4 + T cells melanoma epitopes.*

Melanoma antigen of peptide origin	Sequence residues	HLA restriction	Reference cited
Melan-A/MART-1	51–73	DR4	Zarour *et al.* [23]
gp100	44–59	DR4	Halder *et al.* [24]
tyrosinase	56–70	DR4	Topalian *et al.* [25]
	193–203	DR4	Kobayashi *et al.* [26]
	386–406	DR15	Kobayashi *et al.* [27]
	448–462	DR4	Topalian *et al.* [25]
MAGE-3	114–127	DR13	Chaux *et al.* [28]
	121–134	DR13	Chaux *et al.* [28]
	141–155	DR11	Manici *et al.* [28]
	146–160	DR11	Manici *et al.* [29]
	282–295	DR11	Manici *et al.* [29]

Lisa S. Kierstead et al.

DC-based vaccines: cross-presentation and "epitope spreading"

Animal models have clearly documented the ability of cultured, syngeneic bone marrow-derived dendritic cells or macrophages to serve as effective immunogens of anti-tumor CTL *in vivo* when prepulsed with tumor-derived peptide epitopes [30–32]. The subsequent vaccination and boosting of mice with as few as 10^5 of these epitope-charged DCs, allowed for the animal to reject a re-challenge with a normally lethal challenge dose of a tumor expressing the naturally processed and presented epitope used in the vaccine [32]. Of significant interest, in some cases, animals rejecting such a tumor challenge were also able to then subsequently reject a challenge with an otherwise identical tumor that fails to lack the epitope used in the original vaccination [32]. These data support the concept of "epitope spreading", which may be of crucial interest in the induction of therapeutic immunity against antigenically heterogeous human lesions.

Based on insights gained in these murine tumor systems, a model of effective tumor vaccination may be hypothesized (Fig. 4). In this model, DC that have acquired injected, vaccine-associated tumor antigen, or DC that have been pre-loaded *ex vivo* with tumor antigen (i.e. peptide) and injected as a vaccine, migrate to vaccine site draining lymph nodes and promote the activation of tumor antigen-specific T cells. In the presence of DC-secreted cytokines (i.e. IL-12, IL-15, IL-18), a Th1-type immune response is augmented, resulting in

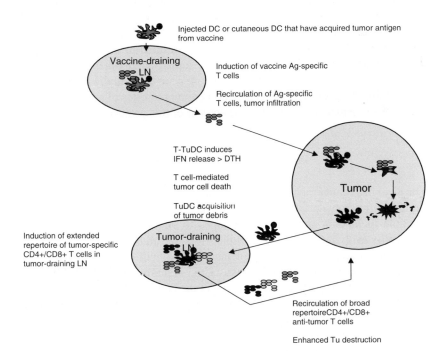

FIGURE 4. *Model of vaccine-induced "epitope spreading". See text for details.*

Dendritic cell-based melanoma vaccines

enhanced antigen-specific CTL generation [33]. These mature CTL may then leave the lymph node, recirculate and recruit to tumor sites. Within the tumor microenvironment, these CTL may mediate the cytolysis or apoptosis of tumor cells that provides a new format of tumor antigen (i.e. tumor "lysate" or apoptotic tumor bodies) that may be acquired by tumor-infiltrating DC [34]. These newly activated DC can then migrate to the draining lymph nodes and facilitate a secondary "wave" of CD4+ and CD8+ T cell induction, resulting in a broadening in the specificity of the anti-tumor effector T cell repertoire (i.e. only a small percentage of T cells will recognize the original vaccine-associated peptide). This phenomenon, termed "epitope spreading" may preclude the generation of "antigen-loss" tumor variants, since an extended range of tumor antigenic epitopes will be targeted by the broadened immune response [35, 36]. This is likely to represent a major mechanism associated with tumor regression in human clinical responders. As such, vaccine protocols designed with a limited series of peptide epitopes or recombinant tumor antigen proteins, should include clinical monitoring that allows for the detection of T cell-mediated immunity directed against not only tumor-relevant, but vaccine-irrelevant (but tumor-associated) specificities.

In the context of our melanoma peptide/DC-based vaccine (Figs 2, 3 and described above), we were able to screen an HLA-A2+/DR4+ melanoma patient (i.e. complete responder #1, CR1) for peripheral blood T cell responses directed against not only the vaccine-associated CD8+ T cells peptides, but against the CD4+ T cell epitope MART-1$_{51-73}$ [23], using IFN-γ ELISPOT. The latter T cell epitope was not a component in the vaccine, yet CD4+ T cell responses directed against this peptide were augmented post-vaccination (Fig. 5). This lends to support of the model outlined in Fig. 4 and suggests that "epitope spreading" occurs in at least some patients that respond clinically to melanoma peptide-based vaccines. We are currently in the process of determining the generality of this phenomenon in a series of additional HLA-A2+/DR4+ patients evaluated in the context of this protocol.

Summary and future directions

The ideal melanoma vaccine designed to effect the systemic eradication of disseminated micrometastatic disease will likely involve the implementation of multiple melanoma antigens and epitopes to circumvent potential immune evasion by evolving melanoma cells placed under immune selective pressure. The immunogenicity of such proteins/peptides will be significantly augmented by DC that promote Th1-associated cellular immunity. While such approaches may be particularly germane in the context of patients with established disease whose general immunocompetency may be reduced, clearly the ideal candidates for melanoma vaccines are those high-risk AJCC stage I/II patients treated surgically who display a high degree of immunocompetency.

Human DC have recently been used successfully in a series of recent clinical protocols, principally for the treatment of melanoma, lymphoma, and

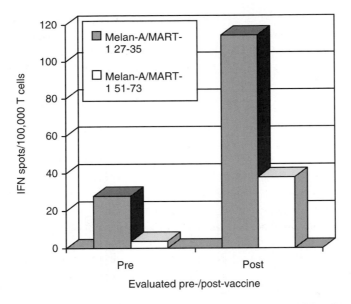

FIGURE 5   *Enhanced CD4+ T cell responsiveness against Melan-A/MART-1 51–73 post-vaccination with CD8+ T cell recognized melanoma epitopes in an HLA-A2+/DR4+ patient: Evidence for "cross-presentation" in vivo. Peripheral blood T cells were harvested from an HLA-A2+ DR4+ patient (i.e. CR1 in Figs 2,3) pre- and one week post-vaccination with autologous DC pulsed with the MART-1 27–35, gp100 280–288, tyrosinase 368–376D, and influenza matrix 58–66 peptides as outlined in Figs 1–3. Twenty hour IFN-γ ELISPOT assays were performed using CD4+ purified T cells as responders and T2.DR4 (HLA-A2+/DR4+) presenting cells in the presence or absence of the indicated peptides. IFN-γ spot number per 100,000 CD8+ or CD4+ T cells is indicated.*

prostate cancer [37–39]. The ability to generate large quantities of autologous dendritic cells from patients with cancer, coupled with the availability of several distinct formats of tumor-associated antigens (i.e. peptides, lysates, apoptotic tumor bodies; Fig. 6) provides the necessary tools to construct highly-immunogenic vaccines. We and others [39,40] have applied these reagents in the setting of cutaneous melanoma, but given commonality of tumor-associated antigens expressed [41–43], it would be particularly interesting to also evaluate the efficacy of such approaches in uveal melanoma, despite the distinct etiologies of these diseases [44].

While the initial clinical results of melanoma peptide/DC-based tumor vaccines engender significant enthusiasm, it would be anticipated that such vaccines will further benefit from the inclusion of an MHC-presented "helper" epitope recognized by CD4+ T cells, in order to optimally activate and maintain the vaccine-dependent CTL response [45]. Such epitopes may direct the generation of CD4+ cytotoxic T cells or a DTH-like immune response mediated by tumor-specific CD4+ T cells within the melanoma lesion (Fig. 4). The clinical efficacy of DC-based vaccination may also be enhanced by the systemic

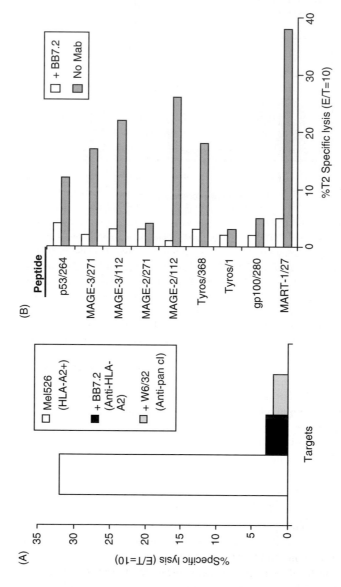

FIGURE 6. *Induction of melanoma-antigen specific CTL by autologous DC + apoptotic tumor (in vitro). Melanoma was resected from an HLA-A2+ patient, made into a single-cell suspension by enzymatic digestion, and the cells γ-irradiated (15,000 rad) to induce apoptosis. These tumor cells were then co-cultured with autologous DC (Tu:DC ratio = 0.1) for 24h at 37°C to allow for DC uptake and processing of apoptotic bodies (DC/Tu), prior to addition of autologous peripheral blood T cells. T cells were agai re-stimulated with DC/Tu on days 7 and 14. T cells were analyzed (on day 21) for their ability to kill HLA-A2 matched melanoma target cells (A) or tumor peptide-pulsed T2 cells (B) in an HLA-A2 restricted manner. The patient's tumor expressed each of the indicated antigens from which the peptides derive based on an RT-PCR analysis using specific primers.*

delivery of cytokines (i.e. IL-2, IL-7, IL-12, IL-15) that promote tumor antigen-specific T cell expansion, effector T cell migration into tumors (i.e. via vascular leak), tumor-infiltrating T cell resistance against tumor-induced apoptosis [46] and Th1-type immunity (i.e. IL-12, IL-18, IFN-α) [47–49].

References

1. Jaffee, E.M., *Ann. N.Y. Acad. Sci.* 886: 67–72, 1999.
2. Kochman, S., and Bernard, J., *Curr. Med. Res. Opin.* 15: 321–326, 1999.
3. Steinman, R., Witmer-Pack, M., and Inaba, K., *Adv. Exp. Med. Biol.* 329: 1–9, 1993.
4. Stingl, G., and Bergstresser, P.R., *Today* 16: 330–333, 1995.
5. Young, J.W., and Inaba, K., *J. Exp. Med.* 183: 7–11, 1996.
6. MacPherson, G.G., and Liu, L., *Adv. Exp. Med. Biol.* 329: 327–332, 1993.
7. Orme, I.M., and Cooper, A.M., *Immunol. Today* 20: 307–312, 1999.
8. Boon, T. and Van der Bruggen, P., *J. Exp. Med.* 183: 725–729, 1996.
9. Celis, E., Tsai, V., Crimi, C., DeMars, R., Wentworth, P.A., Chesnut, R.W., Grey, H.M., Sette, A., and Serra, H.M., *Proc. Natl. Acad. Sci. USA* 91: 2105–2109, 1994.
10. Bakker, A.B., Marland, G., De Boer, A.J., Danen, H., Adema, G.J., and Figdor, C.G., *Cancer Res.* 55: 5330–5339, 1995.
11. Dalerba, P., Ricci, A., Russo, V., Rigatti, D., Nicotra, M.R., Mottolese, M., Bordignon, C., Natali, P.G., and Traversari, C., *Int. J. Cancer* 77: 200–204, 1998.
12. Marchand, M., Weynants, P., Rankin, E., Arienti, F., Belli, F., Parmiani, G., Cascinelli, N., Bourlond, A., Vanwijck, R., Humblet, Y., Canon, J.-L., Laurent, C., Naeyaert, J.-M., Plagne, R., Deraemaeker, R., Knuth, A., Jager, E., Brasseur, F., Herman, J., Coulie, P.G., and Boon, T., *Int. J. Cancer* 63: 883–885, 1995.
13. Mukherji, B., Chakraborty, N.G., Yamasaki, S., Okino, T., Yamase, H., Sporn, J.R., Kurtzman, S.K., Ergin, M.T., Ozols, J., and Meehan, *Proc. Natl. Acad. Sci. USA* 92: 8078–8082, 1995.
14. Pittet, M.J., Valmori, D., Dunbar, P.R., Speiser, D.E., Lienard, D., Lejeune, F., Fleischhauer, K., Cerundolo, V., Cerottini, J.C., and Romero, P., *J. Exp. Med.* 190: 705–715, 1999.
15. Herr, W., Protzer, U., Lohse, A.W., Gerken, G., Meyer zum Buschenfelde, K.H., and Wolfel, T., *J. Infect. Dis.* 178: 260–265, 1998.
16. Herr, W., Linn, B., Leister, N., Wandel, E., Meyer zum Buschenfelde, K.H., and Wolfel, T., *J. Immunol. Methods* 203: 141–152, 1997.
17. Jager, E., Jager, D., and Knuth, A., *Cancer Metastasis Rev.* 18: 143–150, 1999.
18. Topalian, S.L., *Curr. Opin. Immunol.* 6: 741–745, 1994.
19. Pai, T.F., Silva, R.A., Smedegaard, B., Appelberg, R., and Andersen, P., *Immunology* 95: 69–75, 1998.
20. Buchanan, K.L., and Murphy, J.W., *Immunology* 90: 189–197, 1997.
21. Tannenbaum, C.S., Wicker, N., Armstrong, D., Tubbs, R., Finke, J., Bukowski, R.M., and Hamilton, T.A., *J. Immunol.* 156: 693–699, 1996.
22. Pardoll, D.M., and Topalian, S.L., *Curr. Opin. Immunol.* 10: 588–594, 1998.
23. Zarour, H., Kirkwood, J.M., Kierstead, L.S., Herr, W., Brusic, V., Slingluff, C.L. Jr., Sette, A., Southwood, S., and Storkus, W.J., *Proc. Natl. Acad. Sci. USA* 97: 400–405, 2000.
24. Halder, T., Pawelec, G., Kirkin, A.F., Zeuthen, J., Meyer, H.E., Kun, L., and Kalbacher, H., *Cancer Res.* 57: 3238–3244, 1997.

25. Topalian, S.L., Gonzales, M.I., Parkhurst, M., Li, Y.F., Southwood, S., Sette, A., Rosenberg, S.A., and Robbins, P.F., *J. Exp. Med.* 183: 1965–1971, 1996.
26. Kobayashi, H., Kokubo, T., Takahashi, M., Sato, K., Miyokawa, N., Kimura, S., Kinouchi, R., and Katagiri, M., *Immunogenetics* 47: 398–403, 1998.
27. Kobayashi, H., Kokubo, T., Sato, K., Kimura, S., Asano, K., Takahashi, H., Iizuka, H., Miyokawa, N., and Katagiri, M., *Cancer Res.* 58: 296–301, 1998.
28. Chaux, P., Vantomme, V., Stroobant, V., Thielemans, K., Corthals, J., Luiten, R., Eggermont, A.M., Boon, T., and Van der Bruggen, P.J., *J. Exp. Med.* 189: 767–778, 1999.
29. Manici, S., Sturniolo, T., Imro, M.A., Hammerm J., Sinigaglia, F., Noppen, C., Spagnoli, G., Mazzi, B., Bellone, M., Dellabona, P., and Protti, M.P., *J. Exp. Med.* 189: 871–876, 1999.
30. Zitvogel, L., Mayordomo, J.I., Tjandrawan, T., DeLeo, A.B., Clarke, M.R., Lotze, M.T., and Storkus, W.J., *J. Exp. Med.* 183: 87–97, 1996.
31. Mayordomo, J.I., Loftus, D.J., Sakamoto, H., De Cesare, C.M., Appasamy, P.M., Lotze, M.T., Storkus, W.J., Appella, E., and DeLeo, A.B., *J. Exp. Med.* 183: 1357–1365, 1996.
32. Celluzzi, C.M., Mayordomo, J.I., Storkus, W.J., Lotze, M.T., and Falo, L.D. Jr., *J. Exp. Med.* 183: 283–287, 1996.
33. Reid, S.D., Penna, G., and Adorini, L., *Curr. Opin. Immunol.* 12: 114–121, 2000.
34. Albert, M.L., Sauter, B., and Bhardwaj, N., *Nature* 392: 86–89, 1998.
35. Disis, M.L., Grabstein, K.H., Sleath, P.R., and Cheever, M.A., *Clin. Cancer Res.* 5: 1289–1297, 1999.
36. Vanderlugt, C.J., and Miller, S.D., *Curr. Opin. Immunol.* 8: 831–836, 1996.
37. Hsu, F.J., Benike, C., Fagnoni, F., Liles, T.M., Czerwinski, D., Taidi, B., Engelman, E.G., and Levy, R., *Nature Med.* 2: 52–55, 1996.
38. Murphy, G.P., Tjoa, B.A., Simmons, S.J., Jarisch, J., Bowes, V.A., Ragde, H., Rogers, M., Elgamal, A., Kenny, G.M., Cobb, O.E., Ireton, R.C., Troychak, M.J., Salgaller, M.L., and Boynton, A.L., *Prostate* 38: 73–78, 1999.
39. Nestle, F.O., Alijagic, S., Gilliet, M., Sun, Y., Grabbe, S., Dummer, R., Burg, G., and Schadendorf, D., *Nat. Med.* 4: 328–332, 1998.
40. Ranieri, E., Kierstead, L.S., Zarour, H., Kirkwood, J.M., Lotze, M.T., Whiteside, T., and Storkus, W.J., *Immunol. Inv.* 29: 121–125, 2000.
41. Chen, P.W., Murray, T.G., Salgaller, M.L., and Ksander, B.R., *J. Immunother.* 20: 265–275, 1997.
42. Wagner, S.N., Wagner, C., Schultewolter, T., and Goos, M., *Cancer Immunol. Immunother.* 44: 239–247, 1997.
43. Kan-Mitchell, J., Liggett, P.E., Harel-W., Steinman, L., Nitta, T., Oksenberg, J.R., Posner, M.R., and Mitchell, M.S., *Cancer Immunol. Immunother.* 33: 333–340, 1991.
44. Niederkorn, J.Y., *Eye* 11: 249–254, 1997.
45. Pardoll, D.M., and Topalian, S.L., *Curr. Opin. Immunol.* 10: 588–594, 1998.
46. Storkus, W.J., Tahara, H., and Lotze, M.T., in *The Cytokine Handbook* (3rd ed.), Thomson, A.W. (ed.), pp. 391–426, Academic Press, New York, 1998.
47. Macatonia, S.E., Hosken, N.A., Litton, M., Viera, P., Hsieh, C.S., Culpepper, J.A., Wysocka, M., Trinchieri, G., Murphy, K.M., and O'Garra, A., *J. Immunol.* 154: 5071–5079, 1995.
48. Belardelli, F., and Gresser, I., *Immunol. Today* 17: 369–372, 1996.
49. Fallarino, F., Uyttenhove, C., Boon, T., and Gajewski, T.F., *Int. J. Cancer* 80: 324–333, 1999.

MANFRED ZIERHUT, RAINER STIEMER, BERNHARD
WANNKE, ANITA MAYER AND JENS MARTIN ROHRBACH

Immunology of basal cell carcinoma of the lid

Abstract

Basal cell carcinoma (BCC) is a malignant tumor of the skin, leading to
extensive tissue destruction without formation of metastases. With an incidence of 400,000 cases per year in the USA it represents the most common
malignant tumor. In the pathogenesis of BCC, UV-radiation may play a role,
leading to depletion of Langerhans cells around the tumor, resulting in
reduced antigen presentation to effector T cells. A role for genetic factors
and human papilloma virus may exist, leading to point-mutations of tumor
suppressor genes. Regarding its immunological behaviour BCC, can down
regulate expression and consequently induce a Th2-response. So T cells are
detectable in the stroma between the tumor and underneath the epidermis, but
not inside the tumor. Homing mechanisms may play a role in BCC surveillance. Like lymphocytes proliferating cells characterized by proliferation
markers, are mostly found at the edge of tumor tissue in BCC. For treatment,
surgery and interferon-alpha still remain the main stay, but new immunological strategies could be helpful for large invasive BCC's in the future.

Keywords: Basal cell carcinoma, UV-radiation, T cells, tumor escape
mechanisms, interferon-alpha

Introduction

Basal cell carcinoma (BCC) is a malignant tumor of the skin, which can lead
to extensive tissue destruction. BCC has the highest incidence of all malignant tumors, and it represents 80 to 90% of all malignant lid tumors [1].
While BCCs rarely metastasize they may lead to invasion of the central
nerval system if located on the skin of the head, and may eventually result
in death.

While the regular therapy of skin BCC consists of surgical excision, this may create severe cosmetic problems and scaring, especially in delicate structures like the lid. Incompletely resected, recurrences are very often which then lead to additional surgery and loss of more lid tissue. Therefore, new therapeutic ideas like immunological strategies are warranted. This requires the investigation of the immunology of BCC.

Epidemiology

With an incidence of 400,000 cases per year in the USA and 150,000 per year in Germany, BCC is the most common malignant tumor [2]. It is typically a tumor of older age, especially in the age of 60 to 70 years, but it also has been described in children. Interestingly, BCC is only rarely found in coloured people.

Pathogenesis of BCC

There is evidence from epidemiological studies that genetic factors, skin pigmentation, higher age and exposure to ultraviolet (UV) radiation are major risk factors for the development of basal cell carcinoma.

The role of UV-radiation in the pathogenesis of BCC is only partly understood [3–8]. UV-radiation can damage the DNA. It also induces local immunosuppressive effects like depletion and alteration of Langerhans cells. Systemic immunosuppressive effects are initiated leading to induction of T-suppressor cells and a reduction of the immune surveillance. UV-radiation induces highly antigenic proteins in skin cancer which in animal models initiate severe immune reactions, leading to recognition and even control of the growth of these malignancies. But it seems that defects in the immune surveillance may contribute to resistance against cutaneous carcinomas in humans. This has especially been shown in patients with suppressed T cell immunity after immunosuppression for preventing rejection of organ allograft. These patients show a 50- to 100-fold increase in the incidence of skin cancer [9]. They develop almost exclusively BCC on unexposed areas of the body, even at young ages. For the growth of BCC there may exist also a role for human papilloma virus (HPV) which is sometimes found in benign papillomas of the skin associated with squamous cell carcinoma and BCC. It seems that UV-radiation leads to HPV replication [10,11]. Langerhans cells around the tumor are reduced or damaged, and they are not able to express co-stimulatory factors necessary for an intact antigen presenting cell [11–13]. UV-radiation also may lead to local proliferation and influx of CD36+, CD11b+ macrophages which are known to induce T-suppressor cells, finally resulting in less tumor antigen presentation to effector T cells [14].

Genetic factors also seem to be important in the pathogenesis of BCC. There is also a low incidence of BCC in coloured people [15,16] and at non-UV-exposed skin areas which may be a strong sign for genetic factors in the induction of BCC [17,18]. Here immunosuppressor genes and other genes are important. Approximately 50% of the patients with BCC demonstrate point-mutation of the tumor suppressor gene p53 [19–21]. The normal wt (wild-type) p53 protein is a strong inhibitor of cell growth and seems to be a strong inducer of apoptosis [22].

Because of the rapid degradation only low levels of wt p53 are detectable in the normal skin [23]. As mutant p53 has a longer half life, immunohistological p53 detection probably reflects p53 mutation and thus loss of normal p53 function [23,24]. Despite the finding that BCCs in sun-exposed areas show the same amount of p53 mutation as BCCs in less sun-exposed areas [25], it can be supposed that UV radiation plays an important role in p53 mutation (inactivation) [26,27]. Consequently, p53 mutations are usually more frequent in BCCs of older patients than in BCCs of younger patients [26]. Increased immunostaining for p53 was found in 30–90% of non-ocular BCCs [23–27]. The fraction of p53 positive cells ranges from 0% to more than 50% in non-ocular BCCs [23,28]. Our investigations revealed that the majority of ocular BCCs has a p53 positive cell fraction of less than 20% [29] (Tables 1, 2). According to Healy et al. [28] p53 protein expression has no prognostic significance for BCCs. On the other hand p53 upregulation was identified in histologically more aggressive BCC variants [23]. Other tumor suppressor genes are found on chromosome 1q22 [30] and 9q [31,32]. So Bcl-2 can induce extensive cell growth by limiting apoptosis. Overexpression of Bcl-2 gene has been shown in 100% of BCC patients [8].

Typically BCC leads to destruction of the tissue. Basal cell carcinoma has a low metastatic potential of approximately 0.003 to 0.4%. Until today only approximately 250 cases of metastazing BCC have been published [8]. This low rate is probably caused by the strong tumor-connective tissue-relation. Metastasis is possible in all histologic forms. It occurs mainly in large, ulcerating, and recurrent tumors and is associated with a high mortality [33].

TABLE 1. *List of primary antibodies [29].*

Antibody	Specificity	Positive control
CD4	T-helper/inducer cells	lymph node, tonsil
CD8	T-suppressor/cytotoxic cells	lymph node, tonsil
CD45Ro	(activated) T cells	thymus
CD50	monocytes, granulocytes, majority of lymphocytes in peripheral blood	lymph node, tonsil
CD68	macrophages	tonsil
HECA-452	cutaneous lymphocyte-associated antigen (CLA), subset of dendritic cells	cutaneous lymphocytes
Ki67 (MIB1)	proliferating cells	basal epidermal cells
p53	p 53 (mutants)	

TABLE 2. *Intracellular (intratumoral) antibody reactivity for Ki67 (MIB1) and p53 antigen [29].*

Antibody	Degree of staining*	Ocular BCCs	Non-ocular BCCs
Ki67 (MIB1)	<10%	2/10	0/0
	10–20%	7/35	2/22
	20–30%	4/20	2/22
	>30%	3/15	3/33
	inconclusive**	4/20	2/22
p53	<10%	13/65	4/44
	10–20%	2/10	1/11
	20–30%	0/0	2/22
	>30%	0/0	0/0
	inconclusive**	5/25	2/22

*For Ki67 (MIB1) and p53 stained tumour cells were related to all tumor cells thus giving the percentage of cells demonstrating nuclear staining as proposed by Barrett *et al.* [23].
**Inconclusive results because of doubtful staining or insufficient tumor tissue.

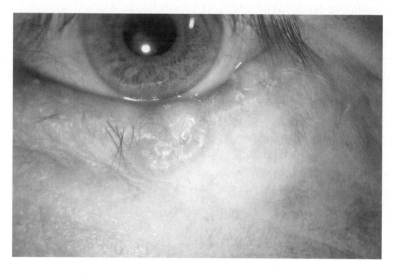

FIGURE 1. *65-year old male patient with solid BCC.*

Histopathology

BCC is characterized by aggregates of atypical basaloid cells which are surrounded by stromal fibrosis and inflammatory cells. From the clinical point of view one can differentiate five types [2,34].

1. *Solid type (75 %) (Figs 1,2)*
   It is characterized by slow growth, sometimes with a central ulceration. Because of mostly clear defined border between malignant tissue and uninvolved tissue, complete excision is easy.

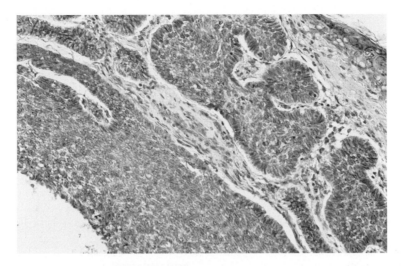

FIGURE 2.   *Histology of solid BCC (HE × 63).*

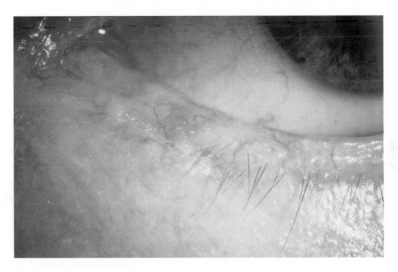

FIGURE 3.   *62-year old female patient with BCC of the morphea-type.*

2. *Pigmented type (10%)*
    The pigmentation of this type seems to result from active pigment uptake of the tumor.
3. *Sclerosing type (morphea-type) (Figs 3,4)*
    Slightly elevated plaque-like tumor, sometimes with nodules, ulceration is rare.
4. *Superficial type*
    This tumor is mostly found on the body, rarely on the lid, characterized by erythematous crusty plaques. This type often is not easy to differentiate from normal tissue.

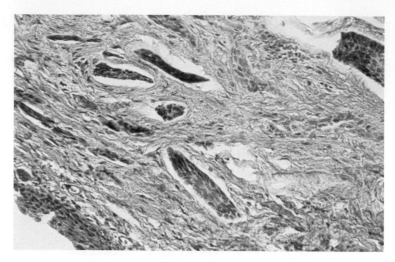

FIGURE 4.   *Histology of morphea-type BCC (HE × 63).*

5. *Mixed types*

These types include metatypical BCCs or carcinomas, which are not easy to differentiate from squamous cell carcinoma clinically, but histologically. They may cause severe ulceration (Ulcus rodens).

Immunohistology of BCC

It seems logical that investigation of tumor infiltrating cells may explain what kind of defects of the host's immune system enable tumor escape and growth. But until today these mechanisms have not been well understood. The reason for this is that BCCs like most other tumors seem to exhibit considerable variation in their lymphocyte cluster probably indicating a different antigenicity between BCCs. Far more investigations have been performed on skin BCC than on lid BCC, but at both locations similar T-cell clusters, the dominating infiltrating lymphocytes, are involved, while B cells are only rarely detectable [11,35–38].

Recently our group has studied the role of CD4+, CD8+, CD45Ro+, CD50+, CD68+ cells in lid BCC, compared to skin BCC (Tables 1 and 3) [29]. Even if there is no uniformity, it seems that these cells are mainly detectable in the stroma between the tumor and underneath the epidermis, but less often in deeper connective tissue. In 82% of ocular and also in 88% of non-ocular BCCs CD4+ cells (Fig. 5) outnumbered CD8+ cells (Fig. 6). More CD4+ cells were usually associated with more CD8+ cells. Intratumoral CD4+ cells were slightly more frequent than CD8+ cells. Tumour islands exhibited only few (invading) immunocompetent cells.

B, NK, Langerhans, and mast cells can also be found to a variable degree. T lymphocytes and mast cells seem to be inversely correlated. Our results indicate that the role of macrophages has probably been underestimated

TABLE 3. *Semiquantitative measurement of immunocompetent cells surrounding tumor islands [29].*

Antibody	Degree of staining*	Ocular BCCs (n = 20) (n/%)	Non-ocular BCCs (n = 9) (n/%)
CD4	0	0/0	0/0
	+	2/10	0/0
	++	10/50	2/22
	+++	7/35	7/78
	inconclusive**	1/5	0/0
CD8	0	2/10	1/11
	+	13/65	4/44
	++	3/15	4/44
	+++	0/0	0/0
	inconclusive**	2/10	0/0
CD4:CD8 ratio	>1	82%	88%
CD45Ro	0	0/0	0/0
	+	4/20	1/11
	++	7/35	4/44
	+++	7/35	3/33
	inconclusive**	2/10	1/11
CD50	0	2/10	0/0
	+	10/50	3/33
	++	4/20	2/22
	+++	3/15	2/22
	inconclusive**	1/5	2/22
CD68	0	0/0	0/0
	+	0/0	0/0
	++	6/30	5/55
	+++	7/35	3/33
	inconclusive**	7/35	1/11
HECA-452***	0	1/7	
	+	6/40	
	++	5/33	1/100
	+++	0/0	
	inconclusive**	3/20	

*Semiquantitative scale: 0 = negative, + = weak, ++ = moderate, +++ = strong.
**Inconclusive results because of doubtful staining or insufficient tumor tissue.
***HECA-452 was investigated in 15 ocular BCCs and one non-ocular BCC only.

(Fig. 7). Cellular infiltrations are probably not correlated with the histological type or the size of BCCs.

Immunohistology after spontaneous BCC regression

Spontaneously regressed BCC tissue has been investigated by Halliday when he characterized immunocompetent cells [39]. These were mainly CD4+

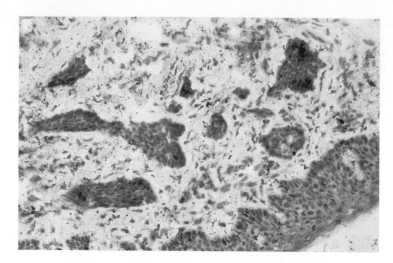

FIGURE 5. *CD4 immunohistology, ocular BCC. CD4+ cells can be localized to a similar amount like in skin BCC between tumor islands. Again, there are no CD4+ cells within BCC islands.*

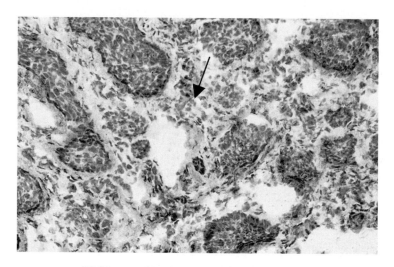

FIGURE 6. *CD8 immunohistology, ocular BCC. Few CD8+ cells (arrows) are scattered between BCC islands which are devoid of CD8+ cells.*

IL-2R+ T cells (Th1 cells), while the numbers of CD8+ cells and antigen-presenting cells with HLA-DR expression was unchanged. B cells were not detectable, and, like NK cells, seem to play a minor role in tumor response.

On the other hand cytotoxic T cells (CTLs) have been shown to be very important in the immune response against various tumours (like melanoma, breast cancer). In skin BCC, the presence of perforin expressing T cells seems to correlate with the infiltration of CD8+ cells, suggesting a role for CTLs in host defense against BCC [36].

M. Zierhut et al.

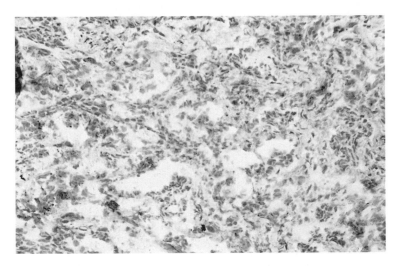

FIGURE 7.   *CD68 immunohistology, ocular BCC. There is a marked infiltration of CD68+ cells (macrophages) around tumor islands.*

Homing of T cells

The mAb HECA-452 identifies the cutaneous lymphocyte-associated antigen (CLA) which is preferentially expressed on cutaneous T cells and a subset of dendritic (Langerhans) cells acting as a homing molecule [40]. HECA-452 reactivity can be detected adjacent to BCCs especially around vessels, probably high endothelial venules, the most important vessels for adhesion and invasion of activated lymphocytes [41] (Table 3) (Fig. 8). This may indicate that homing mechanisms may play a role in BCC surveillance.

Proliferation markers

Non-ocular BCCs have been investigated with cell proliferation markers like Ki67 (MIB1) [23,28,42] or proliferating cell nuclear antigen (PCNA) [23,43,44]. Growth fraction (percentage of proliferating cells) ranges from almost 0% to more than 30% [23,28,42–44]. Thus, the results are also fairly comparable to ocular BCCs (Table 2).

Like lymphocytes, proliferating cells are mostly found at the edge of tumor islands in non-ocular [28,43] as well as in ocular BCCs (Fig. 9). The often high growth fraction contrasts to the usually slow growth of BCCs.

Therefore, it seems reasonable to assume that a greater amount of BCC cells undergoes apoptosis. Investigation of proliferation markers may allow the prediction of clinical recurrences [23,28,44]. Fibrosing (sclerosing) BCCs exhibit usually a higher percentage of Ki67 and PCNA positive cells than solid (nodular) tumors [23]. The PCNA index also correlates to peritumoral TGF-β expression [43].

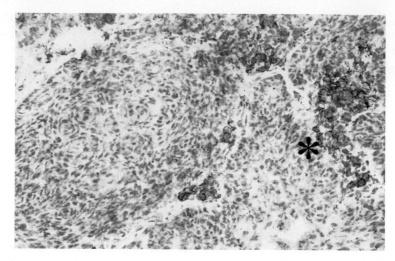

FIGURE 8.   *HECA-452 immunohistology, non-ocular BCC. A considerable peritumoral infiltrate of HECA-452+ cells is visible underneath the epidermis (asterisk) surrounding a vessel. A few HECA-452+ cells are localized within the tumor. Similar results were found for ocular BCCs.*

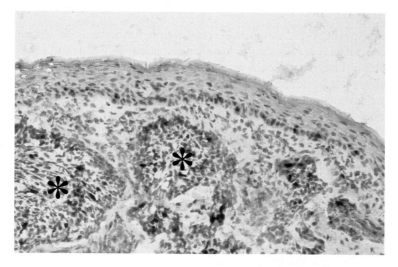

FIGURE 9.   *Ki67 (MIB1) immunohistology, ocular BCC. The growth fraction of tumor islands underneath the epidermis (asterisk) was estimated as approximately 30%. There is an accentuation of Ki67+ cells at the edge of BCC islands indicating an increased proliferative activity at the front of invasion.*

Blood-T-cell levels in BCC patients

In 1975 Dellon *et al.* [45] reported, that T-cell levels in the blood of patients with BCC are reduced, but normalize after excision of the tumor, while

M. Zierhut et al.

became elevated in patients with tumors larger than 2 cm. While these results were not found by Weimar *et al.* [46], Sivkova *et al.* [47] detected a reduced CD4/CD8 relation in their BCC patients. Recently, our group has confirmed these results in part [48].

Tumor escape mechanisms of BCC

Like most tumors, BCC has developed mechanisms to escape detection and destruction of the hosts immune system. Often HLA-class-I-antigen and β-2 microglobulin are not detectable in BCCs, preventing activation of CD8+ cells. Also HLA-class II antigen-expression seems to be downregulated by BCC cells, preventing activation of CD4+ cells [29].

BCC cells also strongly express the mRNA of IL-4, IL-5 and IL-10 [49], Th2-type cytokines, leading probably to inactivation of Th1 cells. Also IL-6 and IL-8 have been demonstrated [50]. Neutralization of tumor-produced IL-10 by mAb and IFN-α treatment could restore anti-tumor T-cell recognition [51]. The production of IL-1α and IL-1β is reduced [8], while the hypersecretion of IL-6 leads to hyperproliferation of cells [8]. IL-8 can act as autocrine growth factor and facilitates tumor cell migration [8]. BCCs have been shown to prevent T-cell response by secreting IL-10, by shedding ICAM-1 (Intercellular Adhesion Molecule 1) or by down-regulation of interferon γ receptors (with reduced HLA-class II antigen-expression) in tumor cells [38].

HLA-Association

An association between HLA-class I and class II genes and the susceptibility of skin cancer has been shown [52]. Our group has failed to demonstrate such an association to HLA-class I- and class II-antigen alleles, which are not found more often in BCC patients than in healty controls (unpublished data).

Treatment of BCC with IFN

Various studies of skin BCC have shown tumor reduction using intralesional injections of IFN [53–58]. While IFN-α has to be injected three times a week (1.5 Mio I.U), IFN-β seems to have a higher tissue affinity so that the lower dose of 0.5–1.0 Mio I.U seems to be as effective as IFN-α. For lid BCC no controlled studies are available.

It remains unclear how IFN works. Interferons are antiproliferative, but are also immuno-modulating, e.g. improving the Th1-cell response by stimulating IL-1 and TNF-α resulting in blocking of Th2-associated cytokines like IL-4 and IL-10. IFNs also induce a higher expression of HLA-antigens and adhesion molecules on tumor cells and surrounding keratinocytes, resulting in a down regulation of tumor escape mechanisms and recruting more tumor infiltrating cells. An elevated rate of apoptosis has also been demonstrated [59].

Conclusion

BCC is the most common malignant tumor which rarely metastazises but grow by invasion. For the pathogenesis UV radiation, probably with still unidentified genetic factors and HPV, are discussed, leading to point mutation of p53 and other tumor suppressor genes. BCC escapes immunocompetent cells like T and Nk cells by down-regulation of the HLA-expression, and probably by inducing a Th2 shift by secretion of IL-4, IL-5 and IL-10, but also of down-regulation of γ-IFN-receptors and shedding ICAM-1. Has the immunsystem successfully encountered BCC, CD4+ IL-2R+ T cells (Th1) are the major tumor-infiltrating cells. For treatment, surgery will continue to be the most important procedure for small BCC. In skin BCC α-IFN has been shown to be effective. The problem for treatment of large tumors remains. Immunological strategies like Langerhans cell – tumor cell – hybridoma-injections, effective in other tumors [60,61], could be helpful.

References

1. Margo, C.E., and Waltz, K., *Surv. Ophthalmol.* 38: 169–192, 1993.
2. Goldberg, L.H., *Lancet* 347: 663–667, 1996.
3. Kricker, A., Armstrong, B.K., and English, D.R., *Cancer Causes Control* 5: 367–392, 1994.
4. Kricker, A., Armstrong, B.K., Englisch, D.R., and Heenan, P.J., *Int. J. Cancer* 60: 482–488, 1995.
5. Kricker, A., Armstrong, B.K., English, D.R., and Heenan P.J., *Int. J. Cancer* 60: 489–494, 1995.
6. Marks, R., *Cancer* (Suppl) 75: 607–612, 1995.
7. Wie, Q., Matanoski, G.M., Farmer, E.R., Hedayati, M.A., and Grossman, L., *J. Invest. Dermatol.* 104: 933–936, 1995.
8. Köhler, D., and Stadler, R. *Klinik und histologie des basalioms.* Springer, Berlin, pp. 135–149, 1997.
9. Birkeland, S.A., Storm, H.H., and Lamm, L.U., *Int. J. Cancer* 60: 183, 1995.
10. McGregor, J.M., and Proby, C.M. in *Cancer surveys, Vol. 26: Skin cancer,* Leigh, I.M., Newton Bishop, J.A., and Kripke, M.L. (eds.), Laboratory Press, Cold Springs Harbor, p. 219, 1996.
11. Strickland, F.M., and Kripke, M.L., *Clin. Plast. Surg.* 24: 637–647, 1997.
12. Aberer, W.G. *et al.*, *J. Invest. Dermatol.* 76: 202, 1981.
13. Azizi, E., Bucana, C., Goldberg, L., *et al.*, *Am. J. Dermatopathol.* 9: 465, 1987.
14. Meunier, L., Bata-Csorgo, Z., and Cooper, K.D., *J. Invest. Dermatol.* 105: 782, 1995.
15. Armstrong, B.K., and Kricker, A., *Dermatol. Clin.* 13: 583, 1995.

16. Scotto, J., Fears, T.R., and Fraumeni, J.F., *NIH Publication* No. 83-2433, National Cancer Institute, Washington, 1983.
17. Kraemer, K.H., *J. Invest. Dermatol.* 105: 887, 1995.
18. Streilein, J.W., *Cancer Surv.* 26: 207, 1996.
19. Lübbe, J., Kleihues, P., and Berg, G., *Hautarzt* 45: 741–745, 1994.
20. Rady, P., Sciinicariello, F., Wagner, R.F. Jr., and Trying, S.K. *Cancer Res.* 52: 3804–3806, 1992.
21. Urano, Y., Asano, T., Yoshimoto, K., *et al.*, *J. Invest. Dermatol.* 104: 928–932, 1995.
22. Williams, G.T., and Smith, C.A., *Cell* 74: 777–779, 1993.
23. Barrett, T.L., Smith, K.J., Hodge, J.J., *et al.*, *J. Am. Acad. Dermatol.* 37: 430–437, 1997.
24. Ro, Y.S., and Kim, J.-H., *J. Korean Med. Sci.* 8: 361–366, 1993.
25. Matsumura,Y., Nishigori, C., Yagi, T., *et al.*, *Int. J. Cancer* 65: 778–780, 1996.
26. D'Errico, M., Calcagnile, A.S., Corona, R., *et al.*, *Cancer Res.* 57: 747–752, 1997.
27. Molès, J.-P., Moyret, C., Guillot, B., *et al.*, *Oncogene* 8: 583–588, 1993.
28. Healy, E., Angus, B., Lawrence, C.M., *et al.*, *Br. J. Dermatol.* 133: 737–741, 1995.
29. Rohrbach, J.M., Stiemer, R., Mayer A. Riedinger, C., Duijvestijn, A. and Zierhut, M., *Graefes Arch. Clin. Exp. Ophthalmol.* in print.
30. Bare, J.W., Lebo, R.V., and Epstein, E.H. Jr., *Cancer Res.* 52: 1494–1498, 1992.
31. Quinn, A.G., Sikkink, S., and Rccs, J.L., *Cancer Res.* 53. 4756–4759, 1994.
32. Stahle-Backdahl, M., *Nord. Med.* 110: 82–84, 1995.
33. Sahl, W.J. Jr., Snow, S.N., and Levine, N.S., *J. Am. Acad. Dermatol.* 30: 856–859, 1994.
34. Betti, R., Inselvini, E., Carducci, M., and Crosti, C., *Int. J. Dermatol.* 34: 174–176, 1995.
35. Deng, J.S., Brod, B.A., Saito, R., *et al.*, *J. Cutan. Pathol.* 23: 140–146, 1996.
36. Deng, J.S., Falo, L.D. Jr., Kim, B., *et al.*, *Am. J. Dermatopathol.* 20: 143–146, 1998.
37. Habets, J.M.W., Tank, B., Vuzevski, V.D., *et al.*, *J. Invest. Dermatol.* 90: 289–292, 1988.
38. Kooy, A.J.W., Tank, B., Vuzevski, V.D., *et al.*, *J. Pathol.* 184: 169–176, 1998.
39. Halliday, G.M., Patel, A., Hunt, M.J., *et al.*, *World J. Surg.* 19: 352–358, 1995.
40. Yasaka, N., Furue, M., and Tamaki, K., *J. Dermatol. Sci.* 11: 19–27, 1996.
41. Duijvestijn, A.M., Horst, E., Pals, S.T., Rouse, B.N., Steere, A.C., Picker, L.J., Meijer, C.J., and Butcher, E.C., *Am. J. Pathol.* 130: 147–155, 1988.
42. Matsuta, M., Kimura, S., Kosegawa, G., *et al.*, *J. Dermatol.* 23: 147–152, 1996.
43. Stamp, G.W.H., Nasim, M., Cardillo, M., *et al.*, *Br. J. Dermatol.* 129: 57–64, 1993.
44. Toth, D.P., Guenther, L.C., and Shum, D.T., *J. Dermatol. Sci.* 11: 36–40, 1996.
45. Dellon, A.L., *Plast. Reconstr. Surg.* 62: 37–48, 1978.
46. Weimar, V.M., Ceilley, R.I., and Goeken, J.A., *J. Am. Acad. Dermatol.* 2: 143–147, 1980.
47. Sivkova, N., Grigorov, L., and Kreissig, I., *Ophthalmologe* 91: 820–823, 1994.
48. Mayer, A., Wannke, B., Rohrbach, J.-M., Stiemer, R.H., Thiel, H.-J., and Zierhut, M., *Invest. Ophthalmol. Vis. Sci.* 40: S153, 1999.
49. Yamamura, M., Modlin, R.L., Ohmen, J.D., *et al.*, *J. Clin. Invest.* 91: 1005, 1993.
50. Yen, H.-T., Chiang, L.-C., Wen, K.-H., Tsai, C.-C., Yu, C.-L., and Yu, H.-S., *Arch. Dermatol. Res.* 288: 157–161, 1996.
51. Rivas, J.M., and Ullrich, S.E., *J. Immunol.* 159: 3865, 1992.

52. Bouwes Bavinck J.N., Vermeer, B.J., Van der Woude, F.J., *et al. N. Engl. J. Med.* 325: 843, 1991.

53. Edwards, L., Tucker, S.B., Perednia, D., Smiles, K.A., Taylor, E.L., Tanner, D.J., and Peets, E., *Arch. Dermatol.* 126: 1029–1032, 1990.

54. Cornell, R.C., Greenway, H.T., Tucker, S.B., Edwards L., Ashworth S., Vance J.C., Tanner, D.J., Taylor E.L., Smiles, K.A., and Peets, E.A., *J. Am. Acad. Dermatol.* 23: 694–700, 1990.

55. Ikic, D., Padovan, I., Pipic, N., Knezevic, M., Djakovic, N., Rode, B., Kosutic, I., and Belicza, M., *Pharmacol. Ther.* 30: 734–737, 1991.

55. Stenquist, B., Wennberg, A.-M., Gisslén, H., and Larkö, O., *J. Am. Acad. Dermatol.* 27: 65–69, 1992.

56. Kowalzick, L., Rogozinski, T., Schober, C., Fierlbeck, G., Mensing, H., Jablonska, S., Remy, W., Rassner, G., Stetter, C., and Brzoska, J., *Eur. J. Dermatol.* 4: 430–433, 1994.

57. Kowalzick, L., *Klinik und histologie des basalioms.* Springer, Berlin, pp. 173–181, 1997.

58. Buechner, S.A., Wernli, M., Harr, T., Hahn, S., Itin, P., and Erb, P., *J. Clin. Invest.* 100: 2691–2696, 1997.

K.P. DINGEMANS[a] AND P.K. DAS[a,b]

CD44 expression and invasiveness in basal cell carcinoma

Abstract

CD44 represents a family of cellular adhesion molecules that interact with different extracellular components and also with a number of growth factors. At the molecular level, the functional diversity of these molecules is associated with extensive alternative splicing and variable degrees of glycosylation. The interrelation of CD44 expression patterns with tumor growth and invasion is exemplified by our work on basal cell carcinoma. The present article represents an overview of the assessment of the varying expression pattern of CD44 (standard and variants) in the various forms of basal cell carcinoma. Our finding that the level of CD44 expression was closely related to the tumor growth pattern (and especially elevated in the thinnest, apparently invasive tumor strands) was greatly facilitated by the application of a simplified classification of basal cell carcinoma. The implications for the interaction of the tumor cells with the extracellular matrix and inflammatory cells are briefly discussed.

Keywords: Tumor, invasion, extracellular matrix, basal cell carcinoma, CD44 isoforms

Introduction

Cancers originating from epithelial cells are termed carcinomas. Most human cancers are carcinomas, presumably due to the facts that epithelia are frequently exposed to different types of physical and chemically induced trauma and that many epithelia undergo continuous cell renewal [1]. One of the carcinomas, basal cell carcinoma (BCC), constitutes the most common form of skin tumors in humans [2]. A wide range of histological growth patterns as well as highly variable rate of invasiveness is seen in BCC [3]. It is particularly this variability of invasive properties of BCC, which present problems to clinicians for treating these tumors effectively. Histopathologically, BCC are

Departments of [a]Pathology and [b]Dermatology, Academic Medical
Centre—University of Amsterdam, Meibergdreef 9, 1105 AZ Amsterdam,
The Netherlands. E-mails: k.p.dingemans@amc.uva.nl; p.k.das@amc.uva.nl

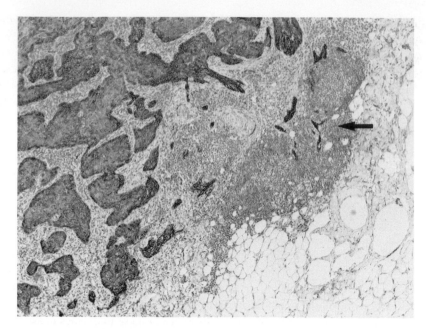

FIGURE 1. *Overview of BCC with predominant nodular growth pattern (left), but with exceedingly thin strands near tumor periphery (right). Notice dense inflammatory infiltrate at tumor periphery, closely associated with thinnest tumor cell strands. Treatment of section with anti-CD44v6 has resulted in heavy labeling of most peripheral strands (arrow), contrasting with weaker labeling of more compact nodules.*

recognised as aggregates of atypical basaloid cells surrounded by fibrous stroma and often a dense inflammatory infiltrate (Fig. 1). In BCC, like any other carcinoma, a basement membrane is often present between the tumor mass and the stroma [4].

The overall invasive process requires continuous modulation of a complex series of interactions between tumor cells and both inflammatory cells and extracellular matrix (ECM) components. In these co-operative processes, adhesion molecules, growth factors and their receptors, and proteolytic enzymes all play a role [5–10]. In this respect, experimental and clinical studies support a role for the family of CD44 glycoprotein adhesion molecules and *in situ* inflammatory responses in tumor invasiveness and prognosis, including that of BCC [10–12]. Several investigators found in BCC only a very low rate of CD44 expression in comparison to the normal epidermis [11–19]. This has been interpreted as indicating a small role (or even no role at all) in invasiveness in BCC and explaining the exceedingly low rate of metastasis in this tumor. In addition to exhibiting a low rate of metastasis, BCC also differs from many other carcinomas in respect to the many histopathological growth patterns that are often seen side by side within an individual tumor. This has led to often complex and controversial histopathological classifications [20]. In this overview, we present an assessment of the interrelation of CD44 expression,

K. P. Dingemans and P. K. Das

tumor growth pattern, and invasiveness. Such an assessment appeared feasible only when we applied a novel simple and straightforward classification encompassing only a limited number of categories.

Family of CD44 isoforms

Molecular aspects

The various forms of CD44 represent a family of cellular adhesive glycoprotein molecules that bind to various ECM components, notably hyaluronan. In fact, it belongs to a larger group of hyaluronan-binding proteins originally designated "hyal-adherins" [21]. The molecules are encoded by a single gene on the human chromosome 11 [22] and are composed of 19 exons as depicted in Fig. 2. This molecular and functional diversity is generated by alternative splicing that results in a number of variant CD44 molecules containing one or

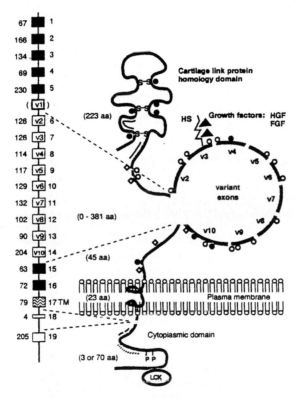

FIGURE 2. *Schematic features of CD44 gene and coded proteins. Note that alternative splicing results into variable sizes of both extracellular and cytoplasmic domains of CD44 isoforms with variable molecular sizes. HS: heparan sulphate; HGF: hepatocyte growth factor; FGF: fibroblast growth factor; round (open and closed) and square structures are sites of glycosylation.*

more different extracellular domains. In addition to exon splicing, glycosylation also contributes to further diversity of this molecule [22–24]. Although all CD44 isoforms contain the hyaluronan-binding domain, their avidity and affinity for hyaluronan varies. Importantly, the CD44 cytoplasmic tail associates with the action cytoskeleton via ankyrin and molecules of the endoplasmic reticulum motility family.

The detailed molecular characteristics of CD44 isoforms and its encoded proteins were reviewed in the literature in relation to the dissemination of cancer [25–30]. Briefly, the extracellular domain of CD44 variants contains putative glycosylation sites, heparan sulphate and chondroitin sulphate binding sites. Particularly, the heparan sulphate binding site in exon V3 also has the important ability to interact with hepatocyte growth factor/scatter factor (HGF/SF) and fibroblast growth factor (FGF). Furthermore, the CD44 isoforms, besides their hyaluronan-binding cytoplasmic domains and ankyrin molecules, contain putative interaction sites for the Src-family kinase p56lek as the transmembrane component. This latter domain is an important link for cellular signalling.

At present, 12 of the CD44 isoforms, containing 19 or 20 exons, are known to be differentially spliced. The membrane-associated CD44 isoforms have five constant spliced exons, at the N-terminus that is linked to 10 alternately spliced exons, two constant membrane-proximal exons, one constant transmembrane exon and two potentially alternately spliced exons coding for cytoplasmic domains. Such alternative splicing has resulted into at least 18 different variant CD44 transcripts carrying combinations of variable exons in addition to the standard exons [29–33]. The heterogeneity of the CD44 molecule appears to arise due to the variability in splicing and the differential N- and O-linked glycosylation that results into different glycosaminoglycan attachment sites [29,30,33,34].

Cellular expression of CD44 and biological function

Since it was reported that an alternatively spliced variant could be associated with the metastatic capacity to rat pancreatic carcinoma cell line [28], numerous studies have been published with regard to the role of CD44 in tumor progression and metastasis [24,26,35–37].

Several of the CD44 isoforms, including the standard type, are expressed in cells of mesenchymal and neuroectodermal origin, including keratinocytes [38] and fibroblasts [39], and haematopoietic cells [23,40], astrocytes and glial cells [41,42].

The vast majority of the cells expressing CD44 show the presence of the "standard" CD44 (CD44s) isoform, which is a product of standard exons [1–5, 23–25,27–31]. This principle isoform is usually expressed in haemopoetic cells whereas the larger sized variant isoforms are expressed in epithelial cells as well as in activated but not in resting lymphocytes [40]. In regard to the expression of CD44 on lymphocytes it is now believed that this family of molecules functions in lymphopoiesis [41], lymphocyte homing [42–45] and lymphocyte activation [9,38,45–49]. Particularly with regard to the latter, CD44 can function as an important co-stimulatory molecule leading to enhanced proliferation and cytokine release which in turn influence the cell surface CD44 expression and their interaction with the ECM [3,22,42–44,46].

It is now well recognised that CD44 functions as an important signalling molecule which is pivotal in both immune interaction and cancer biology [2,30,45]. Particularly, with regard to the expression of epithelial CD44, it has been suggested that this molecular species play an important role in relation to cell proliferation [47] and cell-cell contacts [45].

CD44 expression in human epidermis

Both the intricate interrelation of the epidermis with the underlying dermis and the relatively easy availability of human skin make this tissue an attractive model for studying CD44 expression patterns. Using immunocytochemical techniques, various investigators [11,13,15–18] showed that the stratum basale, the stratum spinosum and usually part of the stratum granulosum of the human epidermis express various CD44 isoforms, whereas the upper stratum granulosum and the stratum corneum are negative. Finally, the basal surface of the stratum basale, facing the basement membrane, was invariably found to be negative. The principle resident cells of human epidermis are the keratinocytes, which form over 90% of the epidermal cells. Langerhans cells and melanocytes are the main cell types found next to the keratinocytes.

Our previous observations (unpublished) showed that all the cells in suspensions of epidermal cells as well as in epidermal cells cultured *in vitro* express CD44 variants. *In situ* studies using immuno-double staining confirmed this observation, albeit that the keratinocytes exhibit a far higher expression than melanocytes and, especially, Langerhans cells [50; Dingemans *et al.*, in preparation]).

CD44 is expressed particularly at the lateral and apical surfaces, whereas no expression is found at the basal cell surface, facing the basement membrane [11]. These findings have been confirmed and extended by electron microscopy [50; Dingemans *et al.*, in preparation], which demonstrated that CD44 expression in the epidermis was virtually confined to the plasma membrane and that the highest expression was found at places where cells are not in close contact but are separated by a wide intracellular space. This suggests that the hyaluronan receptor function of CD44 is important in maintaining the intracellular space within the epidermis, which facilitates intraepidermal cellular motility as well as fluid exchange. Tuhkanen *et al.* [50] found the highest expression on spinous cells, suggesting that regulation of CD44 expression might be related to the detachment of cells from the basement membrane. The alterations in the normal morphogenesis that is associated with malignant transformation of cells also alters the neighbouring cell-matrix and cell-cell adhesion, and ultimately cell motility, which in turn can be related to altered expression patterns of CD44 in skin epithelia [9,38].

Studies on keratinocytes *in vitro* showed CD44 expression in filopodia, but not in focal adhesion sites, structures involved in the regulation of cell migration and adhesion to ECM molecules such as laminin and fibronectin [38]. However, the significance of *in vitro* findings for the *in vivo* situation remains to be established.

Splice variants in association with invasiveness and morphology of BCC

Several authors have reported on the status of CD44 expression by various non-cutaneous epithelia and its relation to cancer invasion and metastasis [e.g. 19,29, 51,52]. However, only very few reports on the expression of cutaneous epithelium are available (see references given above). In a recent publication from our laboratory [11], we quantitatively analysed the relation between CD44 expression in BCC and its histological growth pattern [11], partly because of this lack of data, but especially because of the extraordinary histopathological variability of BCC, outlined above. This variability is reflected in the large numbers of histological growth patterns distinguished in most diagnostic classifications of BCC. Thus, Heenan *et al.* [53] listed 10 patterns and Wade and Ackerman [54] even illustrate no less than 26 different patterns.

In order to take advantage of the superior morphology of paraffin-embedded tissue in comparison to that of frozen material, we collected 27 surgically resected, formalin-fixed and paraffin-embedded BCC from the files of the Department of Pathology of the Academic Medical Center. To increase the chance of finding two or more different growth patterns side by side within one tumor, we left out very small tumors (<4 mm) and biopsy specimens; furthermore, we preferentially selected cases in which the diagnostic report already mentioned the presence of more than one growth pattern. Careful re-examination of the original H&E sections revealed that only 7 of the 27 tumors selected were truly homogeneous.

One of the first requirements for a quantitative analysis as outlined above is a simple, straightforward and reproducible histopathological classification of BCC, encompassing only a limited number of categories. To this end, we first grouped the various histopathological pictures encountered into the three commonly occurring basic patterns, nodular, infiltrative, and superficial. This last pattern is often called "superficial multifocal", but several investigators have pointed out that tumors exhibiting it are not truly multifocal, their apparent multifocality stemming from the erroneous impression presented by two-dimensional histological sections [55]. During the course of the study, aberrant CD44 expression was observed in small tumor areas with an "adenoid" pattern; this pattern was therefore added later as a fourth category.

The criteria for the four histological growth patterns distinguished were as follows:

Nodular growth pattern (Fig. 3a): well-demarcated, but often irregular nodules, usually with regularly palisaded peripheral tumor cells. The nodules

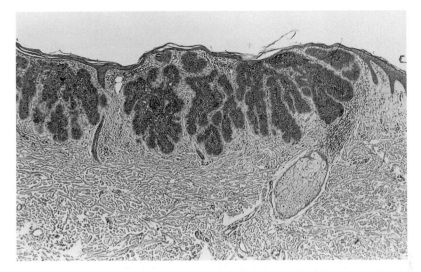

FIGURE 3A. *H&E staining of BCC, demonstrating basic growth patterns distinguished. From [11]. Reproduced by kind permission of the British Association of Dermatologists. Nodular growth pattern: irregular, but well-demarcated nodules. Notice little direct contact with overlying epidermis.*

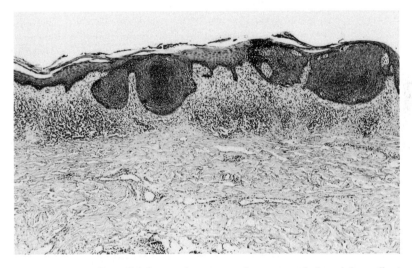

FIGURE 3B. *Superficial growth pattern: large, rounded nodules adhering closely to epidermis.*

had only very little contact with the overlying epidermis or with epidermal adnexes. In total, 22 tumor areas or whole tumors were classified as nodular.

Superficial growth pattern (Fig. 3b): separate (at least in the plane of the section), rounded and compact nodules closely attached to the epidermis or to the epidermal adnexes. Sometimes they were even partly invested by elongated

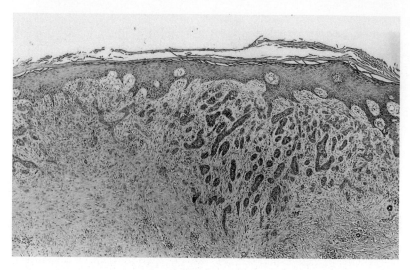

FIGURE 3C.   *Infiltrative growth pattern: tumor tissue made up of many separate, thin strands.*

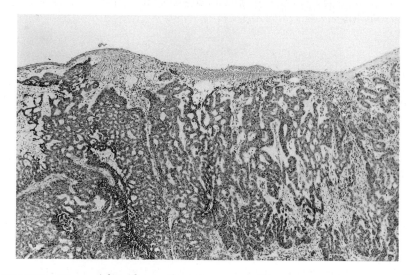

FIGURE 3D.   *Adenoid growth pattern: very thin, anastomosing tumor cell strands, resulting in reticulate pattern. Exceptionally large adenoid area is shown for sake of clarity. Overlying epidermis has disappeared.*

epidermal rete ridges. In total, 6 tumors or tumor areas were classified as superficial.

Infiltrative growth pattern (Fig. 3c): irregular strands lacking a palisading periphery. In total, 13 tumors or tumor areas were classified as infiltrative.

Adenoid growth pattern (Fig. 3d): irregular, very thin strands (frequently only one cell in diameter) in a reticulate pattern. Areas with this growth

K. P. Dingemans and P. K. Das

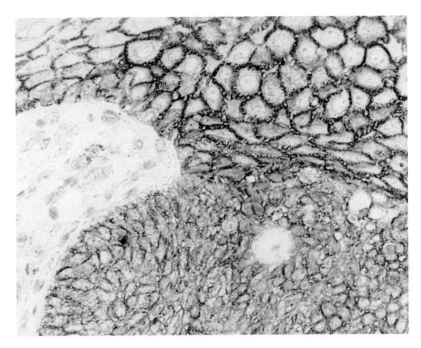

FIGURE 4. *Connection of superficial tumor nodule (bottom) with pre-existing epidermis (top). Labeling with anti-CD44v5 is more intense in epidermis than in tumor. Epidermal keratinocytes have larger size and more pronounced "cell bridges" than tumor cells. Basal surfaces of epidermal keratinocytes and tumor cells, facing surrounding connective tissue, has remained negative.*

pattern were usually small and frequently formed the connection between the epidermis and tumor tissue exhibiting one of the other growth patterns. In total, 12 areas were classified as adenoid.

In accordance with the literature [53], all tumors consisted of cells that were distinctly smaller than the keratinocytes in the normal epidermis and that had less conspicuous intercellular "bridges" (Fig. 4). All tumor cell groups were largely invested by a recognisable basement membrane; however, this was usually more continuous and prominent near the largest, most compact nodules than near the thinnest, most ill-defined strands. Interestingly, a dense lymphocytic or plasmocytic infiltrate was frequently found exactly at the places where such peripheral strands invaded the adjacent tissue (Figs 1, 5). In a number of tumors, thin tumor strands were found to invade adjacent structures like nerve sheaths (Fig. 6), erector pili muscles, and subcutaneous fat and muscle tissue.

We tested antisera against pan-CD44, CD44v3, CD44v5, CD44v6, CD44v7/8, and CD44v10 for their usefulness in immunohistochemical staining of paraffin sections. When a simple antigen-retrieval procedure was applied, most of these antisera produced strong and reliable labelling, *i.e.*: a. with

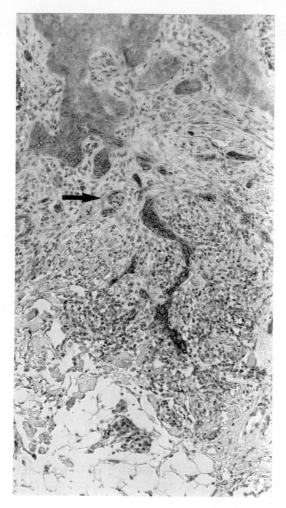

FIGURE 5. *Thin, peripheral, apparently invasive tumor cell strand, heavier labeled with anti-CD44v3 than more compact nodules (top), forming main tumor cell mass. Note dense infiltrate closely associated with thin tumor cell strand. Arrowhead indicates small nerve, shown at higher magnification in Fig. 6.*

a pattern fully identical to that found on frozen sections treated with the same antisera and b. with an identical labelling pattern of the pre-existent epidermis that was present in every tissue block and served as an internal control. Only the results obtained when paraffin sections were treated with the antisera directed against CD44v7/8 and CD44v10 consistently differed from those in frozen material. The value of the latter two antisera was therefore disputable [15] and they were omitted from the present investigation.

Both in the tumor tissue and in the pre-existent epidermis, the labelling of all CD44 isoforms was restricted to the cell surfaces. In the epidermis, all cell

K. P. Dingemans and P. K. Das

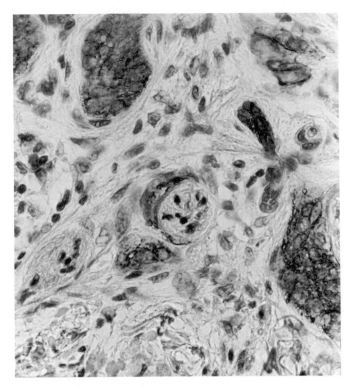

FIGURE 6. *Detail of Fig. 5. Small nerve, largely surrounded by sheath of CD44v3-positive tumor cells, can be seen between irregular tumor cell strands.*

surfaces in the stratum basale, the stratum spinosum and usually part of the stratum granulosum were labelled, with the exception or the basal surface of the cells in the stratum basale, facing the basement membrane; the stratum corneum was always negative. Also in the tumor tissue, the peripheral cell surfaces facing the surrounding stroma were always negative (Fig. 4) (except for the two exceptional situations discussed below). Unexpectedly, the *distribution* of the label obtained with the different isoforms used was fully identical, with the exception of pan-CD44 which was positive not only on epithelial cells, but on many stromal cells as well. With all CD44 isoforms used, the staining *intensity* on the tumor tissue was considerably weaker than that found on the pre-existent epidermis in the same section. Compact tumor nodules (those forming part of the nodular growth pattern as well as those in the superficial growth pattern) were labelled rather homogeneously. There were, however, two intriguing exceptions: (a) palisading peripheral cells were often labelled more intensively than the remainder of the nodule, especially when the nodule was irregularly shaped (Fig. 7); (b) in the nodular growth pattern, but not in the superficial growth pattern, the labelling of tumor areas located very near to the epidermis was usually stronger than that of deeper areas, and sometimes even approached that of the epidermis (Fig. 8).

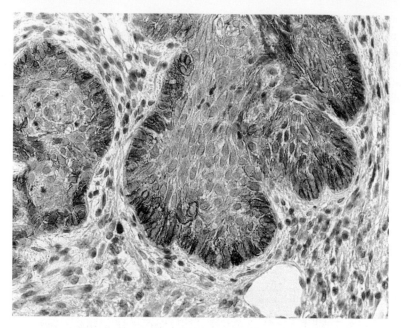

FIGURE 7. *Irregularly shaped tumor nodules, labeled with anti-CD44v3. Note heavy label on peripheral row of palisading tumor cells. From [11]. Reproduced by kind permission of the British Association of Dermatologists.*

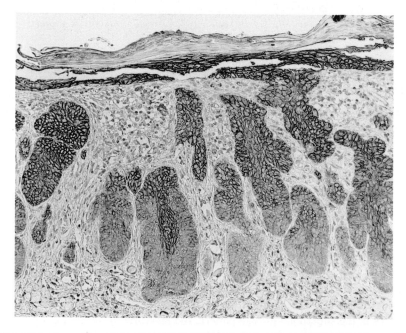

FIGURE 8. *Overview of nodular BCC, labeled with anti-CD44v5. Note relatively strong staining of parts of tumor nodules located near epidermis (top).*

K. P. Dingemans and P. K. Das

Thin tumor strands (those forming part of the infiltrative growth pattern as well as those forming part of the adenoid growth pattern) showed a labelling intensity that was considerably higher than that found on compact nodules (although still far below that in the epidermis). Also here, there was an intriguing phenomenon: the thinnest, most peripheral strands or peripherally located small tumor cell groups, apparently detached from the main tumor mass, were labelled with an intensity that even surpassed that of the other strands (Figs 6, 9).

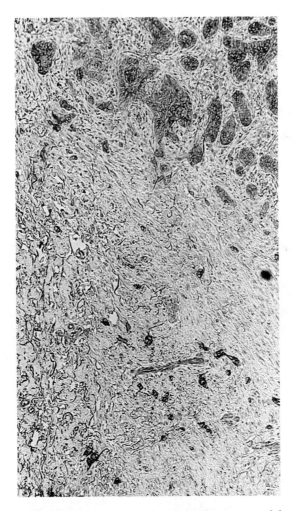

FIGURE 9.   *Most of tumor tissue (top) consists of compact nodules, only weakly stained with anti-CD44v5. However, area at bottom of figure, located at distance of main tumor mass, contains numerous exceedingly small, irregular, and apparently detached tumor cell groups that are stained much heavier. From [11]. Reproduced by kind permission of the British Association of Dermatologists.*

In short, an obvious relation seemed to exist between the degree of compactness of the tumor cell groups and the intensity of the CD44 labelling, the thinnest strands showing the highest intensity. Quantitative analysis of the labelling intensities of all 53 individual tumor areas studied showed that this relation was statistically highly significant.

Apart from their exceptionally strong labelling, the thinnest tumor strands mentioned above also showed an aberrant distribution of the label: in both situations, it seemed to be present not only on cell surfaces facing adjacent tumor cells, but also on those facing the surrounding stroma [11] (Fig. 10).

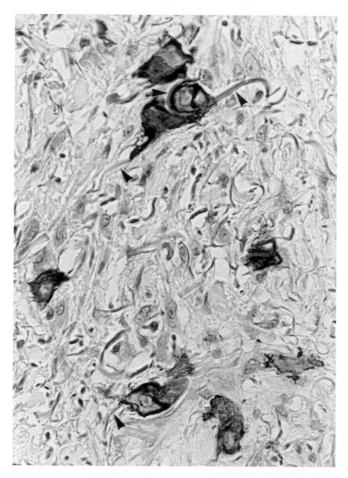

FIGURE 10. *Detail of bottom area of preceding illustration, showing irregularity of tiny tumor cell groups. Note heavy labeling of what seems to be outer tumor cell surface, facing thick collagen fibers (arrow heads) in surrounding connective tissue. From [11]. Reproduced by kind permission of the British Association of Dermatologists.*

K. P. Dingemans and P. K. Das

Concluding remarks

Our results demonstrate that BCC do express CD44 at a significant level. Furthermore, the rate of expression is obviously related to the tumor growth pattern (basically: low in the compact, apparently non-invasive nodules *vs.* high in the thin, apparently invasive strands). These findings strongly suggest an important role of CD44 in BCC invasiveness. However, the underlying mechanism has yet to be detected.

Previous investigators, reporting an insignificant CD44 labelling in BCC, or even no labelling at all, may have been biased by the presence of the far more strongly labelled epidermis in every specimen. A second factor is presumably the fact that many previous authors did not apply an antigen retrieval procedure to visualise CD44 labelling.

One approach to further assess the role of CD44 in BCC invasivity is a detailed ultrastructural study of the distribution of CD44. Our provisional ultrastructural findings are not only in keeping with the light microscopic findings, but they also confirm the increased CD44 expression at the tumor–stroma interface precisely in apparently invasive areas, that could not be proven, but only suspected at the light microscopic level.

Acknowledgements

We would like to convey thanks for the technical assistance to Marja Ramkema, Cynthia Lehé, and for advise on the clinical pathological classification to dr. Allard van der Wal.

This work is part of the research programmes ODP 9 and ODP 10 of the Jan van Loghem Immunology Institute, Academic Medical Centre, University of Amsterdam, The Netherlands.

References

1. Alberts, B., Bray, D., Lewis, J., Roberts, K., and Watson, J.D. (eds.), *Molecular Biology of the Cell*, 3rd ed., Gerland Publishing Inc., 1994.
2. Miller, S.J., *J. Am. Acad. Dermatol.* 24: 1–13, 1991.
3. Mackie, R.M., *Textbook of Dermatology*, 5th ed., Vol. 2, Champion, R.H., Burton, J.L., and Ebling, F.J.G. (eds.), 1488–1495, Blackwell Scientific Publications, Oxford, 1992.
4. Stetler-Stevenson, W.G., Aznavoorian, S., and Liotta, L.A., *Annu. Rev. Cell Biol,* 9: 541–573, 1993.
5. Fishman, D.A., Chilukuri, K., and Stack, M.S., *Gynec. Oncol.* 67: 193–199, 1997.
6. Fligial, S.E.G., and Varani, J., *Invasion Metastasis* 13: 225–233, 1993.
7. Fridman, R., Scott, A.F., Muller, D., Reich, R., and Penno, M.B., *Invasion Metastasis* 10: 208–224, 1990.
8. Varani, J., Perone, P., Inman, D.R., Bumeister, W., Schollenberger, S.B., Fligiel, S.E.G., Sitrin, R.G., and Johnson, K.J., *Am. J. Pathol.* 146: 210–217, 1995.

9. Knudson, C.B., and Knudson, W., *FASEB J.* 7: 1233–1241, 1994.

10. Baum, H.P., Schmidt, T., Shock, G., and Reichrath, J., *Br. J. Dermatol.* 134: 465–468, 1996.

11. Dingemans, K.P., Ramkema, M.D., Koopman, G., van der Wal, A.C., Das, P.K., and Pals, S.T., *Br. J. Dermatol.* 140: 17–25, 1999.

12. Hunt, M.J., Halliday, G.M., Weedon, D., Cooke, B.E., and Barnetson, R.S.C., *Br. J. Dermatol.* 130: 1–8, 1994.

13. Seelentag, W.K.F., Günthert, U., Saremaslani, P., *et al.*, *Int. J. Cancer.* 69: 218–244, 1996.

14. Guttinger, M., Sutti, F., Barnier, C., *et al.*, *Eur. J. Dermatol.* 5: 398–406, 1995.

15. Dietrich, A., Tanczos, E., Vanscheidt, W., *et al.*, *J. Cutan. Pathol.* 24: 37–42, 1007.

16. Hale, L.P., Patel, D.D., Clark, R.E., and Haynes, B.F., *J. Cutan. Pathol.* 22: 536–545, 1995.

17. Seiter, S., Tilgen, W., Herrmann, K., *et al.*, *Virchows Arch.* 428: 141–149, 1996.

18. Terpe, H.J., Stark, H., Prehm, P., and Günthert, U., *Histochemistry* 101: 79–89, 1994.

19. Mackay, C.R., Terpe, H.J., Stauder, R., *et al.*, *J. Cell Biol.* 124: 71–82, 1994.

20. Sexton, M., Jones, D.B., and Haloney, M.E., *J. Am. Acad. Dermatol.* 23: 1118–1126, 1995.

21. Toole, B.P., *Curr. Opin. Cell Biol.* 2: 839–844, 1990.

22. Lesley, J., Hyman, R., and Kincade, P.W., *Adv. Immunol.* 54: 271–335, 1993.

23. Stamenkovic, I., Amiot, M., Pessando, J.M., and Seed, B.A., *Cell* 56: 1057–1062, 1989.

24. Dougherty, G.J., Lansdorp, P.M., Cooper, D.L., and Humpries, R.K., *J. Exp. Med.* 174: 1–5, 1991.

25. Underhill, C., *J. Cell Sci.* 103: 293–298.

26. Herrlich, P., Zöller, M., Pals, S.T., and Ponta, H., *Immunol. Today* 14: 395–401, 1993.

27. Naor, D., Vogt Sionov, R., and Ish-Shalom, D., *Adv. Cancer Res.* 71: 241–259, 1997.

28. Günthert, U., Hofmann, M., Rudy, W., *et al.*, *Cell* 65: 13–21, 1991.

29. Wielenga, V.J.M., Heider, K.H., Offerhaus, G.J.A., *et al.*, *Cancer Res.* 53: 4754–4762, 1993.

30. Drillenburg, P., and Pals, S.T., *Blood* 95: 1900–1910.

31. Screaton, G.R., Bell, M.V., Bell, J.I. and Jackson, D.G., *J. Biol.Chem.* 268: 12235–12243, 1993.

32. Tolg, C., Hofmann, M., Herrlich, P., and Ponta, H., *Nucleic Acids Res.* 21: 1225–1229, 1993.

33. Jalkanen, S., and Jalkanen, N., *J. Cell. Biol.* 116: 817–830, 1992.

34. Jackson, D.G., Bell, J.L., Dickinson, *et al.*, *J. Cell Biol.* 128: 673–685.

35. Günthert, U., Stauder, R., Meyer, B., *et al.*, *Cancer Surv.* 24: 19–30, 1995.

36. Imazaki, F., Yokosuka, O., Yamaguchi, T., *et al.*, *Gastroenterology* 110: 362–372, 1996.

37. Combaret, V., Gross, N., Lasset, *et al.*, *J. Clin. Oncol.* 14: 25–38, 1996.

38. Brown, T.A., Bouchard, T., St. John, T., *et al.*, *J. Cell Biol.* 113: 207–221, 1991.

39. Green, S.J., Tarone, G., and Underhill, C.B., *Exp. Cell Res.* 178: 224–238, 1988.

40. Koopman, G., Heider, K.H., Horst, E., *et al.*, *J. Exp. Med.* 177: 897–904, 1993.

41. Girgrah, N., Lekarte, M., Becker, L.E., *et al.*, *J. Neuropathol. Exp. Neurol.* 50: 779–792, 1991.

42. Vogel, H., Butcher, E.C., and Picker, L.J., *J. Neurocytol.* 21: 363–373, 1992.

K. P. Dingemans and P. K. Das

43. Jalkanen, S., Bargatze, R.F., Herron, L.R., and Butcher, E.C., *Eur. J. Immunol.* 16: 1195–1202, 1986.
44. Denning, S.M., Le, P.T., Singer, L.H., and Haynes, B.F., *J. Immunol.* 144: 7–15, 1990.
45. Picker, L.J., Nakache, M., and Butcher, E.C., *J. Cell Biol.* 109: 927–937, 1989.
46. Taher, T.E.L., Smits, L., Griffioen, A.W., *et al.*, *J. Biol. Chem.* 271: 2863–2867, 1996.
47. Alho, A.M., and Underhill, C.B., *J. Cell Biol.* 108: 1057–1565, 1989.
48. Mulder, J.W.R., Kruyt, P.M., Sewnath, M., *et al.*, *Lancet* 344: 1470–1472, 1994.
49. Wang, C., Tammi, M., and Tammi, R., *Histochemistry* 98: 105–112, 1992.
50. Tuhkanen, A.L., Tammi, M., Pelttari, A., *et al.*, *J. Histochem. Cytochem.* 46: 241–248, 1998.
51. Heider, K.H., Hofmann, M., Horst, E., *et al.*, *J. Cell Biol.* 120: 227–233, 1993.
52. Fox, S.B., Fawcett, J., Jackson, D.G., *et al.*, *Cancer Res.* 54: 4539–4546, 1994.
53. Heenan, P.J., Elder, D.E., and Sobin, L.H., *Histological Typing of Skin Tumors*, 2nd ed., Springer, 1996.
54. Wade, T.R., and Ackerman, A.B., *J. Dermatol. Surg. Oncol.* 4: 23–28, 1978.
55. Madsen, A., *Acta Pathol. Microbiol. Scand. Suppl.* 177: 3–63, 1965.

PAUL FISCH

Recognition of lymphoma cells by human γδ T lymphocytes

Abstract

The biological role of γδ T cells is still unclear. Human lymphocytes expressing the variable region genes Vγ9 and Vδ2 are the major subpopulation of γδ T cells in human blood. Vγ9/Vδ2 T cells are stimulated by non-peptidic antigens contained in some bacterial extracts and by the HLA class I-deficient Burkitt's lymphoma Daudi. Recent data suggest that human Vγ9/Vδ2 T cells recognize most human B-cell lymphomas, but that the γδ T-cell activation following stimulation by HLA class I-expressing lymphoma cells is downmodulated by inhibitory natural killer cell receptors that are expressed by most human Vγ9/Vδ2 T cells. Thus, Vγ9/Vδ2 T cells may represent a natural defense system against B-cell lymphomas that is primed in childhood by the activation and expansion of Vγ9/Vδ2 T lymphocytes in response to non-peptidic bacterial antigens.

Keywords: γδ T lymphocytes, γδ T-cell receptor, natural killer cells, B-cell lymphomas

Introduction

Human T cells expressing the T-cell receptor of γδ-type typically comprise less than 5% of lymphocytes in the peripheral blood. Since their discovery, γδ T cells were known to mediate "lymphokine activated killer" (LAK) activity against tumor cells, comparable to lysis by activated natural killer (NK) cells [1,2]. Strong cytolysis of the MHC class I deficient cell lines K562 and Daudi by IL-2 activated NK cells and γδ T cells could be explained on the basis of the "missing self" hypothesis [3,4]. This hypothesis described the inverse correlation of HLA class I expression and sensitivity to cytolysis. Tumor cells frequently show diminished expression of HLA class I or lose expression of particular HLA class I alleles. The discovery of natural killer cell receptors (NKR) for HLA class I provided the molecular explanation for the "missing self hypothesis" [5]. Most of these NKR function as killer inhibitory receptors (KIR). They transmit

Department of Pathology, University of Freiburg Medical Center,
79114 Freiburg, Germany

inhibitory signals to killer cells upon binding of particular self-HLA class I alleles. It appears that MHC unrestricted killer cells with strong cytolytic potential express at least one KIR for a self-HLA class I molecule, so that autologous cells generally remain unharmed. Killer cells expressing inhibitory NKR will destroy autologous tumor cells that have lost expression of all MHC class I alleles or that have lost a class I allele which is most inhibitory for a given clone of killer cells. NKR have been detected on most NK cells and on many cytotoxic $\gamma\delta$ T lymphocytes, but only rarely on cytotoxic $\alpha\beta$ T cells. Two main subsets of $\gamma\delta$ T lymphocytes can be detected in human blood. Most human $\gamma\delta$ T cells belong to the Vγ9/Vδ2 subset while a minor subset expresses Vδ1 paired with different Vγ genes. NKR are expressed by the vast majority of human Vγ9/Vδ2 T lymphocytes, but rarely by $\gamma\delta$ T cells of the Vδ1 subset [6–8]. This article reviews the current knowledge on the function of human $\gamma\delta$ T lymphocytes and discusses the controversial role of the TCR $\gamma\delta$ in target cell recognition.

Recognition of Daudi and phosphoantigens by Vγ9/Vδ2, but not Vδ1 T cells

In an effort to characterize antigens recognized by $\gamma\delta$ T cells we initially analyzed many $\gamma\delta$ T-cell clones and compared them to NK clones derived from the same individuals [9]. We studied the specificity of these clones against the Burkitt's lymphomas Daudi and Raji. Unexpectedly, the $\gamma\delta$ T-cell clones mediated a different pattern of MHC unrestricted cytotoxic activity than the NK clones: Practically all $\gamma\delta$ T-cell clones were highly cytotoxic against the β_2-microglobulin (β_2m) deficient Burkitt's lymphoma Daudi while they virtually failed to lyse the HLA class I$^+$ Burkitt's lymphoma Raji. In contrast, most NK clones killed Daudi and Raji equally well. Because of the missing-self hypothesis, we first considered that the strong cytolysis by $\gamma\delta$ T cells of Daudi but not Raji cells, might be due to the absence of HLA class I on Daudi. However, most NK clones killed Daudi and Raji equally well and an HLA class I-expressing Daudi variant, transfected with the mouse β_2m gene, was strongly killed by the $\gamma\delta$ T-cell clones. Thus, we first concluded that missing expression of HLA class I by Daudi was probably not the main reason for the peculiar specificity of the $\gamma\delta$ T-cell clones [9]. We thought that the TCR $\gamma\delta$ itself might be involved in the recognition of Daudi cells by human Vγ9/Vδ2 T lymphocytes.

In subsequent experiments we found proliferative responses of the Vγ9/Vδ2 T-cell clones towards Daudi cells *in vitro*, although these clones have never been in contact with Daudi cells before [10]. The type of "feeder cells", i.e. autologous or allogeneic lymphocytes or lymphoblastoid B-cell lines, used to derive such clones did not affect the specificity of the $\gamma\delta$ T-cell clones [9]. These Vγ9/Vδ2 T-cell clones were not "alloreactive". Moreover, when lymphocytes from normal donors were cultured in the presence of irradiated Daudi cells, Vγ9/Vδ2 T cells proliferated in these cultures [10,11]. The specificity for Daudi cells was restricted to Vγ9/Vδ2 T cells because Vδ1

T cells did not proliferate to Daudi and the vast majority of IL-2 expanded Vδ1 T-cell clones failed to kill Daudi cells *in vitro* [11].

All Daudi-reactive Vγ9/Vδ2 T cells, but not the Vδ1 lymphocytes and Vδ1 clones also proliferated to certain preparations of bacterial antigens [10,12]. The response of human Vγ9/Vδ2 T-cell clones to bacterial antigens required antigen presenting cells (APC), but not the expression of HLA class I A, B, C, or HLA class II DR, DP, DQ or the TAP1 and TAP2 peptide transporter genes on the APC [10]. Intracellular antigen processing was not required because fixed APC also presented the bacterial antigens to Vγ9/Vδ2 T cells [10]. Initially, we and other assumed that the mycobacterial antigens recognized by human γδ T cells were heat shock proteins (hsps) [10,13,14], but subsequent studies convincingly demonstrated the non-peptidic organic nature of these molecules that carried phosphate groups [1,15]. Thus, these soluble ligands for γδ T cells within bacterial antigen preparations were designated "phosphoantigens".

Recognition of Daudi-hybrids by Vγ9/Vδ2 T cells

Our hypothesis was that human Vγ9/Vδ2 lymphocytes recognized an undefined ligand expressed by Daudi cells, but not by other lymphoma cells, such as Raji. We asked if this "Daudi-γδ-stimulatory phenotype" represented a dominant or a recessive trait. To address this question, we tested hybrids of Daudi cells, such as Daudi × melanoma or Daudi × Burkitt's lymphoma hybrids for their recognition by human Vγ9/Vδ2 T cells [6,16]. The deficient HLA class I expression of Daudi was restored in all Daudi hybrids because the missing β_2m-synthesis of Daudi cells was complemented by the fusion partners. Thus, the hybrids expressed the HLA class I alleles of Daudi and the fusion partners. To our surprise the "Daudi-γδ-stimulatory phenotype" was suppressed in the Daudi × lymphoma hybrids when analyzing the proliferative responses of fresh human lymphocytes. While after one week of mixed lymphocyte cultures of lymphocytes from particularly responsive donors with irradiated Daudi cells more than 50% of the proliferating T cells expressed the Vγ9/Vδ2 TCR, there were generally less than 10% of γδ T cells in similar cultures stimulated by the Daudi-hybrids. When examining cytolysis, the Daudi-hybrids were generally resistant to lysis by cytotoxic Vγ9/Vδ2 T-cell clones. Similarly, an HLA class I$^+$ Daudi variant transfected with the human β_2m gene was fairly resistant to lysis by the γδ T-cell clones [6]. These HLA class I$^+$ Daudi cells expressed about 10 times higher levels of HLA class I than the mouse β_2m transfected Daudi cells which we had studied earlier [9]. In "mixed lymphocyte-Daudi cell cultures", this HLA class I$^+$ Daudi variant induced expansion of lower percentages of Vγ9/Vδ2 T cells than the parental Daudi cells. Thus, it appeared that the *in vitro* proliferative responses of γδ T cells to Daudi cells, as well as cytolysis by cytotoxic clones depended on the absence of HLA class I on Daudi Burkitt's lymphoma cells: Restoration of HLA class I by fusion to β_2m-expressing cells or by transfection of Daudi cells with β_2m markedly reduced or even virtually abolished the "Daudi γδ-stimulatory phenotype".

Recognition of B-cell lymphomas by Vγ9/Vδ2 T cells

In parallel, we examined γδ T-cell recognition of a large panel of B-cell lymphomas (BL), mostly Burkitt's lymphomas. When these BL were tested for their capacity to expand γδ T cells freshly isolated from human blood, none of a panel of more than 30 BL tested expanded γδ T cells from normal donors at a level comparable to that of Daudi cells [6]. Since all these BL expressed HLA class I, this suggested that the absence of HLA class I at the cell surface of Daudi cells might be related to the "Daudi-γδ-stimulatory phenotype". However, recognition of Daudi cells by human γδ T cells was not merely a consequence of missing $\beta_2 m$ because three other surface HLA class I non-expressing solid tumor cell lines that also lacked $\beta_2 m$, the melanomas FO-1 and SK-MEL-33, as well as the colon carcinoma HCT failed to induce expansion of γδ T cells from freshly isolated lymphocytes *in vitro* [6].

Recognition of Daudi-hybrids and B-cell lymphomas by CD4$^+$ Vγ9/Vδ2 T-cell clones

Rare Vγ9/Vδ2 T-cell clones express CD4 and these clones produce lymphokines upon stimulation with Daudi cells [17]. We derived such "helper" γδ T-cell clones from a normal donor and tested them for recognition of Daudi cells, the Daudi-hybrids and the B-cell lymphomas described above [6]. We found that for these clones the "Daudi-γδ-stimulatory phenotype" seemed to be dominantly expressed in the hybrids: The Daudi-hybrids induced secretion of tumor necrosis factor (TNF) and granulocyte-macrophage colony stimulating factor (GM-CSF) by the helper Vγ9/Vδ2 T-cell clones, comparable to their secretion of TNF and GM-CSF in response to Daudi cells. Thus, the "Daudi-γδ-stimulatory phenotype" was recognized in a dominant fashion in Daudi hybrids by such rare γδ T-cell clones. In addition, these clones secreted TNF in response to most B-cell lymphomas within our large panel of B-cell lymphomas, as well as to HLA class I$^+$ variant Daudi cells. However, these clones did not produce TNF in response to K562 cells and cell lines from solid tumors, including the $\beta_2 m$-deficient cell lines mentioned above. Thus, Daudi cells were not special in their recognition by CD4$^+$ Vγ9/Vδ2 T-cell clones, but that these CD4$^+$ Vγ9/Vδ2 T-cell clones produced lymphokines in response to most, although not all, BL.

Expression and function of natural killer cell receptors by human γδ T lymphocytes

Most cytotoxic Vγ9/Vδ2 T-cell clones showed decreased lysis of HLA class I-expressing Daudi-hybrids and HLA class I$^+$ variant Daudi cells, as compared to the parental $\beta_2 m$-deficient Daudi cell line. Thus, cytolysis by cytotoxic Vγ9/Vδ2 T-cell clones was negatively regulated by HLA class I expression on the target cells (Fig. 1 A–C). Most of the cytotoxic Vγ9/Vδ2 T-cell clones

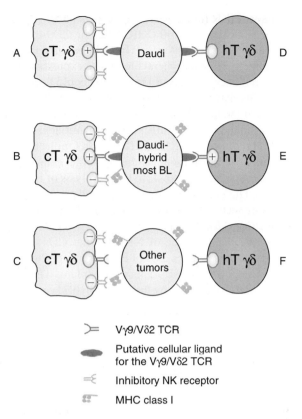

A — cT γδ (+) — Daudi — hT γδ — D

B — cT γδ (+) — Daudi-hybrid most BL — (+) hT γδ — E

C — cT γδ ( ) — Other tumors — hT γδ — F

>= Vγ9/Vδ2 TCR

Putative cellular ligand for the Vγ9/Vδ2 TCR

Inhibitory NK receptor

MHC class I

FIGURE 1.   *Hypothetical model for the recognition of tumor cells by Vγ9/Vδ2 T lymphocytes. (A) The majority of human cytotoxic Vγ9/Vδ2 T cells (cT γδ) express diverse NKR for HLA class I. These T cells kill Daudi and proliferate to Daudi, presumably via TCR mediated recognition of a yet uncharacterized ligand. Lymphoma variants in vivo may show low expression of some or all HLA class I alleles and this would make them susceptible to this NK-like mechanism of immunosurveillance. (B) In vitro derived Daudi-hybrids and most BL cultured in vitro show high level of HLA class I expression. They also express the putative Vγ9/Vδ2 TCR ligand. Since cytotoxic Vγ9/Vδ2 T cells express NKR that transmit negative signals to the killer cells, most of such BL and the Daudi-hybrids are insensitive to lysis by these Vγ9/Vδ2 T-cell clones and they do not stimulate their proliferation. (C) Other tumor cells (solid tumors and perhaps Raji, K562) may not express the putative ligand and, regardless of their HLA class I expression, they are not specifically recognized by Vγ9/Vδ2 T cells (although they may be killed by IL-2 activated clones via an NK-like mechanism in the case of HLA deficient tumor cells). (D, E) CD4+ helper Vγ9/Vδ2 T cells (hT γδ) do not express NKR and do not display cytolytic activity in vitro. They secrete lymphokines after stimulation by Daudi cells and most other B-cell lymphomas, presumably by recognition of the same unknown ligand Since they do not express NKR, these clones are not inhibited by HLA class I expression. (F) They do not recognize tumor cells that do not express the ligand. + and − indicate activating (positive) and inhibitory (negative) signals.*

expressed inhibitory NKR for HLA class I, such as p58.1 (KIR2DL1), p58.2 (KIR2DL3), p70 (KIR3DL1), p140 (KIR3DL2) or CD94 with most clones expressing several different receptors [6]. In addition, unstimulated Vγ9/Vδ2 T cells isolated directly from peripheral blood also expressed NKR [6]. These KIR were functional because lysis of Daudi cells could be strongly inhibited by monoclonal antibodies (mAb) against these KIR. The likely mechanism of this inhibition is that the mAb against KIR are crosslinked by Fc-receptors on Daudi cells. Crosslinked anti-KIR mAb then transmit negative signals to the T cells, similar to binding of the KIR to HLA class I molecules, the "natural" receptor of the KIR [6]. In addition, incubating target cells with certain anti-HLA class I mAb, such as mAb A6-136, induced lysis of target cells such as the Daudi-hybrids, HLA class I$^+$ variant Daudi cells or some BL, suggesting that HLA class I molecules protect such target cells from lysis by cytotoxic Vγ9/Vδ2 T-cell clones [18].

When examining the presence of NKR by the CD4$^+$ Vγ9/Vδ2 T-cell clones, we found that these clones did not express any of the known KIR, nor did they express CD94 (Fig. 1D–F). This may explain, why the CD4$^+$ Vγ9/Vδ2 T-cell clones were stimulated by the Daudi-hybrids and most of the BL, just as they were stimulated by Daudi cells. Similarly to the CD4$^+$ Vγ9/Vδ1 T-cell clones, most γδ T-cell clones expressing Vδ1 did not express NKR. The presence of NKR on most fresh that is, non-activated Vγ9/Vδ2 lymphocytes, may provide an explanation for the peculiar proliferative responses of Vγ9/Vδ2 T cells to Daudi cells. Although yet unproven, these NKR may prevent in vitro proliferation of freshly isolated γδ T cells to the Daudi-hybrids, as well as to HLA class I expressing BL.

Is the specificity of human γδ T cells determined by the T-cell receptor or the NKR?

The specificity for Daudi and the bacterial phosphoantigens correlates with the use of the Vγ9/Vδ2 TCR because Vδ1-expressing γδ T-cell clones generally do not recognize Daudi cells. In addition, CD4$^+$ γδ T-cell clones that are devoid of known NKR also show specificity for Daudi cells, while they do not secrete lymphokines upon stimulation with K562 cells (if tested under "resting conditions" that is, several weeks after the last stimulation with feeder cells). The CDR3 regions of the γ- and δ-chains from Vγ9/Vδ2 T cells in peripheral blood that can be expanded in vitro by Daudi cells and bacterial phosphoantigens have been analyzed in detail and revealed polyclonal junctional segments of the TCR γ- and δ-chains [19]. However, despite this heterogeneity, almost all Vδ2 J-sequences from peripheral, but not thymic Vγ9/Vδ2 clones carry a distinct motif consisting of a hydrophobic residue (Val, Leu, or Ile) at a conserved position ($δ^{97}$) within CDR3 of the δ-chain [20]. This raises the possibility that circulating Vγ9/Vδ2 T cells are selected and expanded by in vivo ligands that may be homologous to those expressed by Daudi cells and/or the bacterial phosphoantigens [8]. TCR mediated specificity for such *in vivo* antigens may explain why Vγ9/Vδ2 T cells are selectively expanded in peripheral blood in the first life decade, as compared to Vδ1 T cells. Importantly, transfer of the Vγ9/Vδ2 TCR in Jurkat cells resulted in specific IL-2 secretion of the transfected Jurkat cells in response to phosphoantigens, Daudi and RPMI 8226 cells [21,22]. Although the IL-2 secretion of these transfectants in response to Daudi and RPMI 8226 was fairly low [21], it appeared to be specific and represents the strongest available hint that the Vγ9/Vδ2 TCR is directly involved in the recognition of Daudi cells and phosphoantigens. Blocking studies with mAb against the Vγ9/Vδ2 TCR cannot prove this direct involvement of the TCR in antigen recognition because of the possibility of transmitting negative signals by binding of non-crosslinked mAb to T-cell activating structures.

In contrast, there is also some basis for the view that the specificity for Daudi cells by human Vγ9/Vδ2 T cells might not depend on the TCR: Vδ1-expressing γδ T-cell clones naturally display lower levels of cytotoxicity, as compared to Vδ2-expressing clones. Thus, lysis of the NK-resistant Daudi cells by Vδ2 T-cell clones might simply reflect the higher cytolytic capacity of these clones. Indeed, a few γδ T-cell clones expressing Vγ9 and Vδ1 also killed Daudi cells [23,24] and it is possible that these rare clones simply had higher cytotoxic abilities, comparable to NK cells that also display Daudi-lysis if activated by IL-2. Thus, it is possible that cytolysis of Daudi, stimulation of proliferation or lymphokine secretion by HLA class I⁻ Daudi cells or phosphoantigens may be unrelated to the Vγ9/Vδ2 TCR itself [8]. Then, the Vγ9/Vδ2 T-cell subset including the rare CD4⁺ Vγ9/Vδ2 T-cell clones, might simply be a T-cell subset that is naturally highly cytotoxic and easily aroused. Upon contact with Daudi cells the NKR⁺ cytotoxic Vγ9/Vδ2 T cells might be stimulated only by the absence of negative signals from the NKR [8]. These cells and the CD4⁺ Vγ9/Vδ2 T-cell clones might be activated by most B-cell lymphomas through B-cell costimulatory molecules. Finally, phosphoantigens might activate T cells by binding to T-cell surface structures distinct from the TCR, but the Vγ9/Vδ2 T-cell population might be more responsive than other T-cell subsets.

Conclusion: NKR on γδ T cells—implications for tumor immunity

γδ T-cell clones with high lytic potential towards Daudi cells express inhibitory NKR while CD4⁺ Vγ9/Vδ2 T-cell clones and Vδ1 T-cell clones that are non-cytolytic do not express KIR. A hypothetical model for the recognition of a common ligand for Vγ9/Vδ2 T cells is presented in Fig. 1. The peculiar proliferative responses of human Vγ9/Vδ2 T cells to Daudi cells appear to be related to the absence of HLA class I molecules at the cell surface of Daudi, presumably, because of the lack of negative signals via the NKR. The Vγ9/Vδ2 TCR might recognize unknown non-polymorphic ligands expressed predominantly at the cell surface of B-cell lymphomas. These ligands might be homologous to bacterial phosphoantigens that stimulate the same Vγ9/Vδ2 T cells. Recognition of such hypothetical "cellular phospho-antigens" might depend on post-translational modification of several or distinct cell surface molecules and these modifications might differ in B-cell lymphomas from that in solid tumors. It is also possible that such ligands can be stress inducible. They could also be expressed at lower levels on normal cells. In order to avoid autoimmunity, Vγ9/Vδ2 T cells express inhibitory NKR to downregulate responses against normal tissues and exogenous antigens. It may not be necessary to lose HLA class I expression completely, but NKR$^+$ Vγ9/Vδ2 T cells might be activated by cells that have decreased expression of HLA class I or cells with reduced expression of certain HLA class I alleles. This has been demonstrated for BL cells and for solid tumors. The CD4$^+$ Vγ9/Vδ2 T cells might function as T-helper cells *in vivo*, that recognize the same antigens as the cytotoxic Vγ9/Vδ2 T-cell clones and that initiate an immune response by secreting lymphokines. It appears that Vγ9/Vδ2 T cells are primed and expanded in the first decade after birth by exogenous phosphoantigens. Then, in the adult they may constitute a system of immunosurveillance against certain tumor cells. The expression of NKR by the majority of Vγ9/Vδ2 T cells implies that these cells are functionally related to NK cells. By TCR mediated recognition of common, but not ubiquitous ligands that are expressed at higher levels on certain hematopoietic tumors, Vγ9/Vδ2 T cells may be a system of killer cells against tumor cells with a different specificity than NK cells.

Acknowledgements

I thank P. Coulie, P. van der Bruggen, G. Klein, M. Malkovsky, R. Handgretinger for discussions, S. Kock for expert technical assistance and O. Viale, E. Meuer, S. Rothenfußer and A. Moris for their contribution to the experimental work.

References

1. Hayday, A.C., *Annu. Rev. Immunol.* 18: 975–1026, 2000.
2. Raulet, D.H., *Annu. Rev. Immunol.* 7: 175–207, 1989.
3. Harel-Bellan, A., Quillet, A., Marchiol, C., DeMars, R., Tursz, T., and Fradelizi, D., *Proc. Natl. Acad. Sci. U.S.A.* 83: 5688–5692, 1986.
4. Kärre, K., Ljunggren, H.G., Piontek, G., and Kiessling, R., *Nature* 319: 675–678, 1986.
5. Moretta, A., Bottino, C., Vitale, M., Pende, D., Biassoni, R., Mingari, M.C., and Moretta, L., *Annu. Rev. Immunol.* 14: 619–648, 1996.
6. Fisch, P., Meuer, E., Pende, D., Rothenfußer, S., Viale, O., Kock, S., Ferrone, S., Fradelizi, D., Klein, G., Moretta, L., Rammensee, H.-G., Boon, T., Coulie, P., and van der Bruggen, P., *Eur. J. Immunol.* 27: 3368–3379, 1997.
7. Halary, F., Peyrat, M.-A., Champagne, E., Lopez-Botet, M., Moretta, A., Moretta, L., Vié, H., Fournié, J.J., and Bonneville, M., *Eur. J. Immunol.* 27: 2812–2821, 1997.
8. Fisch, P., Moris, A., Rammensee, H.-G., and Handgretinger, R., *Immunol. Today* 21:187–191, 2000.

9. Fisch, P., Malkovsky, M., Braakman, E., Sturm, E., Bolhuis, R.L.H., Prieve, A., Sosman, J.A., Lam, V.A., and Sondel, P.M., *J. Exp. Med.* 171: 1567–1579, 1990.

10. Fisch, P., Malkovsky, M., Kovats, S., Sturm, E., Braakman, E., Klein, B.S., Voss, S.D., Morrissey, L.W., De Mars, R., Welch, W.J., DeMars, R., Bolhuis, R.L.H., and Sondel, P.M., *Science* 250: 1269–1273, 1990.

11. Sturm, E., Braakman, E., Fisch, P., Vreugdenhil, R.J., Sondel, P., and Bolhuis, R.L.H., *J. Immunol.* 145: 3202–3208, 1990.

12. Kabelitz, D., Bender, A., Schondelmaier, S., Schoel, B., and Kaufmann, S.H.E., *J. Exp. Med.* 171: 667–679, 1990.

13. Holoshitz, J., Koning, F., Coligan, J.E., De Bruyn, J., and Strober, S., *Nature* 339: 226–229, 1989.

14. Haregewoin, A., Soman, G., Hom, R.C., and Finberg, R.W., *Nature* 340: 309–312, 1989.

15. Constant, P., Davodeau, F., Peyrat, M.A., Poquet, Y., Puzo, G., Bonneville, M., and Fournie, J.J., *Science* 264: 267–270, 1994.

16. Viale, O., van der Bruggen, P., Meuer, E., Kunzmann, R., Kohler, H., Mertelsmann, R., Boon, T., and Fisch, P., *Immunogenetics* 45: 27–34, 1996.

17. Spits, H., Paliard, X., Vandekerckhove, Y., Van Vlasselaer, P., and De Vries, J.E., *J. Immunol.* 147: 1180–1188, 1991.

18. Ciccone, E., Pende, D., Vitale, M., Nanni, L., Di Donato, C., Bottino, C., Morelli, L., Viale, O., Amoroso, A., Moretta, A. and Moretta L., *Eur. J. Immunol.* 24: 1003–1006, 1994.

19. Davodeau, F., Peyrat, M.A., Hallet, M.M., Gaschet, J., Houde, I., Vivien, R., Vie, H., and Bonneville, M., *J. Immunol.* 151: 1214–1223, 1993.

20. Davodeau, F., Peyrat, M.A., Hallet, M.M., Houde, I., Vie, H., and Bonneville, M., *Eur. J. Immunol.* 23: 804–808, 1993.

21. Bukowski, J.F., Morita, C.T., Tanaka, Y., Bloom, B.R., Brenner, M.B., and Band, H., *J. Immunol.* 154: 998–1006, 1995.

22. Bukowski, J.F., Morita, C.T., Band, H., and Brenner, M.B., *J. Immunol.* 161: 286–293, 1998.

23. Fisch, P., Oettel, K., Fudim, N., Surfus, J.E., Malkovsky, M., and Sondel, P.M., *J. Immunol.* 148: 2315–2323, 1992.

24. Handgretinger, R., Geiselhart, A., Moris, A., Grau, R., Teuffel, O., Bethge, W., Kanz, L., and Fisch, P., *N. Engl. J. Med.* 340: 278–284, 1999.

SARAH E. COUPLAND, MICHAEL HUMMEL AND
HARALD STEIN

Somatic mutation analysis of ocular adnexal extranodal marginal zone B-cell lymphomas

Abstract

The most common lymphoma occurring in the ocular adnexa is the extra-nodal marginal zone B-cell lymphoma (EMZL). On the basis of analyses of somatic mutations in the variable region (V) of the immunoglobulin heavy (IgH) chain gene segment, it is thought that the development of EMZL in other locations is dependent on antigen stimulation. This study investigated the presence of somatic hypermutations in clonally rearranged IgH chain V genes of ocular adnexal EMZL, to estimate whether the mutation pattern is compatible with antigen selection.

Twenty-six ocular adnexal EMZL were diagnosed on the basis of morphology, histology and immunohistology according to the REAL Classification. A nested polymerase chain reaction (PCR) was performed on DNA extracted from paraffin sections. The isolated PCR products were sequenced and compared with published VH-germ line segments to determine the number of somatic mutations in the complementarity-determining region (CDR) 2 and framework region (FW) 3.

The number of somatic mutations in the EMZL varied between 0 and 24: 5 cases had 0–3 somatic mutations, while 4–24 mutations were observed in the remaining 21 cases. Based on the ratio of replacement to silent mutations in the CDR2 or FW3 regions, antigen selection appears to have occurred in 60% of ocular adnexal EMZL. The VH3 family was the most commonly expressed germline VH family (54%), followed by VH4 (23%) with biased usage of the latter. Some germline VH genes used included DP-8, DP-10, DP-53, DP-63 (VH4.21) and DP49 which are frequently employed by autoantibodies such as rheumatoid factors and natural autoantibodies.

EMZL of the ocular adnexa have an IgH chain mutation pattern which supports the current concept that they represent a clonal expansion of post-germinal centre memory B cells. In two thirds of ocular adnexal EMZL,

Department of Pathology, University Hospital Benjamin Franklin,
Free University, Berlin, D-12203, Germany

antigen selection appears to have occurred; autoantibodies may have a role in their development.

Keywords: EMZL, ocular adnexa, lymphoma, somatic mutation, antigen selection

Extranodal marginal zone B-cell lymphomas of the ocular adnexa

Lymphomas of the ocular adnexa—i.e. the conjunctiva, lids, orbit and the lacrimal gland—represent approximately 8% of all extranodal lymphomas [1]. Recent studies have demonstrated that the majority of lymphomas occurring in these tissues are non-Hodgkin B-cell lymphomas and that the most common lymphoma subtype is the extranodal marginal zone B-cell lymphoma (EMZL) [2–4]. This term was proposed by the Revised European-American Lymphoma (R.E.A.L.) Classification [5] as EMZL are thought to arise from marginal zone B cells, due to the similarity of the cell populations both morphologically and immunophenotypically [5]. It incorporates both the so-called "M.A.L.T." lymphomas, arising from mucosa-associated lymphoid tissue [6], and those of so-called "M.A.L.T type", arising in locations where neither M.A.L.T. nor a mucosa is present. Due to the minimal amount of organised lymphatic tissue in the ocular adnexa, in particular in the orbit, the term EMZL is the most appropriate for the description of this lymphoma entity.

In general, EMZL are commonly occurring, low grade B-cell lymphomas, although a high grade transformation has been described [7,8]. They differ from their nodal counterparts in that they often remain localised to their sites of origin for many years prior to dissemination. EMZL develop in a variety of locations, such as the ocular adnexa, normally possessing minimal lymphoid tissue [9,10]. The most common site is the stomach [5,9]; others include the thyroid [11] and salivary glands [12].

Histologically, these tumors consist of small cells and occasional blasts surrounding reactive B-cell follicles, the presence of which is reflected by CD21-staining for follicular dendritic cells. The cytology of the tumor cells varies, resembling centrocytes, monocytoid B cells or small lymphocytes (Fig. 1). Plasmacellular differentiation is often apparent. Infiltration of adjacent epithelium by tumor cells, such as in some conjunctival specimens or in orbital cases with lacrimal gland involvement, results in the formation of so-called "lymphoepithelial lesions". Furthermore, "follicular colonisation" [13], or secondary infiltration of the follicle centres, can be observed. The tumor cells typically have the following immunophenotype: CD45+, CD20+, BCL-2+, CD10−, CD5−, cyclin D1−. Monotypic light- or heavy-chain restriction (Fig. 2) can be demonstrated, particularly in those with plasmacellular differentiation. The growth fraction of the tumor (Ki-67 antigen) cells usually reflects the low-grade nature of the lymphoma.

Although their pathogenesis remains unclear, recent cytogenetic studies have demonstrated the translocation t(11;18) in 45% of stomach EMZL, as

Sarah E. Coupland, Michael Hummel and Harald Stein

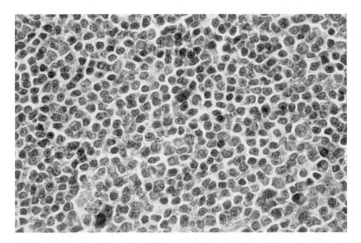

FIGURE 1. *Histology of an orbital EMZL demonstrating the tumor infiltrate consisting of cells with variable morphology resembling centrocytes, monocytoid B cells or small lymphocytes, as well as plasma cells and ocassional blasts (Giemsa staining; ×40 objective).*

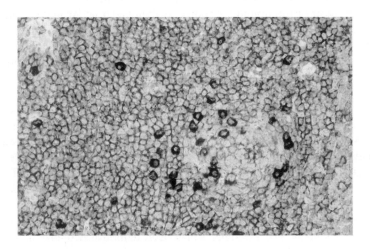

FIGURE 2. *IgM positivity of the tumor cells and scattered reactive plasma cells (PAP immunohistochemistry; ×20 objective).*

well as trisomy 3 in EMZL of different locations [14–18] Further, the development of EMZL in the stomach, the salivary gland and the thyroid gland has been associated with auto-immune disease or bacterial infection prior to tumor development [19]. For example, salivary gland EMZL are associated with Sjögren's syndrome [12,20], thyroid gland EMZL with Hashimoto's thyroiditis [11], and those of the stomach, with *Helicobacter pylori* infection [21–23]. Indirect evidence suggests that the development of EMZL in these locations is dependent on antigen stimulation provided by the associated immune reactions [24,25]. This evidence includes the analysis of *somatic mutations* in the variable region of the immunoglobulin heavy chain (IgH) gene segment of these tumors [21,26,27].

Immunoglobulin diversity and somatic hypermutation

IgH genes, located on chromosome 14, consist of variable (VH), diversity (D) and joining (JH) gene segments. A functional VH–D–JH complex is formed in the bone marrow during B-cell ontogeny when one of the D segments is combined with a JH segment and, subsequently, combined with a VH gene segment [28]. Further, "N" segments of varying lengths and random composition are introduced at the junctions through the activity of Tdt during this process. In this way, B cells are capable of producing an extensive and diverse range of antibodies with varying specificities [29,30]. The repertoire of germline VH segments can be grouped into seven "families" (VH1 to VH7) based on the similarity of the nucleotide sequences [31–34]. Members of the same VH family are usually more than 80% homologous, while homology between VH genes from different families is less than 70%.

Maturation of the immune response is thought to occur in the germinal centres, during a "follicle centre response", upon antigenic challenge by a process of "somatic hypermutation" of the VH region [29,35–37]. *Somatic hypermutation* non-randomly introduces predominantly single base changes into the IgV genes via a mechanism which is to date not completely understood. B cells with mutated IgV genes are then selected according to the affinity of the encoded antibody for antigen retained on the follicular dendritic cells, resulting in an increase in the affinity of the humoral response [35]. Mutations occur mainly in the complementarity determining regions (CDRs) of the VH regions, thought to constitute the antigen-binding site [38]. A clustering of replacement (R) (versus silent, S) mutations in the CDRs is considered to be an indicator of antigenic selection [39,40]. The identification of mutated IgV genes has been applied to the study of normal B cells to determine either follicle cell ancestry, or continued influence of the follicle centre microenvironment. For example, it has been demonstrated that naive pre-germinal centres B cells carry non-mutated VH genes, whereas germinal centre B cells and germinal-centre-derived memory cells express mutated VH region genes [29,35,36,41]. This information has been useful in the subtyping of B-cell lymphomas, dividing these malignancies into those descended from pre-germinal B cells (e.g. B-CLL [42,43] and mantle cell lymphoma [44]), and others descended from germinal or post-germinal centre B cells (e.g. follicle centre lymphoma [44], multiple myeloma [45], endemic Burkitt's lymphoma [46,47]). The continued accumulation of mutations ("ongoing mutations") in tumors resulting in intraclonal heterogeneity has been reported in follicle centre lymphoma [48], EMZL [21,49] and Burkitt's lymphoma [46].

Sarah E. Coupland, Michael Hummel and Harald Stein

Somatic mutations in the VH region of ocular adnexal EMZL

We recently analysed twenty-six cases of ocular adnexal EMZL for the presence of somatic hypermutations in clonally rearranged IgH chain genes [50]. The DNA sequence analysis was performed using an automated DNA sequencer (Applied Biosystems 377A) by applying the DyeDeoxy Terminator Method. Isolated polymerase-chain-reaction (PCR) amplified products for IgH were sequenced in both directions utilising the re-amplification primers, FR2FS and VLJH, respectively. Only those cases with a complete homology between both sequences were chosen for comparison with published VH germline sequences (VBASE; German Cancer Research Centre, Heidelberg, Germany) [51].

For n random mutations, the number of expected R mutations in the CDR2– or FW3 region was calculated according to the formula $Rcdr = n \times Acdr \times Rfcdr$, where $Acdr$ is the relative size of the CDR or FWR and $Rfcdr$ is the frequency of R mutation for the CDR or FWR [40,52]. The expected number of S mutations was obtained for CDR2 and FW3 using the same formula with Rf replaced by $1-Rf$. Rf values are typically different for CDRs and FWRs and can vary among different genes depending on the nucleotide sequence. The R:S mutation ratios in the CDR and FW3 were compared as described by Jukes and King [53]. The probability that the R mutations observed in the CDR occurred by chance were calculated according to Chang *et al.*: $n!/(k!(n-k)!)qk(1-q)n-k = p$ where n = total number of mutations, k = number of R mutations in the CDR, and q = proportion of CDR [52].

The closest VH germline utilised and the expected and observed number of R and S mutations in the CDR2 and FW3 regions of the V-region as well as p values for the CDR2 are summarised for each case in Table 1.

The process of somatic hypermutation in IgH genes appears to have occurred in 60% of ocular adnexal EMZL during their development. An intermediate number of mutations (average, 11) was observed in the VH region of these post-germinal centre tumor cells in the majority of the ocular EMZL. This number of mutations is similar to those observed in IgH genes (CDR2 and FR3) in EMZL of other sites [26,27,49] and supports their proposed derivation from post-germinal centre cells. Interestingly, there was no relationship between the number of somatic mutations and the location of the lymphoma, i.e. those mucosally-related and non-mucosally related (orbital) EMZL.

Some of the ocular adnexal EMZL examined were unusual in that they either demonstrated germline configuration or mutation rates similar to those observed in follicle centre lymphomas [47] and diffuse large cell B-cell lymphomas. VH genes with no or only a few somatic mutations are usually observed in lymphomas derived from pre-germinal centre B cells, such as B-CLL [42,43] and mantle cell lymphoma [44]. The three ocular adnexal EMZL with germline configuration lacked "pseudofollicles" (usually present in B-CLL), were negative for CD23 and demonstrated loose, ill-defined meshwork of follicular dendritic cells seen in the majority of EMZL but usually absent from B-CLL [54,55]. Furthermore, the tumor cells were negative

TABLE 1. *Clinical details, mutation number, growth fraction and immunophenotype of the investigated EMZL of the ocular adnexa.*

Case	Age	Gender	Site	Stage	Mutation number	Growth fraction	Phenotype
1	77	F	Orbit	II	24	10	IgM+, K−, L−
2	60	F	Orbit; LG	I	5	5	IgM+, K−, L−
3	66	M	Orbit	I	17	10	IgM−, K−, L−
4	71	F	Orbit	IV	0	30	IgM+, K+
5	52	F	Orbit	II	12	10	IgM+, K+
6	66	F	Orbit	III	15	40	IgM+, K+
7	52	F	Orbit	I	18	20	IgM+, K+
8	58	F	Conj	I	0	5	IgM+, K+
9	74	F	Orbit	I	6	15	IgM+, K+
10	71	F	Conj	I	24	5	IgM−, K−, L−
11	62	M	Conj	IV	15	40	IgM−, K−, L+
12	15	M	Orbit	III	15	30	IgM+, IgD+, L+
13	23	M	Conj	I	8	40	IgM+, K+
14	68	M	Conj	IV	4	50	IgM+, K+
15	77	F	Conj	I	16	20	IgM+, K−, L−
16	48	F	Conj	I	14	5	IgM+, K+
17	69	M	Conj	II	3	15	IgM+, K−, L−
18	92	F	Conj	I	24	5	IgM+, L+
19	82	F	Orbit	I	17	10	IgM+, K−, L−
20	75	F	Orbit	I	7	60	IgM+, K+
21	64	F	Orbit	I	13	15	IgM+, K−, L−
22	40	F	Conj	II	10	15	IgM+, L+
23	53	M	Orbit; LG	II	3	10	IgM+, K+
24	88	F	Conj	III	14	10	IgM+, L+
25	60	F	Orbit; LG	I	0	10	IgM+, L+
26	34	M	Conj	I	21	15	IgM+, K+

Abbreviations: F = female; M = male; Conj = conjunctiva; LG = lacrimal gland; Growth fractions are determined with the antibody MIB-1 and are given as percentages.

Sarah E. Coupland, Michael Hummel and Harald Stein

for CD5, cyclin D1 and IgD, normally observed in mantle cell lymphomas [5]. It could be postulated that the precursor cells of these tumors were post-germinal centre memory cells, which had been subject to a process of negative selection [56] during their passage through the germinal centre.

The highly mutated ocular adnexal EMZL, in contrast, did not have the characteristic follicular architecture observed in follicle centre lymphomas nor the immunophenotype characteristic for these tumors (i.e. CD10 and BCL-6 positivity) [5]. Further, morphological characteristics of diffuse large cell B-cell lymphomas were not present. It is possible that a process of ongoing IgH gene hypermutation, as reported in follicular centre lymphomas as well as salivary gland EMZL [49], is present in these tumors to explain their high mutation rates. The histologically observed follicular colonisation of EMZL [13] could result in re-entry of the tumor cells into the germinal centre and, therefore, re-exposure to the process of somatic hypermutation. Whether post-germinal centre memory B cells, however, can accumulate additional Ig gene mutations and the mechanism whereby this may occur remains controversial.

An antigen selection process appears to have occurred in the development of approximately 60% of ocular adnexal EMZL. This implication is under-scored by the fact that in these cases either: (1) the observed number of R and silent mutations in the CDR2 was greater and in the FW3 regions lower than expected; (2) the R/S ratio in the CDR regions was >2.9 and in the FW3 region <1.5; and (3) the probability of the observed R mutations occurring by chance in the CDR2 region by chance was low (Table 2). Further, this antigen selection process did not appear to be dependent upon the presence of a mucosa, occurring with a similar frequency in orbital EMZL as those in the conjunctiva. Interestingly, eight EMZL (30%) expressed VH genes frequently associated with auto-antibodies: DP-8, DP-10 (alternative name 51p1 gene), DP-53, DP-63 (also called VH4.21) and DP49 (Table 2) [57–59]. Auto-antibodies using the germline DP-53 and DP49 have been described in Alzheimer's disease [60] and rheumatoid arthritis [61], respectively. Those using the DP-63 germline gene—the most frequently rearranged gene over-all—have been shown to possess unique auto-immune properties and have been associated with various diseases such as idiopathic cold agglutinin disease [59,62] and collagen vascular diseases such as SLE [63,64] and rheumatoid arthritis [61]. A relationship between DP-10 and B-CLL has been demonstrated in previous studies, whereby 51p1 underlies an auto-antibody associated cross-reactive idiotype expressed in up to 20% of B-CLL [65]. Recently, 3 of 5 cases of EMZL of the parotid gland were demonstrated to have closest homology to DP-10 [49]. The above results would suggest that, in some ocular adnexal EMZL, the epitope possibly responsible for direct stimulation is self-antigen. Similar observations have been reported by previous authors investigating EMZL in other locations [21,26,27].

A variety of germline VH gene usage was seen in the development of ocular adnexal EMZL, although tumors expressing heavy chain genes from the VH2, VH6 or VH7 families were not detected. This may be due to the small size of these families relative to the number of cases analysed. The largest of

TABLE 2. *Germline usage (V_H)*, number of silent and replacement mutations observed and expected in the CDR2 and FR3.*

Case	Germline usage (V_H)*		Homology (%)	Mutations (n)	CDR2 expected			CDR2 observed			FR3 expected			FR3 observed			CDR2 p
					R	S	R:S	R	S	R:S	R	S	R:S	R	S	R:S	
1	V5-51	DP-73	79.4	24	5.99	2.10	2.85:1	4	3	1.3:1	11.7	4.13	2.83:1	11	6	1.8:1	0.1317
2	V3-48	DP-51	94.2	5	1.3	0.4	3.25:1	0	0	0	2.5	0.8	3.13:1	2	3	0.67:1	0.232
3	V3-74	DP-53	87.1	17	4.5	1.59	2.83:1	8	2	4:1	8	3	2.6:1	7	0	inf	0.0195
4	V3-53	DP-42	100	0			0			0			0			0	
5	VH4	DP-70	92.4	12	3.07	1.07	2.87:1	4	3	1.3:1	5.80	2.03	2.85:1	3	2	1.5:1	0.198
6	V3-21	DP-58	89.4	15	4.1	1.45	2.82:1	7	5	1.4:1	6.96	2.37	2.94:1	2	1	2:1	0.56
7	V4-21	DP-63	86.6	18	4.7	1.66	2.83:1	6	1	6:1	8.60	3.02	2.85:1	5	6	0.83:1	0.156
8	V1-69	DP-10	100	0			0			0			0			0	
9	V3-11	DP-35	92.7	6	1.52	0.53	2.86:1	1	1	1:1	2.9	1.0	2.9:1	4	0	inf	0.35
10	V4-4	DP-70	86.2	24	11.8	4.16	2.83:1	6	2	3:1	5.92	2.08	2.85:1	8	8	1:1	0.009
11	V1-18	DP-14	91.6	15	3.8	1.33	2.85:1	3	2	1.5:1	7.3	2.57	2.84:1	7	3	2.3:1	0.221
12	V3-7	DP-54	86.4	15	6.33	2.22	2.85:1	5	5	1:1	12.1	4.27	2.83:1	8	7	1.14:1	0.1618
13	V3-7	DP-54	94.5	8	2.05	0.72	2.84:1	4	2	2:1	3.87	1.36	2.85:1	2	0	inf	0.091
14	V3-74	DP-53	97.7	4	1.02	0.36	2.83:1	0	1	0	1.93	0.67	2.88:1	3	0	inf	0.305
15	V3-15	DP-38	91.8	16	4.35	1.53	2.84:1	5	2	2.5:1	7.48	2.63	2.84:1	6	3	2:1	0.1977
16	V3-30	DP-49	90.5	14	3.59	1.26	2.84:1	6	1	6:1	6.76	2.37	2.85:1	3	4	0.75:1	0.0799
17	VH3-74	DP-53	96.3	3	0.77	0.27	2.85:1	3	0	inf	1.44	0.51	2.82	0	0	0	0.0172
18	V4-39	DP-79	85.4	24	6.29	2.02	3.11:1	7	3	2.3:1	11.4	4.02	2.84:1	10	4	2.5:1	0.167
19	V3-30.3	DP-46	86.9	17	3.92	1.37	2.86:1	10	0	inf	7.84	2.75	2.85:1	3	4	0.75:1	0.00132
20	VH1	DP-8	95.8	7	1.78	0.63	2.83:1	v1	2	0.5:1	3.40	1.19	2.85:1	0	4	0	0.305
21	VH4	DP-71	91.9	13	2.99	1.05	2.84:1	4	1	4:1	6.00	2.10	2.85:1	5	3	1.67:1	0.189
22	V5-51	DP-73	94.7	10	2.66	0.94	2.84:1	6	0	inf	4.7	1.66	2.83:1	4	0	inf	0.003
23	VH4.21	DP-63	96.4	3	0.77	0.27	2.85:1	3	0	inf	1.44	0.50	2.88:1	0	0	0	0.0169
24	VH4	DP-79	91.4	14	3.59	1.26	2.84:1	6	1	6:1	1.44	0.50	2.88:1	4	3	1.3:1	0.07
25	V3-23	DP-47	100	0			0			0			0			0	
26	V3-7	DP-54	86.8	21	4.84	1.67	2.89:1	7	1	7:1	9.68	3.40	2.84:1	9	4	2.3:1	0.102

* According to GenBank, release 79 using FASTA or VBASE for data bank comparison.

TABLE 3. *VH family usage in ocular adnexal EMZL and comparison with adult peripheral B cells.*

VH family	Ocular adnexal EMZL		PBL [66] (%)
	Number	%	
VH1	3	11.5	16
VH2	–	–	8
VH3	14	53.8	65
VH4	7	26.9	5
VH5	2	7	4
VH6	–	–	2
VH7	–	–	ng

Abbreviation: ng = not given.

the seven germline families, the VH3 family [66], was the most commonly germline VH family used in the present study (14 of the 26 cases, 54%), in agreement with Kon *et al.*, who examined VH usage in three ocular adnexal tumors, diagnosed as small lymphocytic lymphoma according to the Working Formulation [67]. The second most commonly expressed VH family in the present study was VH4 (7 cases, 27%). When compared with adult peripheral B cells (Table 3) and marginal zone cells (unpublished results), a slightly biased usage of VH4 and possibly of VH5 (but not of VH3) by ocular adnexal EMZL becomes apparent. In contrast to the extensive VH3 family, the VH4 and VH5 gene repertoires are small but are frequently rearranged throughout B-cell ontogeny, in auto-antibodies and in B-cell malignancies [59,68,69]. Overrepresentation of VH4 has been reported in follicle centre lymphoma [68] and in diffuse large cell lymphomas [70]; biased usage of VH5, in CLL [69].

In summary, the majority of ocular adnexal EMZL, similar to their counterparts at other sites, are derived from post-germinal centre B cells. Antigen selection—possibly that of endogenous antigens—appears to have a role in promoting the development of the majority of EMZL at these sites. Further investigations are required to determine (a) what these stimulating antigens are; (b) if ongoing mutations are present in highly mutated ocular adnexal EMZL; and (c) the pathogenesis of the remaining EMZL where antigen selection did not appear to have an essential role. This work could provide further insight into the development of lymphomatous diseases in these tissues, possibly having an influence on their future treatment strategies.

References

1. Freeman, C., Freeman, L.N., Berg, J.W., and Cutler, S.J, *Cancer* 29: 252–260, 1972.
2. Coupland, S.E., Krause, L., Delecluse, H.J., Anagnostopoulos, I., Foss, H.D., Hummel, M., Bornfeld, N., Lee, W.R., and Stein, H., *Ophthalmology* 105: 1430–1441, 1998.

3. White, W.A., Ferry, J.A., Harris, N.L., and Grove, A.S., *Ophthalmology* 102: 1994–2006, 1995.
4. Wotherspoon, A.C., Diss, T.C., Pan, L.X., Schmid, C., Kerr Muir, M.G., Lea, S.H., and Isaacson, P.G., *Histopathology* 23: 417–424, 1993.
5. Harris, N.L., Jaffe, E.S., Stein, H., Banks, P.M., Chan, J.K., Cleary, M.L., Delsol, G., De Wolf Peeters, C., Falini, B., Gatter, K.C., *et al.*, *Blood* 84: 1361–1392, 1994.
6. Isaacson, P.G., Spencer, J., and Finn, T., *Hum. Pathol.* 17: 72–82, 1986.
7. Isaacson, P.G., *Br. J. Biomed. Sci.* 52: 291–296, 1995.
8. Du, M., Peng, H., Singh, N., Isaacson, P.G., and Pan, L., *Blood* 86: 4587–4593, 1995.
9. Isaacson, P.G., Banks, P.M., Best, P.V., McLure, S.P., Muller-Hermelink, H.K., and Wyatt, J.I., *Am. J. Surg. Pathol.* 19: 571–575, 1995.
10. Jakobiec, F.A., Iwamoto, T., and Knowles, D.Md., *Arch. Ophthalmol.* 100: 84–98, 1982.
11. Hyjek, E., and Isaacson, P.G., *Hum. Pathol.* 19: 1315–1326, 1988.
12. Hyjek, E., Smith, W.J., and Isaacson, P.G., *Hum. Pathol.* 19: 766–776, 1988.
13. Isaacson, P.G., Wotherspoon, A.C., Diss, T., and Pan, L.X., *Am. J. Surg. Pathol.* 15: 819–828, 1991.
14. Brynes, R.K., Almaguer, P.D., Leathery, K.E., McCourty, A., Arber, D.A., Medeiros, L.J., and Nathwani, B.N., *Mod. Pathol.* 9: 995–1000, 1996.
15. Dierlamm, J., Pittaluga, S., Wlodarska, I., Stul, M., Thomas, J., Boogaerts, M., Michaux, L., Driessen, A., Mecucci, C., Cassiman, J.J., *et al.*, *Blood* 87: 299–307, 1996.
16. Dierlamm, J., Michaux, L., Wlodarska, I., Pittaluga, S., Zeller, W., Stul, M., Criel, A., Thomas, J., Boogaerts, M., Delaere, P., Cassiman, J.J., de Wolf-Peeters, C., Mecucci, C., and Van den Berghe, H., *Br. J. Haematol.* 93: 242–249, 1996.
17. Ott, G., Katzenberger, T., Greiner, A., Kalla, J., Rosenwald, A., Heinrich, U., Ott, M.M., and Muller-Hermelink, H.K., *Cancer Res.* 57: 3944–3948, 1997.
18. Wotherspoon, A.C., Finn, T.M., and Isaacson, P.G., *Blood* 85: 2000–2004, 1995.
19. Isaacson, P.G., and Spencer, J., *J. Clin. Pathol.* 48: 395–397, 1995.
20. Schmid, U., Helbron, D., and Lennert, K., *Virchows Arch. [Pathol. Anat.]* 395: 11–43, 1985.
21. Du, M., Diss, T.C., Xu, C., Peng, H., Isaacson, P.G., and Pan, L., *Leukemia* 10: 1190–1197, 1996.
22. Parsonnet, J., Hansen, S., Rodriguez, L., Gelb, A.B., Warnke, R.A., Jellum, E., Orentreich, N., Vogelman, J.H., and Friedman, G.D., *N. Engl. J. Med.* 330: 1267–1271, 1994.
23. Wotherspoon, A.C., Ortiz Hidalgo, C., Falzon, M.R., and Isaacson, P.G., *Lancet* 338: 1175–1176, 1991.
24. Greiner, A., Marx, A., Heesemann, J., Leebmann, J., Schmausser, B., and Muller-Hermelink, H.K., *Lab. Invest.* 70: 572–578, 1994.
25. Hussell, T., Isaacson, P.G., Crabtree, J.E., Dogan, A., and Spencer, J., *Am. J. Pathol.* 142: 285–292, 1993.
26. Qin, Y., Greiner, A., Trunk, M.J., Schmausser, B., Ott, M.M., and Muller-Hermelink, H.K., *Blood* 86: 3528–3534, 1995.
27. Qin, Y., Greiner, A., Hallas, C., Haedicke, W., and Muller-Hermelink, H.K., *Lab. Invest.* 76: 477–485, 1997.
28. Tonegawa, S., *Nature* 302: 575–581, 1983.
29. Jacob, J., Kelsoe, G., Rajewsky, K., and Weiss, U., *Nature* 354: 389–392, 1991.

30. Kelsoe, G., *Semin. Immunol.* 8: 179–184, 1996.
31. Berman, J.E., Mellis, S.J., Pollock, R., Smith, C.L., Suh, H., Heinke, B., Kowal, C., Surti, U., Chess, L., Cantor, C.R., *et al.*, *Embo. J.* 7: 727–738, 1988.
32. Cook, G.P., and Tomlinson, I.M., *Immunol. Today* 16: 237–242, 1995.
33. Lee, K.H., Matsuda, F., Kinashi, T., Kodaira, M., and Honjo, T., *J. Mol. Biol.* 195: 761–768, 1987.
34. Pascual, V., and Capra, J.D., *Adv. Immunol.* 49: 1–74, 1991.
35. Berek, C., Berger, A., and Apel, M., *Cell* 67: 1121–1129, 1991.
36. Betz, A.G., Neuberger, M.S., and Milstein, C., *Immunol. Today* 14: 405–411, 1993.
37. Liu, Y.J., Joshua, D.E., Williams, G.T., Smith, C.A., Gordon, J., and MacLennan, I.C., *Nature* 342: 929–931, 1989.
38. Amit, A.G., Mariuzza, R.A., Phillips, S.E., and Poljak, R.J., *Nature* 313: 156–158, 1985.
39. Levy, N.S., Malipiero, U.V., Lebecque, S.G., and Gearhart, P.J., *J. Exp. Med.* 169: 2007–2019, 1989.
40. Shlomchik, M.J., Marshak-Rothstein, A., Wolfowicz, C.B., Rothstein, T.L., and Weigert, M.G., *Nature* 328: 805–811, 1987.
41. Kuppers, R., Zhao, M., Hansmann, M.L., and Rajewsky, K., *Embo. J.* 12: 4955–4967, 1993.
42. Aoki, H., Takishita, M., Kosaka, M., and Saito, S., *Blood* 85: 1913–1919, 1995.
43. Meeker, T.C., Grimaldi, J.C., O'Rourke, R., Loeb, J., Juliusson, G., and Einhorn, S., *J. Immunol.* 141: 3994–3998, 1988.
44. Hummel, M., Tamaru, J., Kalvelage, B., and Stein, H., *Blood* 84: 403–407, 1994.
45. Bakkus, M.H., Heirman, C., Van Riet, I., Van Camp, B., and Thielemans, K., *Blood* 80: 2326–2335, 1992.
46. Chapman, C.J., Zhou, J.Z., Gregory, X., Rickinson, A.B., and Stevenson, F.K., *Blood* 88: 3562, 1996.
47. Tamaru, J., Hummel, M., Marafioti, T., Kalvelage, B., Leoncini, L., Minacci, C., Tosi, P., Wright, D., and Stein, H., *Am. J. Pathol.* 147: 1398–1407, 1995.
48. Bahler, D.W., Zelenetz, A.D., Chen, T.T., and Levy, R., *Cancer Res.* 52: 5547s–5551s, 1992.
49. Bahler, D.W., Miklos, J.A., and Swerdlow, S.H., *Blood* 89: 3335–3344, 1997.
50. Coupland, S.E., Foss, H.D., Anagnostopoulos, I., Hummel, M., and Stein, H., *Invest. Ophthalmol. Vis. Sci.* 40: 555–562, 1999.
51. Tomlinson, I.M., Cook, G.P., Walter, G., Carter, N.P., Riethman, H., Buluwela, L., Rabbitts, T.H., and Winter, G., *Ann. N. Y. Acad. Sci.* 764: 43–46, 1995.
52. Chang, B., and Casali, P., *Immunol. Today* 15: 367–373, 1994.
53. Jukes, T.H., and King, J.L., *Nature* 281: 605–606, 1979.
54. Stein, H., Gerdes, J., and Mason, D.Y., *Clin. Haematol.* 11: 531–559, 1982.
55. Stein, H., Lennert, K., Feller, A.C., and Mason, D.Y., *Adv. Cancer Res.* 42: 67–147, 1984.
56. Nossal, G.J., *Cell* 76: 229–239, 1994.
57. Deane, M., Mackenzie, L.E., Stevenson, F.K., Youinou, P.Y., Lydyard, P.M., and Mageed, R.A., *Scand. J. Immunol.* 38: 348–358, 1993.
58. Kipps, T.J., *Blood Cells* 19: 615–625; 631–632, 1993.
59. Pascual, V., Victor, K., Lelsz, D., Spellerberg, M.B., Hamblin, T.J., Thompson, K.M., Randen, I., Natvig, J., Capra, J.D., and Stevenson, F.K., *J. Immunol.* 146: 4385–4391, 1991.

60. Fang, Q., Kannapell, C.C., Fu, S.M., Xu, S., and Gaskin, F., *Clin. Immunol. Immunopathol.* 75: 159–167, 1995.
61. Williams, D.G., and Taylor, P.C., *Eur. J. Immunol.* 27: 476–485, 1997.
62. Silberstein, L.E., Jefferies, L.C., Goldman, J., Friedman, D., Moore, J.S., Nowell, P.C., Roelcke, D., Pruzanski, W., Roudier, J., and Silverman, G.J., *Blood* 78: 2372–2386, 1991.
63. Isenberg, D., Spellerberg, M., Williams, W., Griffiths, M., and Stevenson, F., *Br. J. Rheumatol.* 32: 876–882, 1993.
64. Stevenson, F.K., Longhurst, C., Chapman, C.J., Ehrenstein, M., Spellerberg, M.B., Hamblin, T.J., Ravirajan, C.T., Latchman, D., and Isenberg, D., *J. Autoimmun.* 6: 809–825, 1993.
65. Kipps, T.J., and Carson, D.A., *Blood* 81: 2475–2487, 1993.
66. Zouali, M., and Theze, J., *J. Immunol.* 146: 2855–2864, 1991.
67. Kon, H., Sato, T., Suzuki, J.I., and Kon, S., *Path. Res. Pract.* 192: 523–531, 1996.
68. Bahler, D.W., Campbell, M.J., Hart, S., Miller, R.A., Levy, S., and Levy, R., *Blood* 78: 1561–1568, 1991.
69. Logtenberg, T., Schutte, M.E., Inghirami, G., Berman, J.E., Gmelig Meyling, F.H., Insel, R.A., Knowles, D.M., and Alt, F.W., *Int. Immunol.* 1: 362–366, 1989.
70. Hsu, F.J., and Levy, R., *Blood* 86: 3072–3082, 1995.

CHI-CHAO CHAN, DE FEN SHEN, AND RONALD R. BUGGAGE

Immunopathology and molecular biology of primary intraocular lymphoma

Abstract

Immunopathology of primary intraocular lymphoma reveals a B-cell lymphoma with monoclonal immunoglobulin light chain on the surface. Molecular pathology of primary intraocular lymphoma demonstrates monoclonality with rearrangements of the immunoglobulin heavy chain gene and translocation of bcl-2. HHV-8 and EBV gene may associate with primary intraocular lymphoma and play a role in oncogenesis. Elevation of interleukin-10 level with an IL-10 to IL-6 greater than 1 is found in the vitreous of primary intraocular lymphoma.

Keywords: Primary intraocular lymphoma, monoclonality, immunoglobulin gene, interleukin-10, virus

Introduction

Primary intraocular lymphoma, a subset of primary central nervous system (CNS) lymphoma is a large B-cell, non-Hodgkin's lymphoma [1–3]. The vitreous, retina, and optic nerve are the usual ocular tissues involved [4]. Systemic spread outside the CNS and the eye is rare [5,6].

Although a relatively rare tumor, the incidence of the tumor has increased dramatically coincident with the AIDS epidemic in the past 15 years [7]. A threefold increase in the incidence of primary non-Hodgkin's CNS lymphoma has also been noted in the United States during the last decade [1,8]. This rise parallels the increase in cases of primary intraocular lymphoma in both immunocompetent and immunocompromised patients [7,9]. Primary intraocular lymphoma frequently masquerades as chronic vitritis [2,3,6,10]. Initially, it may be "responsive" to corticosteroid therapy [9]. The persistent "vitritis" frequently proceeds to form large cellular clumps in the vitreous and multifocal subretinal infiltrates with overlying retinal pigment epithelial

Laboratory of Immunology, National Eye Institute, National Institutes of Health,
Bethesda, Maryland, USA
223

detachment which is pathognomonic for primary intraocular lymphoma. Primary intraocular lymphoma may present similar to viral retinitis with retinal vasculitis, hemorrhages, detachment, and necrosis [11,12]. In addition to vitreous cells and infiltrates beneath the retina, other clinical manifestations of this tumor include decreased visual acuity, keratic precipitates, anterior chamber cells and flare, and increased intraocular pressure. The CNS symptoms and signs, whether as the initial presentation or subsequent to ocular disease, soon develop and progress.

The disease is aggressive with a five-year survival rate of less than 33% [13]. Early diagnosis and prompt, aggressive treatment may improve prognosis [2]. Because appropriate treatment of intraocular lymphoma often involves radiation therapy and/or chemotherapy, a definitive pathologic diagnosis is required. Interpretation of the pathology, particularly the cytology, often requires a highly experienced ophthalmic pathologist and/or cytopathologist [14].

Histology

Vitreous and cerebrospinal fluid (CSF)

Because many patients with intraocular lymphoma have CNS involvement at the time of presentation, a thorough history and neurologic examination including CSF evaluation are critical. Occasionally, repeat lumbar punctures are needed with at least 10 ml of CSF sent for cytology. If there are no malignant cells in the CSF, a full diagnostic vitrectomy on the eye with the most severe "vitritis" or poorest visual acuity should be performed [2].

Because the lymphoma cells often are fragile and easily degenerate, it is essential that diagnostic samples (CSF and vitreous) be immediately processed. We recommend the surgical fluids be mixed in cell culture medium in the operating room and hand carried to the cytology laboratory for processing without delay. In the laboratory, the fluid is cytospined as reported previously [2,15–17]. The cell pellet is collected and placed on coated slides for cytology and immunohistochemistry. The supernatant can be analyzed for cytokine levels, particularly interleukin (IL)-10 and IL-6 using ELISA.

Examination of the vitreous and CSF for lymphoma cells requires perseverance and expertise. Typical lymphoma cells are large, pleomorphic cells with scanty basophilic cytoplasm and round, oval, bean-shaped, or clover leaf-shaped nuclei [15,18–21]. Hypersegmented nuclei with fingerlike projections (Fig. 1), prominent nucleoli, and multiple mitoses are diagnostic. The morphologic features of the lymphoma cells are often easier to recognize from CSF specimens because there is less surrounding necrotic debris and vitreal fibrin; however, fewer cells typically are obtained for examination. In contrast, more lymphoma cells are present in the vitrectomy samples of primary intraocular lymphoma. Additionally, the vitreous often contains considerable numbers of reactive lymphocytes, macrophages, degenerative cells, necrotic debris and fibrous material, making cytological diagnosis difficult.

Chi-Chao Chan, De Fen Shen and R. N. Buggage.

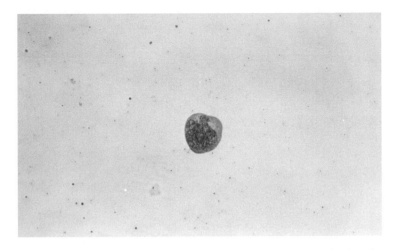

F I G U R E 1 .   *Photomicrograph showing a typical primary intraocular lymphoma cell in the vitreous. (Giemsa, ×1,000).*

Eye

A characteristic feature of primary intraocular lymphoma is tumor detachment of the retinal pigment epithelium [20,22,23]. Tumor cells infiltrate between the retinal pigment epithelium and Bruch's membrane. The neoplastic cells are large, pleomorphic, and hyperchromatic with prominent to conspicuous nucleoli (Fig. 2). Mitosis and necrosis are frequently observed. Usually they lack cellular cohesion or cytoplasmic processes a cytologic finding that discriminates this tumor from metastatic carcinoma and other CNS neoplasms. Tumor cells are often clustered in a perivascular arrangement in the retina and optic nerve head. Diffuse infiltration of the retina and vitreous as well as hemorrhagic retinal necrosis may occur. Areas of retinal pigment epithelial depigmentation, atrophy, and disciform scars may result from tumor detachment of the retinal pigment epithelium.

Primary intraocular lymphoma rarely infiltrates the uvea, although reactive lymphocytic infiltration is a common manifestation in the choroid. In the National Eye Institute we have observed two cases of iris infiltration by lymphoma cells (unpublished data). Orbital involvement by primary intraocular lymphoma has been reported in patients with AIDS [24,25]. In some of the cases neoplastic spread has involved the retina, optic nerve, and sclera, and even choroid [26,27].

Immunohistochemistry

Immunostaining

Primary intraocular lymphoma like primary CNS lymphoma is almost always a monoclonal B-cell lymphoma. Immunopathologic evaluations of surgically enucleated and autopsy eyes have confirmed that ocular lymphoma is of B-cell

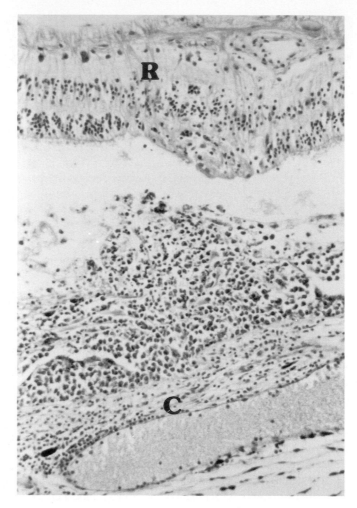

FIGURE 2. *Photomicrograph showing primary intraocular lymphoma cells located in the subretinal space. Most of the infiltrating inflammatory cells are in the choroid (R, retina, C, choroid; hematoxylin and eosin, ×160).*

lineage [4,22,23], composed of CD19 positive cells with either κ or λ light chain restriction (Fig. 3A). The accompanying inflammatory response is predominantly normal appearing non-malignant reactive T lymphocytes. These T cells are found in the choroid, the retina, and the vitreous cavity. Interestingly, the T cells adjacent to tumor cells are predominantly CD8 positive cells (Fig. 3B). Scattered macrophages may be distributed among the tumor cells.

Immunocytochemical evaluation of vitrectomy specimens has yielded variable results [14,28–30]. Brown and associates reviewed 57 cases of primary intraocular lymphoma in which cell marker studies were performed,

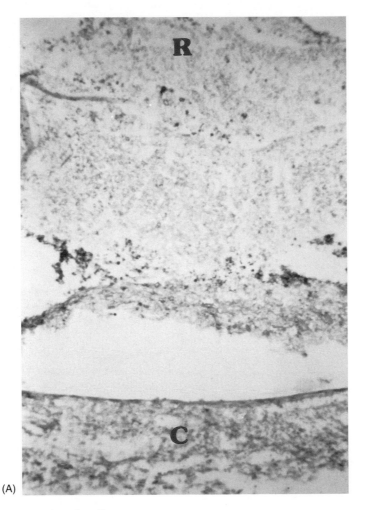

(A)

FIGURE 3   *(continued).*

and noted that 53% were B-cell lymphomas, 21% were T-cell derived, 10% were null-cell, and 16% were polyclonal or untypeable [28]. However, our experience and that of others is that vitreal primary intraocular lymphoma typically bares B-cell markers [2,12,15,29,31]. Monoclonality of either κ or λ light chain for the tumor cells is required to confirm the definitive diagnosis of primary intraocular lymphoma.

Flow cytometry

Recently, the immunophenotype of vitreous cells obtained by diagnostic vitrectomy has been identified successfully using flow cytometry with antibodies against specific surface antigens including B-lymphocyte and T-lymphocyte markers [31]. Cytofluorography may be recommended in the cases containing

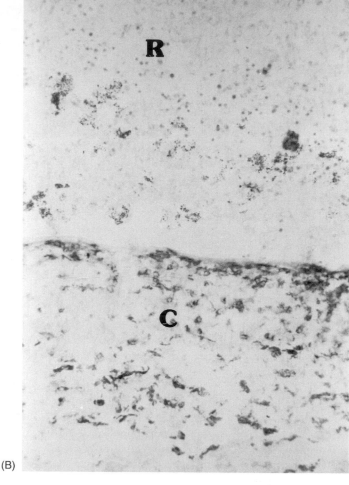

(B)

FIGURE 3. *Photomicrograph showing (A) positive κ light chain staining of the subretinal primary intraocular lymphoma cells, and (B) CD8 T-cells near the tumor in the choroid (R, retina, C, choroid; avidin–biotin complex immunoperoxidase, ×100).*

large number of cells in the vitreous samples and where the cytopathologists and ophthalmic pathologists are lacking. This technique may become an alternative method for the detection of intraocular lymphoma cells in the vitreous.

Cytokines

Interleukin-10 (IL-10)

Cytokine production has been evaluated in various lymphoid tumors. IL-10 is a growth and differentiation factor for B lymphocytes, and induces activated

Chi-Chao Chan, De Fen Shen and R. N. Buggage.

B cells to secrete large amounts of immunoglobulin [32,33]. IL-10 has been associated with the presence of malignant lymphoid neoplasm [34,35]. We have published that high IL-10 levels exist in the vitreous and cerebral spinal fluid of most patients with primary intraocular lymphoma [16,17]. From 1994 to 1998, 13 vitrectomy specimens with primary intraocular lymphoma were collected at the National Eye Institute. Using ELISA, IL-10 levels were detected in all specimens with a range from 13.5 to 8,127 pg/ml that correlated with the number of malignant cells in the vitreous. In contrast, there are no or barely detectable IL-10 levels in the vitreous of non-malignant and non-inflamed control samples. Recently, Ongkosuwito reported elevated vitreal IL-10 levels in patients with early stage of acute retinal necrosis and acute ocular toxoplasmosis [36]. In these cases, IL-10 appears to be produced by the infiltrating Th2 cells.

Interleukin-6 (IL-6)

Many cells produce IL-6. They include T and B lymphocytes, monocytes, epithelia, endothelia, and fibroblasts [37]. Elevated IL-6 has been reported in the aqueous humor and vitreous of patients with uveitis [36,38–40]. Although B lymphoma cells are capable of IL-6 production [41-43], the ratio of IL-10 to IL-6 in the vitreous of patients with primary intraocular lymphoma is often greater than 1 [17]. However, the vitreal ratio of IL-10 to IL-6 is frequently less than 1 in patients with uveitis [36]. In the 13 vitreous samples with primary intraocular lymphoma diagnosed at the National Eye Institute, only one had an IL-10 to IL-6 ratio less than 1. In this case, malignant cells were identified only in the retina but not in the vitreous. To date, we have analyzed cytokine levels on 52 vitrectomy specimens from 50 patients with infectious and non-infectious uveitis. Elevated IL-6 was found in 31 samples (59%) but elevated IL-10 in only six (12%), in all IL-10:IL-6 was less than 1 (Buggage, submitted). Measurement of vitreal IL-10 and IL-6 levels and their ratio have become a helpful adjunct in the diagnosis of intraocular lymphoma.

Both IL-10 and IL-6 message RNAs have been transcribed by the B-lymphoma cells [44]. We have also demonstrated IL-10 and IL-6 mRNA in primary intraocular lymphoma cells (Fig. 4) [45]. Under direct microscopic visualization malignant cells were procured from the histological and cytological slides of five patients. Expression of IL-6 mRNA and IL-10 mRNA were found in lymphoma cells by reverse transcription PCR.

Molecular pathology

Immunoglobulin gene rearrangement

Immunoglobulin gene rearrangement does not occur at any significant frequency during normal B-cell differentiation [46]. In contrast, the immunoglobulin gene sequence is rearranged in B-cell lymphomas and results in the monoclonality of their lymphoid neoplasm. Consequently, DNA sequences at the junction of V (variable), D (diversity), J (joining) segments can be used as clone-specific markers in individual patients with lymphoma [47–50]. The heavy chain immunoglobulin (IgH) gene rearrangement has been reported in systemic non-Hodgkin's lymphoma and leukemia of B-cell lineage [51–55].

Recently we have identified IgH gene rearrangement in primary intraocular lymphoma [27,56]. To date we have demonstrated aberrant IgH gene rearrangement at the V–D–J joint of the third framework region (FR3A) in the neoplastic cells by microdissecting the malignant cells from the histological and cytological slides of 20 patients with primary intraocular lymphoma (Fig. 4). Tumor cells in every patient contained FR3A PCR products. Examination of the PCR product, FR3A of the IgH gene is now becoming another useful adjunct for the diagnosis of primary intraocular lymphoma.

Apoptosis plays an important role in tumor survival. The Bcl-2 family members are closely associated with programmed cell survival [57]. The Bcl-2 protein suppresses apoptosis [58]. The high levels of Bcl-2 promote cancer by

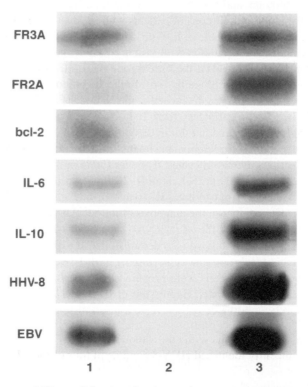

FIGURE 4. *PCR amplification showing various gene products in a case with AIDS related primary intraocular lymphoma: positive FR3A, negative FR2A, positive bcl-2 translocation, positive IL-10 and IL-6 mRNA, and positive HHV-8 and EBV genomes. Lane 1, primary intraocular lymphoma; lane 2, negative control; lane 3, positive control.*

Chi-Chao Chan, De Fen Shen and R. N. Buggage.

inhibiting apoptosis, thereby prolonging cell survival. The bcl-2 gene, located on chromosome 18, is near to the IgH gene locus on chromosome 14 [59]. The reciprocal t(14;18) chromosomal translocation brings the bcl-2 gene into juxtaposition with the IgH promoter. The resultant fusion gene causes bcl-2 gene deregulation and high level expression of Bcl-2 protein. Insertion of bcl-2 into the pre-B cell line has been shown to prolong survival of these cells independent of growth factors [60]. Approximately 85% follicular non-Hodgkin's lymphoma and approximately 20% diffuse large B-cell lymphomas have found a t(14;18) translocation [61,62].

Among the 20 cases of primary intraocular lymphoma that we have analyzed, 15 have shown a bcl-2/IgH gene translocation and each of these cases had aggressive clinical presentations (Fig. 4). Although there is a discrepancy between the frequency of the disease prognosis and the Bcl-2 protein/bcl-2 gene rearrangement in systemic B-cell lymphoma, a correlation between bcl-2 gene translocation and prognosis is found in our series [27].

Viral genome

In vitro, Epstein-Barr virus (EBV) efficiently transforms human B lymphocytes, causing them to proliferate continuously [63]. EBV is known to be strongly associated with Burkitt's lymphoma. EBV and the latent membrane protein can be detected in tumor cells of almost all AIDS-related CNS lymphoma. Signaling of the latent membrane protein through aggregation with TNF-α receptor-associated factor molecules has an important role in pathogenesis of the EBV-positive, AIDS-related lymphoma [64–67]. However, EBV is not frequently found in the immunocompetent patients with CNS lymphoma [68,69].

Using microdissection and PCR, we have also examined the EBV genome in 17 lymphoma cases which include two AIDS patients. Among the 17 cases, only one AIDS case who had a diffuse lymphoma involving the CNS, eye and orbit harbored EBV DNA (Fig. 4). Most of the cases at the National Eye institute represent early stage primary intraocular lymphoma.

In the past three years, it has been suggested that human herpesvirus-8 (HHV-8), a virus known to contribute to Kaposi's sarcoma, is associate with lymphomagenesis in humans [63]. The base sequence of the viral DNA fragments and their flanking sequences have partial homology to the human EBV and monkey herpesvirus saimiri [70–72]. HHV-8 is reported in a high percentage of primary effusion lymphoma [73], Castleman's disease [74,75], and multiple myeloma [76,77]. HHV-8 genome has been reported in primary CNS lymphoma of patients with and without AIDS [78].

We have recently identified HHV-8 genome in four of the 17 cases of primary intraocular lymphoma (Fig. 4). Using microdissection, we separately selected malignant cells and reactive lymphocytes [79]. We found that HHV-8 DNA was only in the neoplastic cells but not normal lymphocytes by PCR amplification and Southern hybridization. Of particular note, HHV-8 genome was detected in both cases with AIDS-related lymphoma suggesting that HHV-8 does indeed play a role in lymphomagenesis.

Pathogenesis

Monoclonality

Immunoglobulins manufactured by B lymphocytes consist of two identical pairs of light and heavy chains. They are formed by a variable and a constant domain. The genes for the variable (antigen-binding) domains are generated by recombination between separate types of gene segments, termed V, D, and J. In normal B cells, a random recombination will produce numerous gene products resulting in a polyclonality. However, rearranged IgH genes will produce a single clone resulting in B-lymphocytic lineage and clonal nature.

By all counts, the overwhelming majority of primary intraocular lymphoma exhibit a B-cell immunophenotype. Monoclonality of B cells can be illustrated with either κ or λ light chain restriction. Primary intraocular lymphoma is often accompanied by a conspicuous complement of admixed T lymphocytes and macrophages that can confound interpretation of the histological and immunohistochemical picture. These reactive elements usually appear as small, well-differentiated lymphocytes and foamy macrophages that are readily distinguished from the large, atypical B cells.

Lymphomagenesis

The exact mechanism leading to malignant transformation of B lymphocytes is still an enigma. Our findings of expression of HHV-8 gene, IL-10 and its mRNA in cells of primary intraocular lymphoma [17,45,79] agree with recent reports of viral oncogene (EBV and HHV-8) and cytokine homologues (IL-6 and IL-10) in association with primary effusion lymphoma and multicentric Castleman's disease [75,80,81]. Viral transcripts that encode oncogene and chemokine homologues are important for HHV-8 tumorigenicity.

Although the pathogenetic role of the virus in lymphoid malignancy is controversial, the tropism of HHV-8 for B cells is well established [82]. The HHV-8 genome encodes homologs of cyclin D1, a cell-cycle control element; certain cytokines, regulators, and receptors; and Bcl-2, an anti-apoptotic protein, among others [83]. The infected viral genome could therefore contribute to cellular growth and transformation through activation of the cell cycle. We speculate that the non-neoplastic B lymphocytes in those AIDS patients who eventually develop primary intraocular lymphoma may be infected with HHV-8, HIV, or other viruses in the eye, where ultimate transformation into malignant cells occurs. Another possibility may be promotion of a second, oncogenic virus.

Nine EBV genes are expressed as proteins in EBV-trasformed B lymphoblastoid cell lines, which are immortalized as a result of EBV infection [64]. One of the latent membrane proteins of EBV engages members of the tumor necrosis factor receptor-associated factor family of signaling molecules, then activates NF-κB expression of multiple viral and cellular genes. Certain subsets of AIDS-non-Hodgkin's lymphoma appear to be EBV-related

Chi-Chao Chan, De Fen Shen and R. N. Buggage.

although a high frequency of EBV is reported in AIDS-primary CNS lymphoma [84]. However, we found EBV genome in only one of the 17 cases with primary intraocular lymphoma suggesting this virus may not play a major role in malignant transformation.

IL-10 is reported to promote *in vitro* proliferation of normal B cells or EBV-transformed B lymphocytes [44,85]. In EBV associated lymphoma, the EBV open reading frame (BCRF-1) expresses IL-10-like activity [86]. This gene is critical for initiation and maintenance of EBV-driven B-cell transformation [87]. In our primary intraocular lymphoma cases we have shown a close association between the level of IL-10 and the number of malignant cells in the eye [16]. One may postulate that IL-10 is a key factor leading to dysregulation of B-cell growth and function in patients with certain subtypes of B-cell lymphoma.

Masood *et al.* have demonstrated that addition of IL-10 antisense oligonucleotide *in vitro* inhibited IL-10 mRNA expression of all tumor-derived B-cell lines regardless of their EBV status [88]. Recombinant IL-10 abrogated this inhibitory effect when given to the same B-cell lymphoma lines that were pretreated with antisense oligonucleotide. The autocrine IL-10 production may contribute to transformed B cells, promoting tumor survival and growth relatively independent of host-derived factors.

However, whether IL-10 exerts a direct effect on malignant B cells is still questionable. It is possible that IL-10 influences the growth of B-cell lymphoma by suppressing the antitumoral immune responses. IL-10 also impairs the ability of cytotoxic cells to kill their target. The precise role of IL-10 in primary intraocular lymphoma thus remains to be determined. Further examination of virus associated malignancies, identification of new viral pathogens, and cytokine homologues in primary intraocular lymphoma will provide clues to the complicated process of oncogenesis and bring us a step closer to more effective treatment of this malicious tumor.

References

1. Hochberg, F.H., and Miller, D.C., *J. Neurosurg.* 1988: 835–853, 1988.
2. Whitcup, S.M., de Smet, M.D., Rubin, B.I., *et al.*, *Ophthalmology* 100: 1399–1406, 1993.
3. Merchant, A., and Foster, C.S., *Int. Ophthalmol. Clin.* 37: 101–115, 1997.
4. Qualman, S.L., Mendelsohn, G., Mann, R.B., and Green, W.R., *Cancer* 52: 878–886, 1983.
5. Henry, J.M., Heffner, R.R., Jr., Dillard, S.H., Earle, K.M., and Davis, R.I., *Cancer* 34: 1293–1302, 1974.
6. Freeman, L.N., Schachat, A.P., Knox, D.L., Michels, R.G., and Green, W.R., *Ophthalmology* 94: 1631–1639, 1987.
7. Eby, N.L., Grufferman, S., Flannelly, C.M., Schold, S.C., Jr., Vogel, F.S., and Burger, P.C., *Cancer* 62: 2461–2465, 1988.
8. O'Sullivan, M.G., Whittle, I.R., Gregor, A., and Ironside, J.W., *Lancet* 338: 895–896, 1991.

9. Peterson, K., Gordon, K.B., Heinemann, M.H., and DeAngelis, L.M., *Cancer* 72: 843–849, 1993.

10. Augsburger, J.J., and Greatrex, K.V., *Trans. Pa. Acad. Ophthalmol. Otolaryngol.* 41: 796–808, 1989.

11. Ridley, M.E., McDonald, H.R., Sternberg, P., Jr., Blumenkranz, M.S., Zarbin, M.A., and Schachat, A.P., *Ophthalmology* 99: 1153–1160; discussion 1160–1161, 1992.

12. de Smet, M.D., Nussenblatt, R.B., Davis, J.L., and Palestine, A.G., *Int. Ophthalmol.* 14: 413–417, 1990.

13. DeAngelis, L.M., Yahalom, J., Thaler, H.T., and Kher, U., *J. Clin. Oncol.* 10: 635–643, 1992.

14. Blumenkranz, M.S., Ward, T., Murphy, S., Mieler, W., Williams, G.A., and Long, J., *Retina*, 12: S64–S70, 1992.

15. Davis, J.L., Solomon, D., Nussenblatt, R.B., Palestine, A.G., and Chan, C.C., *Ophthalmology* 99: 250–256, 1992.

16. Chan, C.C., Whitcup, S.M., Solomon, D., and Nussenblatt, R.B., *Am. J. Ophthalmol.* 120: 671–673, 1995.

17. Whitcup, S.M., Stark-Vancs, V., Wittes, R.E., *et al.*, *Arch. Ophthalmol.* 115: 1157–1160, 1997.

18. Klingele, T.G., and Hogan, M.J., *Am. J. Ophthalmol.* 79: 39–47, 1975.

19. Michels, R.G., Knox, D.L., Erozan, Y.S., and Green, W.R., *Arch. Ophthalmol.* 93: 1331–1335, 1975.

20. Parver, L.M., and Font, R.L., *Arch. Ophthalmol.* 97: 1505–1507, 1979.

21. Char, D.H., Ljung, B.M., Miller, T., and Phillips, T., *Ophthalmology* 95: 625–630, 1988.

22. Dean, J.M., Novak, M.A., Chan, C.C., and Green, W.R., *Retina* 16: 47–56, 1996.

23. Lopez, J.S., Chan, C.C., Burnier, M., Rubin, B., and Nussenblatt, R.B., *Am. J. Ophthalmol.* 112: 472–474, 1991.

24. Schanzer, M.C., Font, R.L., and O'Malley, R.E., *Ophthalmology* 98: 88–91, 1991.

25. Font, R.L., Laucirica, R., and Patrinely, J.R., *Ophthalmology* 100: 966–970, 1993.

26. Matzkin, D.C., Slamovits, T.L., and Rosenbaum, P.S., *Ophthalmology* 101: 850–855, 1994.

27. Shen, D.F., Zhuang, Z., LeHoang, P., *et al.*, *Ophthalmology* 105: 1664–1669, 1998.

28. Brown, S.M., Jampol, L.M., and Cantrill, H.L., *Surv. Ophthalmol.* 39: 133–140, 1994.

29. Wilson, D.J., Braziel, R., and Rosenbaum, J.T., *Arch. Ophthalmol.* 110: 1455–1458, 1992.

30. Char, D.H., Ljung, B.M., Deschenes, J., and Miller, T.R., *Br. J. Ophthalmol.* 72: 905–911, 1988.

31. Davis, J.L., Viciana, A.L., and Ruiz, P., *Am. J. Ophthalmol.* 124: 362–372, 1997.

32. Banchereau, J., Briere, F., Liu, Y.J., and Rousset, F., *Stem. Cells (Dayt)* 12: 278–288, 1994.

33. Benjamin, D., *Cancer Treat. Res.* 80: 305–319, 1995.

34. Benjamin, D., Park, C.D., and Sharma, V., *Leuk. Lymphoma* 12: 205–210, 1994.

35. Blay, J.Y., Burdin, N., Rousset, F., *et al.*, *Blood* 82: 2169–2174, 1993.

36. Ongkosuwito, J.V., Feron, E.J., Van Doornik, C.E., *et al.*, *Invest. Ophthalmol. Vis. Sci.* 39: 2659–2665, 1998.

37. Lotz, M., *Cancer Treat. Res.* 80: 209–233, 1995.

38. Murray, P.I., Hoekzema, R., Van Haren, M.A., De Hon, F.D., and Kijlstra, A., *Invest. Ophthalmol. Vis. Sci.* 31: 917–920, 1990.

39. Feys, J., Emond, J.P., Salvanet-Bouccara, A., and Dublanchet, A., *J. Fr. Ophtalmol.* 17: 634–639, 1994.

40. de Boer, J.H., Van Haren, M.A., De Vries-Knoppert, W.A., *et al.*, *Curr. Eye Res.* 11: 181–186, 1992.
41. Kato, H., Kinoshita, T., Suzuki, S., *et al.*, *Leuk. Lymphoma* 29: 71–79, 1998.
42. Voorzanger, N., Touitou, R., Garcia, E., *et al.*, *Cancer Res.* 56: 5499–5505, 1996.
43. Preti, H.A., Cabanillas, F., Talpaz, M., Tucker, S.L., Seymour, J.F., and Kurzrock, R., *Ann. Intern. Med.* 127: 186–194, 1997.
44. Emilie, D., Zou, W., Fior, R., *et al.*, *Methods* 11: 133–142, 1997.
45. Shen, D., Zhuang, Z., Matteson, D.M., *et al.*, *Invest. Ophthalmol. Vis. Sci.* 39: S290, 1998.
46. Lewis, S.M., *Adv. Immunol.* 56: 27–150, 1994.
47. Ramasamy, I., Brisco, M., and Morley, A., *J. Clin. Pathol.* 45: 770–775, 1992.
48. Trainor, K.J., Brisco, M.J., Story, C.J., and Morley, A.A., *Blood* 75: 2220–2222, 1990.
49. Calvert, R.J., Evans, P.A., Randerson, J.A., Jack, A.S., Morgan, G.J., and Dixon, M.F., *J. Pathol.* 180: 26–32, 1996.
50. Armes, J.E., Southey, M., Eades, S., *et al.*, *Pediatr. Pathol. Lab. Med.* 16: 435–449, 1996.
51. Chen, Y.-T., Whitney, K.D., and Chen, Y., *Mod. Pathol.* 7: 429–434, 1994.
52. Linke, B., Bolz, I., Fayyazi, A., *et al.*, *Leukemia* 11: 1055–1062, 1997.
53. Rockman, S.P., *Leukemia* 11: 852–862, 1997.
54. Jeffers, M.D., McCorriston, J., Farquharson, M.A., Stewart, C.J., and Mutch, A.F., *Cytopathology* 8: 114–121, 1997.
55. Achille, A., Scarpa, A., Montresor, M., *et al.*, *Diagn. Mol. Pathol.* 4: 14–24, 1995.
56. Chan, C.C., Shen, D., Nussenblatt, R.B., Boni, R., and Zhuang, Z., *Diagn. Mol. Pathol.* 7: 63–64, 1998.
57. Adams, J.M., and Cory, S., *Science* 281: 1322–1326, 1998.
58. Hockenbery, D.M., Zutter, M., Hickcy, W., Nahm, M., and Korsmeyer, S., *Proc. Natl. Acad. Sci. USA* 88: 6961–6969, 1991.
59. Weiss, L.M., Warnke, R.A., Sklar, J., and Cleary, M.L., *N. Engl. J. Med.* 317: 1185–1189, 1987.
60. Vaux, D.L., Cory, S., and Adams, J.M., *Nature* 335: 440–444, 1988.
61. Jacobson, J.O., Wilkes, B.M., Kwaiatkowski, D.J., Medeiros, L.J., Aisenberg, A.C., and Harris, N.L., *Cancer* 72: 231–236, 1993.
62. Pezzella, F., Ralfkiaer, E., Gatter, K.C., and Mason, D.Y., *Br. J. Haematol.* 76: 58–64, 1990.
63. Lyons, S.F., and Liebowitz, D.N., *Semin. Oncol.* 25: 461–475, 1998.
64. Liebowitz, D., *N. Engl. J. Med.* 338: 1413–1421, 1998.
65. Cinque, P., Brytting, M., Vago, L., *et al.*, *Lancet* 342: 398–401, 1993.
66. De Luca, A., Antinori, A., Cingolani, A., *et al.*, *Br. J. Haematol.* 90: 844–849, 1995.
67. Yu, G.H., Montone, K.T., Frias-Hidvegi, D., Cajulis, R.S., Brody, B.A., and Levy, R.M., *Diagn. Cytopathol.* 14: 114–120, 1996.
68. Bergmann, M., Blasius, S., Bankfalvi, A., and Mellin, W., *Gen. Diagn. Pathol.* 141: 235–242, 1996.
69. Bashir, R., Luka, J., Chelohia, K., Chamberlain, M., and Hochberg, F., *Neurology* 43: 2358–2362, 1993.
70. Moore, P.S., Gao, S.J., Dominguez, G., *et al.*, *J. Virol.* 70: 549–558, 1996.
71. Karcher, D.S., and Alkan, S., *Hum. Pathol.* 28: 801–808, 1997.
72. Cesarman, E., Nador, R.G., Bai, F., *et al.*, *J. Virol.* 70: 8218–8223, 1996.
73. Asou, H., Said, J.W., Yang, R., *et al.*, *Blood* 91: 2475–2481, 1998.
74. Kikuta, H., Itakura, O., Taneichi, K., and Kohno, M., *Br. J. Haematol.* 99: 790–793, 1997.

75. Teruya-Feldstein, J., Zauber, P., Setsuda, J.E., *et al.*, *Lab. Invest.* 78: 1637–1642, 1998.
76. Chauhan, D., Bharti, A., Raje, N., *et al.*, *Blood* 93: 1482–1486, 1999.
77. Rettig, M.B., Ma, H.J., Vescio, R.A., *et al.*, *Science* 276: 1851–1854, 1997.
78. Corboy, J.R., Garl, P.J., and Kleinschmidt-DeMasters, B.K., *Neurology* 50: 335–340, 1998.
79. Chan, C.C., Shen, D.F., Whitcup, S.M., *et al.*, *Blood* 1999.
80. Cesarman, E., and Knowles, D.M., *Semin. Diagn. Pathol.* 14: 54–66, 1997.
81. Gessain, A., Briere, J., Angelin-Duclos, C., *et al.*, *Leukemia* 11: 266–272, 1997.
82. Mesri, E.A., Cesarman, E., Arvanitakis, L., *et al.*, *J. Exp. Med.* 183: 2385–2390, 1996.
83. Russo, J.J., Bohenzky, R.A., Chien, M.C., *et al.*, *Proc. Natl. Acad. Sci. USA* 93: 14862–14867, 1999.
84. MacMahon, E.M., Glass, J.D., Hayward, S.D., *et al.*, *Lancet* 338: 969–973, 1991.
85. Khatri, V.P., and Caligiuri, M.A., *Cancer Immunol. Immunother.* 46: 239–244, 1998.
86. Vieira, P., de Waal-Malefyt, R., Dang, M.N., *et al.*, *Proc. Natl. Acad. Sci. USA* 88: 1172–1176, 1991.
87. Miyazaki, I., Cheung, R.K., and Dosch, H.M., *J. Exp. Med.* 178: 439–447, 1993.
88. Masood, R., Zhang, Y., Bond, M.W., *et al.*, *Blood* 85: 3423–3430, 1995.

CHARLES E. THIRKILL

Immunology of paraneoplastic syndromes

————

Abstract

Cancers inflict numerous and dire effects upon the host through the production and release of a variety of biochemicals, many of which are natural compounds produced in unnatural quantities within abnormal anatomical locations. There is often an impressive immune reponse to cancerous growth which in many cases fails to defend the host, and occasionally increases the complexity of the disease. If during its uncontrolled proliferation the cancer should coincidentally express a potent autoantigen the organ in which that antigen is normally expressed may come under immune-mediated attack.

This paradox may result from the cancer's ability to block the host's immunologic activity within its immediate location while the affected organ located elsewhere has no such capacity. Some preexisting flaw such as prior trauma to the organ involved may prove a requirement that provides access to hitherto 'immunologically privileged sites'. The resultant loss of tolerance results in autoimmune reactions that are often the first indication of a health problem prompting the patient to seek medical help.

A growing collection of paraneoplasias have been found to appear in association with a series of biologically distinct cancers. This chapter decribes those that are best documented in published accounts of cancers that not only avoid elimination by the host's immune response, but also incite damaging autoimmune reactions through the coincidental expression of key autoantigens.

The intent here is to discuss immune-mediated paraneoplasia in which a growing number of reports have led to furthering understanding of the nature of the phenomena, and to encourage further inquiry into the use of these peculiar immunologic reactions in the detection and treatment of the cause.

Keywords: Cancer-induced autoimmunity, ectopic expressions

Ocular Immunology, Research Building One, U.C. Davis Medical Center, California, 95817, USA

237

Introduction

Cancers inflict numerous and dire effects upon the patient through the production and release of a variety of biochemicals, many of which are natural compounds produced in unnatural quantities within abnormal anatomical locations. Along with mutated cancer components, the appearance of specific cell associated products outside of normal distribution can evoke an immune response comparable to that of a transplant. The resultant loss of homeostasis precipitates numerous signs and symptoms, often the first indication of a health problem prompting the patient to seek medical help.

The descriptive names given to the so called 'immune-mediated' paraneoplasias are a collection of 'umbrella terms' encompassing groups of syndromes with similar signs and symptoms, but differing immunologically [1–3]. Autoimmunity is implicated from observations of patients displaying abnormal immunologic activity focused upon specific antigens located at the site of paraneoplastic activity. The individuality of the patient ensures considerable diversity in the immune response to any given malignancy, but the appearance of common immunologic reactions in different patients with the same type of malignancy indicates a common pathway of sensitization. The logical assumption that the cancer incites the immunologic reactions is based upon observations of malignancies expressing the protein involved in the abnormal immunologic reaction [1,4–10]. The antigens involved are organ-specific, and identify immunologically distinct subgroups. Acceptance of this 'immunologic connection' in many forms of paraneoplasia led to the use of serologic assays to detect antibody activity with key 'paraneoplasia-associated' antigens that were found to share distinctive relationships with specific types of cancers [11–13].

Surgical removal of the causal neoplasm has in some cases resulted in amelioration of immune-mediated paraneoplasia [2,14–18], gamma globulin treatment is reported to have beneficial results in some [19], plasmapheresis and immunosuppression may provide symptomatic relief [3,13,15,20,21], but no single approach is universally successful. This failure may result from the initiation of self perpetuating immunologic reactions involving specific host antigens to which tolerance has been permanently broken. Successful treatment of immune-mediated paraneoplasia may require combination therapy aimed at eliminating the patients cancer, and immunologic desensitization addressing the abnormal hypersensitivity that may prove as debilitating and life-threatening as the malignancy.

There are many immunologic aspects to the paraneoplasias, and each type of neoplasm can produce a variety of secondary effects. The intent here is to describe those in which consistent reports of specific antigen/antibody reactions have led to furthering understanding of the pathogenesis of paraneoplasia, and how they assist in the recognition of the type of neoplasm involved.

Charles E. Thirkill

Brain

From the earliest published descriptions the secondary effects of cancer were, and continue to be found most often in patients with small cell carcinomas, the archetype inducer of immune-mediated paraneoplasia usually located in the lungs of heavy smokers [22,23]. Other neoplasias such as thymomas, lymphomas, adenomas, ductal carcinomas, and melanomas represent additional causes of cancer-induced immunologic abnormalities, but the greater proportion of autoimmune reactions continue to be reported in association with, and sometimes preceding the recognition of small cell carcinomas [12,13]. The high prevalence of neurological disorders occurring with this malignancy may result from its surmised neuroendocrine origins, the kulchitsky cell [24–28]. Loss of control of such influential cells can have an immediate and deleterious effect upon homeostasis, often inducing an impressive immune response as the transformed cells begin the inappropriate translation of genes not normally expressed within the organ in which the cancer emerges [29].

Paraneoplastic Cerebellar Degenerations (PCD) were the first paraneoplasia to be described and occur in a wide range of different types of neoplasia such as lymphomas, carcinomas of the ovaries, uterus, breast, and adenocarcinomas, in addition to the most frequently culpable small cell carcinoma. The pathologic process involves changes in, and loss of specific brain cells. The selective destruction of Purkinje cells brought attention to the syndrome, but an increasing collection of other brain components were subsequently found to succumb to immune-mediated attack [3,30,31]. The resultant loss of cognisance may initially be confused with other diseases before the syndrome is recognized, and the inciting cancer identified [13,32–34].

Once it was recognized as a distinct clinical entity PCD was immediately suspected to involve immunologic reactions [35], and has since been shown to include abnormal antibody activity with a series of distinct neuronal proteins.

The earliest immunologic 'cancer-connection' was established in paraneoplastic cerebellar degenerations when in some cases, the cause of the sensitization could be traced to small cell carcinomas expressing the putative autoantigens involved in the patients immunologic reactions [36]. This mode of sensitization represents a frequent theme in the pathogenesis of paraneoplasias, and in time may be found the cause of all that are shown or suspected to be immune-mediated.

The growing list of brain proteins involved in the syndromes are identified by their relative mass observed in Western blot reactions upon an extract of brain. Examples include the Yo, Hu and Ri antigens but are not limited to these proteins since some patients develop central nervous system (CNS) syndromes in the absence of immunoreactivity with any of the three. The list of immunoreactive neuronal proteins continues to grow but these three represent recognized disease-associated cancer markers, and antibody activity with either one is reason to suspect occult neoplasia in a patient presenting with an unexplained CNS disorder.

The Yo antigen is located within the cytoplasm of Purkinje cells and is associated with some types of PCD. The Yo syndrome may manifest in association with breast, ovarian, transitional cell carcinomas, or adenocarcinomas, and in some cases the antigen has been found expressed in the causal cancer [37]. However, PCD can also occur in patients with Hodgkin's lymphoma, lung cancer and other types of malignancies in the absence of antibody reactions with the Yo antigen [3,38,39]. This immunologic disparity suggests that PCD patients who produce an immune response to the Yo antigen are collectively experiencing the same antigenic stimulus. Those who do not may be reacting to a closely related member of the same family of proteins, since clinical presentations are very similar.

The Hu antigen is a member of the family of RNA-binding proteins located in neurons of the central and peripheral nervous system. Antibody reaction with this protein are associated with the appearance of paraneoplastic encephalomyelitis (PEM) [40]. At autopsy, antibody complexes and activated lymphocytes recognizing the Hu antigen may be found within the brain of the affected individual [41]. Paradoxically, the response to treatment and survival of small cell carcinoma patients is increased in those who produce high titers of antibodies to the Hu antigen [42]. It could be surmised that benefit ensues from the inhibition of the activity of the carcinoma expressing the Hu antigen, a possibility that provides added encouragement for continued efforts at immune-mediated suppression of malignancies [11,43].

The immune response to the Ri antigen is associated with the induction of paraneoplastic opsoclonal-ataxia in breast and lung cancer patients. The antigen is also a member of the family of RNA-binding proteins located within the brain and spinal cord, and has been described as an aberrant expression in the patients neoplasm. Like many other suspected autoantigens, the Ri antigen is highly conserved in nature, and shares homology with components of yeast and retroviral proteins [44].

While cytotoxic antibody activity is suspected in paraneoplastic brain syndromes, unlike the Lambert–Eaton myasthenic syndrome and paraneoplastic pemphigus, efforts at passive transfer to experimental animals with antibodies reactive with the Hu, Yo and Ri antigens have failed to reproduce the signs and symptoms of the disease [45]. Nevertheless, these antibody reactions represent an immunologic connections with cancer that serves to prompt further inquiry when encountered in patients for whom no other explanation for a loss of cognisance is apparent [13].

Muscle

The *Lambert–Eaton Myasthenic Syndrome (LEMS)* is one of the most studied paraneoplasia and is linked with small cell carcinomas expressing the specific neurotransmitter protein involved in the myasthenia [46]. Current doctrine

Charles E. Thirkill

advocates that the ectopic appearance of immunologic epitopes of the voltage-gated calcium channels prompts a related and pathologic immune response that cross-reacts with the corresponding component in the muscle presynaptic nerve terminal [2,47]. The pathologic significance of autoantibodies in the production of LEMS is supported by passive transfer experiments in which antibodies from affected individuals were shown to produce similar myasthenic effects in neonatal mice following intraperitoneal infusion of the patient's immunoglobulins [48].

Thymoma associated myasthenia gravis

A variant of the phenomenon of 'aberrant expression' occurs in some rare malignant thymomas that have been shown to express neurofilaments sharing antigenic epitopes with (1) the acetylcholine receptor (AChR), a key component of the autoimmune reactions of Myasthenia Gravis (MG), and (2) Titin, a muscle-specific protein [49–51]. These observations immediately invite acceptance of this coincidental expression as the mode of sensitization. However, laboratory animals given transplants of thymomas have failed to produce antibodies that typify either paraneoplastic or classic MG [52], a paradox that requires further inquiry since it is essential that the sensitizing cause in each be identified and compared. The expression of only part; an epitope of the molecule of interest contrasts with that described in small cell carcinomas in which the whole molecular autoantigen appears in the cancer. The immunologic analysis of epitope recognition must include an appreciation of the need to match epitopes since those expressed by the malignancy may not be those involved in the patient's immune response [49,52,53]. These differences are not apparent in Western blot analyses, and require the more sensitive technique of molecular matching using specific synthesized epitopes to resolve the questions [54].

The recognition that some well recognized autoantigens and component epitopes are actively expressed by dendritic cells within the normal thymic medulla is probably of great relevance to the induction, and avoidance of autoimmunity [55,56]. The thymus is considered to be a repository of immunologic instruction, the locus of surveillance where immune cell education occurs. The 'learning' process may require close contact with host autoantigens to induce the tolerance required for natural survival. Loss of tolerance is avoided in the normal individual where active immunologic suppressor functions are intact. Autoimmune reactions in cancer patients may accordingly be restricted to those with faulty suppressor function, making them genetically predisposed to succumb to sensitization [32].

The production of autoantibodies reactive with key muscle components has in some cases diminished following early and complete surgical removal of the thymoma, a result that coincides with the increased survival rate of MG patients following thymectomy [2,53]. But this does not exclude the occasional example of the appearance of MG subsequent to thymectomy [14,15]. The immunologic complexities of the myasthenias slowly unravel as pieces of information on the pathogenicity of each fall into place, and a little more of the workings of this collection of diseases is understood.

The association of neurofilaments with autoimmune diseases and paraneo-palsia continues to grow. Different classes of thymomas differ in the expression of neurofilaments, and the consequential induction of related autoantibodies [49,51]. A spectrum of severity of thymic transformations occurs ranging from gross to barely recognizable, a situation that has provoked supposition that MG proper evolves from the benign, less recognized thymic changes which almost always accompany this disease [50]. In this respect, the nature of para-neoplastic and classic myasthenia gravis tend to converge.

Paraneoplastic stiff man syndrome (PSMS)

Rheumatologic disorders are not uncommonly the first indication of occult cancers that continue to be found with an impressive incidence in patients with unclarified rheumatic complaint [57]. The intermittent muscle spasms that characterize the Stiff Man Syndrome are precipitated by noise, fear or touch, and may initially be confused with other diseases involving muscular rigidity. Antibody production to amphiphysin was originally thought pathognomonic for PSMS [58,59]. Amphiphysin is a neuronal protein associated with synap-tic vesicles and found in different isoforms in the nodes of Ranvier of the brain, and around tubules within skeletal muscle. Expression of amphiphysin by small cell and breast carcinomas indicates one possible pathway leading to loss of tolerance, and complies with the theory of 'aberrant expression' as the sensitization process [1]. However, more recent studies reveal immunoreac-tivity with this potential autoantigen can develop in association with breast, ovarian and small cell carcinomas in the absence of stiffness [60,61]. And the same abnormal hypersensitivity also occurs in association with many other paraneoplasia, such as sensory neuropathy, encephalomyelitis, cerebellar degenerations and the Lambert–Eaton myasthenic syndrome [3,60,62]. This apparent confusion may result from multiple paraneoplasias superimposed, probably resulting from mixed malignancies that may pass unrecognized in the complex process of diagnosis and tumor classification. While immunore-activity with amphiphysin is abnormal, and sufficient reason to arouse suspi-cion of an underlying neoplasm, it is not representative of any specific type of malignancy. The implication of amphiphysin as an autoantigen in immune-mediated paraneoplasia is therefore far from clear, but serves to prompt further studies into questions concerning genetic susceptibility to loss of tolerance to this important and widespread tissue component.

An immunologic connection occurs between paraneoplastic stiff man syn-drome, the classic stiff man syndrome [63,64], and that developing in some cases of insulin-dependent diabetes mellitus (IDDM) [65]. All three involve endocrine imbalance resulting from autoimmune interference with different pathogenesis, but include the coincidental production of antibodies to glu-tamic acid decarboxylase (GAD). Although different epitopes of the GAD molecule are involved in each disease [66,67], the commonality involving the same molecule may prove exceedingly interesting when the cause of the auto-immune reactions in the three syndromes is eventually identified. Until this is understood the coincidence continues to represent another example of immuno-logic overlap between paraneoplasia, and diseases unrelated to cancer.

Skin

Paraneoplastic pemphigus (PNP)

Skin disorders may be the most common form of paraneoplasia, and on first encounter can easily be mistaken for a multitude of other problems. However, when bulbous pemphigus appears in a patient the possibility of an occult neo-plasia should be included in deliberations of the cause. This insidious syndrome has been described in patients with both malignant, and benign neoplasia, with an obvious survival bias towards that induced by benign growths [68–70].

The appearance of pemphigus ranks as one of the strongest stimuli prompt-ing the patient to seek medical attention. Occurring most often in patients with lymphocytic leukemia or malignant lymphomas no direct immunologic connection between the patient's neoplasia and the eruption of the dermatol-ogic disorder has been discovered. The pattern of sensitization may follow the path of other paraneoplasia and result from 'aberrant expression', but a thorough analysis of this possibility has yet to be made.

There are several distinct skin-related immunologic reactions associated with the appearance of cancer-induced pemphigus, some of the antigens invol-ved are recognized as the cytoplasmic components desmoplakin, envoplakin and periplakin, but also include members of the desmoglein family of cell surface proteins [71,72]. Antibody activity with these skin keratinocyte compo-nents is classically demonstrated by immunoprecipitation assays, Western blot analyses, and indirect immunofluorescence in which antibodies of the IgG subclass predominate [70,73].

Blistering oral lesions commonly accompany those of the skin and provide easily biopsied samples for direct immunofluorescence in which abnormal antibody, and complement aggregates are found localized within intercellular spaces. Confirmation can be made using the well established technique of indi-rect immunofluorescence on sections of rodent urinary bladder when related antibodies are found to localize upon epithelial cell surface antigens [70,74,75]. Western blot reactions on extracts of normal human skin reveal antibody inter-actions with any or all of five paraneoplastic pemphigus-related proteins which have relative molecular weights of 170, 190, 210, 230 and 250 kd [76,77].

Tissue cultures of human keratinocytes labelled with any convenient iso-tope and mixed with serum samples from the PNP patient result in the immunoprecipitation of PNP-related skin proteins, demonstrable by poly-acrylamide gel analysis with subsequent autoradiography [72,77,78].

Passive transfer of comparable skin lesions to neonatal mice with anti-bodies from PNP patients provides another example of the cytotoxic immunoglobulins encountered in the paraneoplasia. As with other types of paraneoplasias, the pathogenesis of PNP appears founded in antibody-mediated autoimmunity resulting from cancer-induced sensitization to specific, disease related proteins [72,79].

Eye

Early inquiries into the immunologic aspects of vision loss in cancer patients described the remote ocular effects of cancer as the 'Visual Paraneoplastic Syndrome' (VPS), and included evidence of abnormal immunologic activity directed at the various cell types that compose the neurosensory retina [80,81]. Different immunologic reactions reported by separate groups of researchers gave advanced warning of the need to organize continuing studies in order to understand the full scope of what were immediately suspected to be cancer-induced autoimmune retinopathies [82–84]. From the very beginning, the small cell carcinoma appeared as the most frequently encountered cause of cancer-induced blindness [23,34].

The implication of autoantibodies in the production of paraneoplastic retinopathies was first suspected when immunoglobulins reactive with retinal ganglion cells were demonstrated in a patients with small cell carcinoma-associated retinal degenerations [80,84,85]. This aberrant immune response was shown to hold the potential for harm when it was found that an intraocular injection of rabbit antibodies reactive with retinal ganglion cells produced an experimental, retinal ganglion cell ablation in cats [86,87]. The results of these experiments illustrated how the selective loss of specific ocular components can occur through antibody-mediated reactions in sensitized individuals [87,88]. Immunologic similarities between host neurofilaments and antigens expressed by small cell carcinoma gave evidence of the sensitization process [89,90], a situation comparable to the epitope cross-reactivity reported in the autoimmune reactions of patients with thymomas in which parts of, but not the whole antigen are expressed [51,53].

Subsequent research uncovered a series of single retinal proteins involved in the antibody reactions of patients with small cell carcinoma-associated retinal degenerations. The first description was that of the 23 kd photoreceptor component, later identified as 'recoverin', a photoreceptor protein essential to the functions of rhodopsin [91]. The recombinant equivalent of this protein is now used routinely as the test antigen in the serologic identification of recoverin hypersensitivity, a specific immunologic subclass of paraneoplastic retinopathy, and a clinically distinctive form of retinal degeneration [92].

The signs and symptoms contributing to retinal degenerations caused by cancers distant from the eye led to the designation; 'Cancer-Associated Retinopathy', the CAR syndrome [34,93,94]. The preponderance of cancer-induced vision loss in small cell carcinoma patients again demonstrates the relatively high frequency of paraneoplasia induced by this particular type of malignancy.

The pathologic significance of antibodies in the pathogenesis of CAR was established in passive transfer experiments using guinea pigs in which the retro-orbital instillation of the patient's serum was shown to demyelinate the optic nerve [95]. This finding emphasized the complexities of the CAR syndrome revealing that, in addition to the anti-retinal antibodies that identify and participate in the retinopathy, the patient's sera contains factors and/or antibodies reactive with and detrimental to optic nerve functions [96,97].

Ensuing inquiries into the damaging properties of anti-recoverin antibodies illustrated an apoptosis-inducing activity upon *in vitro* cultivated monolayers of rat retina cells [98], and antibody-mediated retinal degenerations *in vivo* following intraocular injection of these immunoglobulins into the genetically prone Lewis rat. This animal is exquisitely sensitive to the induction of auto-immune reactions within the eye, and provides a useful model to demonstrate both the pathologic processes involved in retinal degenerations [99,100], and the need for inherited susceptibility [101].

Entry of immunoglobulins to the inner workings of the neuronal retina may depend on leaks induced into the blood-retina barrier by the biochemical influence of the cancer, with subsequent access to the intracellular CAR antigen(s) through means comparable to those proposed to occur in other autoimmune diseases in which autoantibodies react with cytoplasmic and nuclear components [102,103].

As acceptance of the sight-robbing characteristics of the CAR syndrome increased reports on the pathologic consequences of immunologic reactions with the 23 kd CAR antigen (recoverin) began to appear in the literature with increasing frequency. The correlation of the 23 kd antigen/antibody reaction with loss of photoreceptor cells in which the antigen is located, and the coincidental expression of the same retinal protein by the patient's small cell carcinoma was proposed as the immunologic 'cancer-connection' responsible for initiating the events that lead to an immune-mediated retinal degeneration [4,7–10].

Three additional small cell carcinoma-associated CAR antigens have since been discovered, with relative molecular weights of 40, 45 and 60 kd, and there are undoubtedly more. The link with small cell carcinoma was strengthened by the demonstration of an experimental, cancer-induced retinopathy in guinea pigs through the intraperitoneal propagation of viable small cell carcinoma cells. This model is based upon the discovery of a specific culture of small cell carcinoma expressing the 40 kd CAR antigen which is located within the outer plexiform layer of the retina [104]. Following intraperitoneal propagation of this culture a 'quiet' retinal degeneration ensued, similar to that observed and described in clinical observations of the syndrome, and was accompanied by antibodies reactive with the 40 kd CAR antigen. However, attributing the retinal degeneration solely to these antibodies is presumptions, since contributions from the many other cancer components and products the animals were exposed to cannot be excluded from the production of the experimental retinopathy. Propagating viable cancer cells in experimental animals results in a profusion of influences from the expression of a multitude of antigenic components and biologically active products. Although more difficult to interpret, the practice of evaluating the influences of viable cancer cells *in vivo* permits a close replication to the complexities of the patient's predicament.

The 45 and 60 kd CAR antigen are both located within the photoreceptor cells of the retina, but the latter is also demonstrable within the optic nerve, cerebellum and spinal cord. Autoimmune reactions with this widely disseminated CNS component may be responsible for the few reports on cancer-associated retinal degenerations accompanied by optic neuropathy [105–107].

Melanoma associated retinopathy (MAR)

Intraocular melanomas are not included in this syndrome which develops as a remote effect of cutaneous malignant melanoma, usually many years after seemingly successful treatment. Onset suggest a recurrence and metastasis, if not already recognized. Electroretinograph findings are described as resembling those of congenital stationary night blindness [108], with diminished b-wave activity that coincides with the immunologic findings of a focus of antibody activity upon cells in the bipolar region of the retina [109–113]. No specific protein has yet been identified in the immunologic idiosyncrasy of this rare syndrome that may instead involve lipid or carbohydrate antigens. Visual fields, like those in other types of paraneoplastic retinopathies, can resemble those of retinitis pigmentosa sharing the same characteristic of a 'quiet' non-inflammatory and progressive degeneration [114]. Optic nerve involvement is common, and could represent a major contributing factor to immune-mediated vision loss in the MAR syndrome, possibly including demyelinating effects comparable to those of other types of vision loss.

Chronic demyelinating polyneuropathy in melanoma patients has been attributed to immunologic cross-reactivity between the melanoma and Schwann cells, both originating from neuroectodermal cells. These immunologic similarities compare with those of other immune-mediated paraneoplasia, and could involve antibody-mediated damage like that associated with the vitiligo which may also complicate melanoma [115].

Paraneoplastic optic neuropathy (PON)

Cancer-induced demyelinization is yet another characteristic of paraneoplasia and may be the presenting signs and symptoms in a variety of different malignancies [116–118]. That encountered in lymphomatous optic neuritis was among the first paraneoplasia to be linked with autoimmunity [119,120]. Confusion may arise with that resulting from treatment [121,122], but demyelination occurring as a remote effect of cancer may be identified by distinct immunologic reactions such as those described in the 23 and 60 kd CAR syndromes [95,105,107]. The 'patchy' demyelination compares with that typical of multiple sclerosis and has been shown transmissible with serum antibodies to experimental animals [95].

Charles E. Thirkill

Cancer-induced demyelination can occur at any stage in the development of the malignancy. As with the majority of paraneoplasia, paraneoplastic demyelination occurs primarily in association with small cell carcinoma [95,107], but has been reported in patients with a variety of different types of neoplasia [117,120,123–126].

Breast cancer associated retinopathies (BCAR)

The immunologic features of Breast Cancer-Associated Retinopathy (BCAR) develop late in the history of the cancer, and may indicate a recurrence in a seemingly 'cured' patient. The few that have been encountered exhibit a focus of antibody activity upon retinal photoreceptors, but the antigen(s) involved are not yet identified. There is a clear need to learn more of the immunologic nature of the BCAR syndrome due to the equally rare occurrence of treatment related ocular toxicity in breast cancer patients that may be confused with this type of paraneoplasia [121,122].

Lymphoma-associated retinopathy (LAR)

A rare form of retinal degeneration appearing in lymphoblastic, Hodgkin's and non-Hodgkin' lymphoma patients. The immunologic reactions of Hodgkin's patients is unusual in that it includes a focus of antibody activity upon retinal cone pedicles, but the antigen(s) participating in this anomalous immunologic reactivity are currently unknown. Detailed reports of the clinical features of each type of LAR have appeared in the literature, accompanied by descriptions of accompanying optic nerve involvement, but the events that initiate the immunologic peculiarities of these syndromes remain unidentified, and may differ from those attributed to ocular sensitization induced by solid tumors.

Onset of vision loss in paraneoplastic retinopathies can be sudden and rapid or delayed and slow, characteristics that appear dependant upon the type of malignancy involved. It is significant that the antibody reactions so clearly defined in small cell carcinoma-associated retinopathies do not appear in the other forms of paraneoplastic vision loss. Since each appears to present with distinct immunologic characteristics, it can be predicted that in time the antigens involved in MAR, BCAR, LAR and PON will be recognized, and provide clues to the events that initiate these pathologic immune-mediated reactions.

Paraneoplastic vasculitis

Little is known about cancer-associated vascular disorders that can include mild hardly noticeable lesions, to the production of life-threatening emboli. In many cases they resemble those that appear in connection with other types of disease unrelated to cancer. Specific immunologic characteristics are not yet recognized, so the blockages and inflammations may result from cancer-induced biochemical imbalance such as the influence of cancer procoagulant, or a direct immunologic influence upon vascular endothelium [127–129].

Cutaneous leukocytoclastic vasculitis, if recognized early, can prompt the search for occult neoplasia due to a strong association with cancer. However, attributing the cancer patient's vascular changes directly to a malignancy is sometimes questionable since an aging individual may be suffering from a collection of unrelated diseases, and present with different types of vasculitis emanating from superimposed health problems, such as polyarteritis nodosa [130], thromboembolism [131], and Henoch-Schonlein purpura [132].

Most recognized cancer-associated vasculopathies occur disseminated in both arteries and veins, and resistant to conventional therapy [131,133–135]. The 'cancer-connection' is formulated in some cases by the correlation of disappearing vasculitis with successful cancer treatment, and recurrence with reappearance of the growth. This implication of paraneoplasia illustrates a real cancer-induced pathologic effect which in many cases involves inflammation, but has yet to be shown to emanate from the type of cancer-induced immunologic confusion comparable to that proposed with other paraneoplasia.

Summary

Genetic susceptibility

In an increasing number of cases, aberrant immunologic reactions in paraneoplasia are traced to the patient's cancer expressing the same 'autoantigen' involved in the pathologic response [4–8,104]. Sensitization is proposed to result from such abnormal exposure, but this line of reasoning is not without flaws [3,12]. In the case of paraneoplastic encephalomyelitis (PEM) antibody production to the cerebral protein designated the Hu antigen is used to identify the syndrome, and expression of the Hu antigen can be demonstrated in the patient's malignancies [43,45]. However, an immunologic response to the Hu antigen can be found in cancer patients without symptoms of the Hu syndrome [42]. Why some succumb and others do not is not understood, but could involve the need for disruptions in the blood/brain barrier such as that demonstrated in animal models od cancer-induced neuropathies [42,45,104,136,137].

Small cell carcinomas are known to express numerous CNS components, but the so called 'immune-mediated paraneoplasias' appear with low incidence relative to the total number of cases reported annually. Sensitization cannot therefore be attributed simply to exposure to 'sequestered' proteins, other factors must be involved. If expression of neurologic proteins in the wrong place at the wrong time is the mechanism whereby some rare individuals lose tolerance to specific cellular components a predisposition to abnormal hypersensitivity may be responsible, analogous to that recognized in other autoimmune diseases [1,32].

Inadvertent translations

The production of antibodies to the same antigen in different individuals with the same type of paraneoplasia supports the proposal of an immunologic 'cancer-connection' as the common mode of sensitization, and suggests the antigenic stimulation may be traced to the same site on the same chromosome in each patient. If the chromosomal location of the 'autoantigen' is adjacent to a transformation site, expression could conceivably result from coincidental translation during tumorigenesis. Co-translation due to genomic proximity would ensure that specific transformation sites will dictate precisely which potential autoantigen the host will be exposed to. Moreover, the 'paraneoplastic autoantigen' would probably be the product of a single gene, and all those recognized to date are.

The scarcity of immune-mediated paraneoplasias could be due to the need for multiple transformation sites to be influenced before cancer formation occurs, and a gradient of decreasing relevance to carcinogenesis could prevail [138]. The transformation site associated with the gene encoding the autoantigen(s) could be of minor importance, not entirely essential to cancerous growth, and may not always be included. This gradient of decreasing importance to the transformation process could contribute to explaining the variance in expression of different neuronal proteins in paraneoplasia, with recognized cancer markers associated with transformation sites essential to carcinogenesis [139,140].

Future trends

If the theory of co-translation proves correct, the immune-mediated paraneoplasias will provide an opportunity to learn more about the chromosomal transformation sites involved in carcinogenesis. Once the chromosomal location of the autoantigens involved is established, an 'upstream and downstream' search of adjacent genes could identify the related transformation site, and possibly even the specific carcinogen required to influence its activity [34]. This pursuit is encouraged by the finding that the autoimmune response in the Lambert–Eaton Myasthenic Syndrome involves the expression of an antigen encoded at a chromosomal region close to one that undergoes rearrangements in the transformation to small cell carcinoma [141].

Paraneoplasias provide examples of autoimmune reactions for which the cause may be readily identified, a rare occurrence in nature. Most recognized autoimmune diseases have no known cause but some may emanate from a combination of genetic susceptibility and the appearance of 'transient neoplasia'. Short lived neoplasia can appear and succumb to the actions of immune surveillance. In ridding the host of the transformed cell immunologic confusion could occur, and a key cellular component recognized as alien. Once tolerance is broken the response might persist through continued exposure to the native tissue component involved in the ensuing autoimmune disease.

Studies on the immunology of paraneoplastic diseases continue to reveal much about the events that occur in the production of abnormal hypersensitivity involving single proteins. The similarities shared between paraneoplastic syndromes and other autoimmune diseases are sometimes quite striking. Inquiries into commonalities may bring a better understanding of the means whereby specific antigens become the target of misdirected immunologic reactions in immune-mediated diseases unrelated to cancer.

Acknowledgement

This study was supported by unrestricted funding from Research to Prevent Blindness (RPB) only and NEI core grant 1 P30 EY12576-01.

References

1. Dropcho, E.J., *Ann. Neurol.* 39: 659–667, 1996.
2. Gripp, S., Hilgers, K.,Wurm, R., and Schmitt, G., *Cancer* 83: 1495–1503, 1998.
3. Dropcho, E.J., *Ann. Neurol.* 37 (Suppl. 1): S102-S113, 1995.
4. Matsubara, S., Yamaji, Y., Sato, M., Fujita, J., and Takahara, J., *B. J. Cancer* 74: 1419–1422, 1996.
5. Yamaji, Y., Matsubara, S., Yamadori, I., Sato, M., Fujita, T., Fujita, J., and Taka, J., *Int. J. Cancer* 65: 671–676, 1996.
6. Matsubara, S., Yamaji, Y., Fujita, T., Kanayama, T., Yamadori, I., Sato, M., Fujita, J., Shiotani, T., and Takahara, J., *Lung Cancer* 14: 265–271, 1996.
7. Polans, A.S., Witkowski, D., Haley, T.L., *et al.*, *Proc. Nat. Acad. Sci. U.S.A.*, 92: 9176–9180, 1995.
8. Yamaji, Y., Matsubara, S., Yamadori, I., Sato, M., Fujita, T., Fujita, J. and Takahara, J., *Int. J. Cancer* 65: 671–676, 1996.
9. Thirkill, C.E., Tait, R.C., Tyler, N.K., Roth, A.M., and Keltner, J.L. *Arch. Ophthalmol.* 111: 974–978, 1993.
10. Thirkill, C.E., Tait, R.C., Tyler, N.K., Roth, A.M., and Keltner, J.L., in *Proceedings of the Third International Symposium on Uveitis*, J.P. Dernouchamps (ed.), pp. 133–135, Kugler Publications, Amsterdam/New York, 1993.
11. King, P.H., and Dropcho, E.J., *Ann. Neurol.* 39: 679–681, 1996.
12. Dropcho, E.J., *J. Neurol. Sci.* 153: 264–278, 1998.
13. Oh, J., Dropcho, E.J., and Claussen, G.C., *Muscle Nerve* 20: 1576–1582, 1997.
14. Ruffini, E., *et al.*, *J. Thorac. Cardiovasc. Surg.* 113: 55–63, 1997.
15. Yoshitake, T., *et al.*, *Kyobo Geka* 48: 447–451, 1995.
16. Paone, J.F., and Jeyasingham, K., *N. Engl. J. Med.* 302: 156, 1980.
17. Kearsley, J.H., Johnson, P., and Halmagyi, G.M., *Arch. Neurol.* 42: 1208–1210, 1985.
18. Chalk, C.H., Murray, N.M., Newsom-Davis, J., O'Neill, J.H., and Spiro, S.G., *Neurology* 40: 1552–1556, 1990.
19. Guy, J., and Aptsiauri, N., *Arch. Ophthalmol.*, 117: 471–477, 1999.
20. Thirkill, C.E., Keltner, J.L., Tyler, N.K., and Roth, A.M., *Arch. Ophthalmol.* 111: 931–937, 1993.
21. Cher, L.M., *et al.*, *Cancer* 75: 1678–1683, 1995.
22. Brain, W.R., Daniel, P.M., and Greenfield, J.G., *J. Neurol. Neurosurg. Psychiatry*, 14: 59–75, 1951.
23. Thirkill, C.E., *Lung Cancer* 14: 253–264, 1996.
24. Greco, F.A., Oldham, R.K., and Bunn, P.A., *Small Cell Lung Cancer*, Grune & Stratton, New York, 1981.

Charles E. Thirkill

25. Weiss, W., in *Comparative Respiratory Tract Carcinogenesis*, Reznik-Schuller, H. (ed.), pp. 1–17, CRC Press, Boca Raton, 1983.
26. Weiss, W., in *Small Cell Lung Cancer*, Greco, F.A., Oldham, R.K., and Bunn, P.A. (eds.), pp. 1–34, Grune & Stratton, New York, 1981.
27. Greco, F.A., Hainsworth, J., Sismani, A., Richardson, R.L., Hande, K.R., and Oldham, R.K., in *Small Cell Lung Cancer*, Greco, F.A., Oldham, R.K., and Bunn, P.A. (eds.), pp. 177–224, Grune & Stratton, New York, 1981.
28. Li, W.H., *Chin. J. Path.* 21: 262–265, 1992.
29. Thirkill, C.E., *Br. J. Biomed. Sci.* 53: 227–234, 1996.
30. Sodeyama, N., *et al.*, *J. Neurol.* 66: 97–99, 1999.
31. Sherer, Y., and Shoenfeld, Y., *Oncol. Rep.* 6: 665–668, 1999.
32. Moll, J.W., *et al.*, *J. Neurol.* 243: 51–56, 1996.
33. Lafeuillade, A., Quilichini, R., Chiozza, R., Pellegrino, P., and Thirkill, C.E., *Presse Med.* 22: 35, 1993.
34. Thirkill, C.E., *Neuro-Ophthalmology* 14: 297–323, 1994.
35. Brain, L., and Wilkinson, M., *Brain* 88: 465–478, 1965.
36. Budde-Steffen, C., Anderson, N.E., Rosenblum, M.K., and Posner, J.B., *Cancer Res.* 48: 430–434, 1988.
37. Greenlee, J.E., Dalmau, J., Lyonsm T., Clawson, S., Smith, R.H., and Pirch, H.R., *Ann. Neurol.* 45: 805–809, 1999.
38. Iwahashi, T., Inoue, A., Koh, C.S., Yanagisawa, N., *J. Neurol. Neurosurg. Psychiatry* 63: 516–519, 1997.
39. Honnorat, J., *et al.*, *J. Neuropathol. Exp. Neurol.* 57: 311–322, 1998.
40. Benyahia, B., Liblau, R., Merle-Beral, H., Tourani, J.M., Dalmau, J., and Delattre, J.Y., *Ann. Neurol.* 45: 162–167, 1999.
41. Voltz, R., Dalmau, J., Posner, J.B., and Rosenfeld, M.R., *Neurology* 5: 1146–1150, 1998.
42. Dalmau, J., Graus, F., Cheung, N.K., Rosenblum, M.K., Ho, A., Canete, A., Delattre, J.Y., Thompson, S.J., and Posner, J.B., *Cancer* 75: 99–109, 1995.
43. Graus, F., *et al.*, *J. Clin. Oncol.* 15: 2866–2872, 1997.
44. Buchanovich, R.J., Posner, J.B., and Darnell, R.B., *Neuron* 11: 657–672, 1993.
45. Sillivis Smitt, P., Manley, G., Dalmau, J., and Posner, J., *J. Neuroimmunol.* 7: 199–206, 1996.
46. Lennon, V.A., and Lambert, E.H., *Mayo Clin. Proc.* 64: 1498–1504, 1989.
47. Levin, K.H., *Neurol. Clin.* 15: 597–614, 1997.
48. Kim, Y.I., *Muscle Nerve* 9: 523–530, 1986.
49. Marx, A., Wilisch, A., Schultz, A., *et al.*, *Am. J. Pathol.* 148: 1839–1850, 1996.
50. Marx, A., Schultz, A., Wilisch, A., Nenninger, R., and Muller-Hermelink, H.K., *Verh. Detsch. Ges. Pathol.* 80: 116–126, 1996.
51. Wilish, A., Schultz, A., Greiner, A., Kirchner, T., Muller-Hermelink, H.K., and Marx, A., *Ver. Detsch. Ges. Pathol.* 80: 261–266, 1996.
52. Spuler, S., Sarropoulos, A., Marx, A., Hohlfeld, R., and Wekerle, H., *Am. J. Pathol.* 148: 1359–1365, 1996.
53. Marx, A., Schultz, A., Wilisch, A., Helmreich, M., Nenninger, R., and Muller-Hermelink, H.K., *Dev. Immunol.* 6: 129–140, 1998.
54. Nagvekar, N., Jacobson, L.W., Willcox, N., and Vincent, A., *Clin. Exp. Immunol.* 112: 17–20, 1998.
55. Charukamnoetkanok, P., Fukushima, A., Whitcup, S.M., Gery, I., and Egwuagu, C.E., *Curr. Eye Res.* 17: 788–792, 1998.

56. Egwaugu, C.E., Charukamnoetkanon, P., and Gery, I., *J. Immunol.* 159: 3109–3112, 1997.
57. Naschitz, J.E., Yeshurun, D., and Rosner, I., *Cancer* 75: 2954–2958, 1995.
58. Butler, M.H., *et al.*, *J. Cell Biol.* 137: 1355–1367, 1997.
59. Yamamoto, R., Li, X., Winter, S., Francke, U., and Killimann, M.W., *Hum. Mol. Gen.* 4: 265–268, 1995.
60. Antoine, J.C., *et al.*, *Arch. Neurol.* 56: 172–177, 1999.
61. Floyd, S., *et al.*, *Mol. Med.* 4: 29–39, 1998.
62. Saiz, A., *et al.*, *J. Neurol.* 66: 214–217, 1999.
63. McEvoy, K.M., *Mayo Clin. Proc.* 66: 300–304, 1991.
64. Gorin, F., Baldwin, B., Tait, R., Pathak, R., and Seyal, M., *Ann. Neurol.* 28: 711–714, 1990.
65. Roll, U., Christie, M.R., Standl, E., and Ziegler, A.G., *Diabetes* 43: 154–160, 1994.
66. Bjork, E., Velloso, L.A., Kampe, O., and Karlsson, A., *Diabetes* 43: 161–165, 1994.
67. Kim, J., *et al.*, *J. Exp. Med.* 180: 595–606, 1994.
68. Cohen, P.R., and Kurzrock, R., *Semin. Oncol.* 24: 334–359, 1997.
69. Kurzrock, R., and Cohen, P.R., *Am. J. Med.* 99: 207–216, 1995.
70. Anhalt, G.J., *Adv. Dermatol.* 12: 77–96, 1997.
71. Moll, R., and Moll, I., *Virchows Arch.* 432: 487–504, 1998.
72. Amagai, M., Nishikawa, T., Nousari, H.C., Anhalt, G.J., and Hashimoto, T., *J. Clin. Invest.* 102: 775–782, 1998.
73. Amagai, M., Hashimoto, T., Green, K.J., Shimizu, N., and Nishikawa, T., *J. Invest. Dermatol.* 104: 895–901, 1995.
74. Schoen, H., Foedinger, D., Derfler, K., Amann, G., Rappersberger, K., Stingl, G., and Volc-Platzer, B., *Arch. Dermatol.* 134: 706–710, 1998.
75. Sklavounou, A., and Laskaris, G., *Oral Oncol.* 35: 437–440, 1998.
76. Jiao, D., and Bystryn, J.C., *J. Eur. Acad. Dermatol. Venereol.* 11: 169–172, 1998.
77. Hashimoto, T., *et al.*, *J. Invest. Dermatol.* 104: 829–834, 1995.
78. Nishikawa, T., Hashimoto, T., Shimizu, H., Ebihara, T., and Amagai, M., *J. Derm. Sci.* 12: 1–9, 1996.
79. Liu, Z., Diaz, L.A., Troy, J.L., Taylor, A.F., Emery, D.J., Fairley, J.A., and Giudice, G.J., *J. Clin. Invest.* 92: 2480–2488, 1993.
80. Kornguth, S.E., Klein, R., Appen, R., and Choate, J., *Cancer* 50: 1289–1293, 1982.
81. Grunwald, G.B., Klein, R., Simmonds, M.A., and Kornguth, S.E., *Lancet* 1: 658–661, 1985.
82. Kornguth, S.E., Kalinke, T., Grunwald, G.B., Schutta, H., and Dahl, D., *Cancer Res.* 46: 2588–2595, 1986.
83. Grisold, W., Drlicek, M., Popp, W., and Jellinger, K., *Acta Neuropathol. (Berl.)* 75: 199–202, 1987.
84. Grunwald, G.B., Kornguth, S.E., Towfighi, J., *et al.*, *Cancer* 60: 780–786, 1987.
85. Kornguth, S.E., *N. Engl. J. Med.* 312: 1607–1608, 1989.
86. Kornguth, S.E., Spear, P.D., and Langer, E., *Brain Res.* 245: 35–45, 1982.
87. Williams, R.W., Crabtree, J.W., Chalupa, L.M., Spear, P.D., and Kornguth, S.E., *Brain Res.* 336: 57–66, 1985.
88. Spear, P.D., Miller, S., Veilhuber, K., and Kornguth, S.E., *Brain Res.* 368: 154–157, 1986.
89. Grunwald, G.B., Klein, R., Simmonds, M.A., and Kornguth, S.E., *Lancet* 1: 658–661, 1985.

Charles E. Thirkill

90. Kornguth, S.E., Kalinke, T., Grunwald, G.B., Schutta, H., and Dahl, D., *Cancer Res.* 46: 2588–2595, 1986.
91. Thirkill, C.E., Tait, R.C., Tyler, N.K., Roth, A.M., and Keltner, J.L., *Invest. Ophthalmol. Vis. Sci.* 33: 2768–2772, 1992.
92. Whitcup, S.M., Vistica, B.P., Milam, A.H., Nussenblatt, R.B., and Gery, I., *Am. J. Ophthalmol.* 126: 230–237, 1998.
93. Thirkill, C.E., Roth, A.M., and Keltner, J.L., *Arch. Ophthalmol.* 105: 372–375, 1987.
94. Jacobson, D.M., Thirkill, C.E., and Tipping, S.J., *Ann. Neurol.* 28: 162–167, 1990.
95. Thirkill, C.E., FitzGerald, P.J., Sergott, R.C., Roth, A.M., Tyler, N.K., and Keltner, J.L., *N. Engl. J. Med.* 321: 1589–1594, 1989.
96. Adamus, G., Guy, J., Schmeid, J.L., Arendt, A., and Hargrave, P.A., *Invest. Ophthalmol. Vis. Sci.* 34: 626–2633, 1993.
97. Thirkill, C.E., in *Autoantibodies*, Peter, J.B., and Shoenfeld, Y. (eds.), pp. 694–699, Elsevier, Amsterdam, 1997.
98. Adamus, G., Machnicki, M., and Seigel, G.M., *Invest. Ophthalmol. Vis. Sci.* 38: 283–291, 1997.
99. Igal Gery Chanaud, N., and Pand Anglade, E., *Invest. Ophthalmol. Vis. Sci.* 35: 3342–3345, 1994.
100. Adamus, G., Ortega, H., Witkowska, D., and Polans, A., *Exp. Eye Res.* 59: 447–456, 1994.
101. Adamus, G., Machnicki, M., Elerding, H., Sugden, B., Blocker, Y.S., and Fox, D.A., *J. Autoimmunity* 11: 523–533, 1998.
102. Alarcon-Segovia, D., Ruiz-Arguelles, A., and Llorente, L., *Immunol. Today*, 17: 163–164, 1996.
103. Alarcon-Segovia, D., Llorente, L., and Ruiz-Arguelles, A., in *Autoantibodies*, Peter, J.B., and Shoenfeld, Y. (eds.), Elesevier, Amsterdam, 1997.
104. Thirkill, C.E., *Ocul. Immunol. Inflamm.* 5: 55–65, 1997.
105. Murphy, M.A., Thirkill, C.E., and Hart, W.M., *J. Neuro-Ophthalmol.* 17: 77–83, 1997.
106. Keltner, J.L., Thirkill, C.E., Tyler, N.K., and Roth, A.M., *Arch. Ophthalmol.* 110: 48–53, 1992.
107. Luiz, J.E., Lee, A.G., Keltner, J.L., Thirkill, C.E., and Lai, E.C., *J. Neuro-Ophthalmol.* 18: 178–181, 1998.
108. Berson, E.L., and Lessell, S., *Am. J. Ophthalmol.* 106: 307–311, 1988.
109. Kirath, H., Thirkill, C.E., Bilgic, S.S., Eldem, B., and Kececi, A., *Eye* 11: 889–892, 1997.
110. Boeck, K., Hofmann, S., Klopfer, M., Ian, U., Schmidt, T., Engst, R., Thirkill, C.E., and Ring, J., *Br. J. Dermatol.* 134: 457–460, 1997.
111. Milam, A.H., Saari, J.C., Jacobson, S.G., Lubinski, W.P., Feun, L.G., and Alexander, K.R., *Invest. Ophthalmol. Vis. Sci.* 34: 91–100, 1993.
112. Milam, A.H., Dacey, D.M., and Dizhoor, A.M., *Vis. Neurosci.* 10: 1–12, 1993.
113. Okel, B.B., Thirkill, C.E., and Anderson, K., *Ocul. Immunol. Inflamm.* 3: 121–127, 1995.
114. Thirkill, C.E., Roth, A.M., Takemoto, D.J., Tyler, N.K., and Keltner, J.L., *Am. J. Ophthalmol.* 112: 132–137, 1991.
115. Bird, S.J., Brown, M.J., Shy, M.E., and Scherer, S.S., *Neurology* 46: 822–824, 1996.
116. Boghen, D., Sebag, M., and Michaud, J., *Arch. Neurol.* 45: 353–356, 1988.

117. Susac, J.O., Lawton-Smith, J., and O'Powell, J.O., *Am. J. Ophthalmol.* 76: 672–679, 1973.
118. Pillay, N., Gilbert, J.J., Ebers, G.C., and Brown, J.D., *Neurology* 34: 788–791, 1984.
119. Kraus, A.M., and O'Rourke, J., *Arch. Ophthalmol.* 70: 173–175, 1963.
120. Kattah, J.C., Suski, E.T., Killen, J.Y., Smith, F.P., and Limaye, S.R., *Am. J. Ophthalmol.* 89: 431–436, 1980.
121. Rubin, P., *et al.*, *Bone Marrow Transplant.* 18: 253–256, 1996.
122. Scaioli, V., *et al.*, *J. Neuro-Oncol.* 25: 221–225, 1995.
123. Anderson, N.E., *Aust. NZ J. Med.* 17: 539, 1987.
124. Waterston, J.A., and Gilligan, B.S., *Aust. N.Z. J. Med.* 16: 703–704, 1986.
125. Boghen, D.R., Sebag, M., and Michaud, J., *Arch. Neurol.* 45: 353–356, 1988.
126. Rudge, P., *Proc. R. Soc. Med.* 66: 1106–1107, 1973.
127. Ponge, T., Boutoille, D., Moreau, A., Germaud, P., Dabouis, G., Baranger, T., and Barrier, J., *Eur. Resp. J.* 12: 1228–1229, 1998.
128. Stashower, M.E., Rennie, T.A., Turiasky, G.W., and Gilliand, W.R., *J. Am. Acad. Dermatol.* 40: 287–289, 1999.
129. Sweeney, S., Utzschneider, R., and Fraire, A.E., *Ann. Diagnostic Pathol.* 2: 247–249, 1998.
130. Yamada, T., *et al.*, *J. Clin. Gastro.* 25: 535–537, 1997.
131. Naschitz, J.E., Yeshurun, D., Eldar, S., and Lev, L.M., *Cancer* 77: 1759–1767, 1996.
132. Maestri, A., Malacarne, P., and Santini, A., *Angiology* 46: 625–627, 1995.
133. Suzuki, T., Obara, Y., Sato, Y., Saito, G., Ichiwata, T., and Uchiyama, T., *Am. J. Ophthalmol.* 122: 125–127, 1996.
134. Oh, S.J., *Neurol. Clin.* 15: 849–863, 1997.
135. Fortin, P.R., *Curr. Opin. Rheumatol.* 8: 30–33, 1996.
136. Greenlee, J.E., Burns, J.B., Rose, J.W., Jaeckle, K.A., and Clawson, S., *Acta Neuropath.* 89: 341–345, 1995.
137. Sillevis Smitt, P.A., Manley, G.T., and Posner, J.B., *Neurology* 45: 1873–1878, 1995.
138. Schifeling, D.J., Horton, J., and Tafelski, T.J., *Dis. Month.* 43: 681–742, 1997.
139. Gazdar, A.F., and Carbone, D.P., *The Biology and Molecular Genetics of Lung Cancer*, pp. 16–26, R.G. Landes Company, CRC Press, Austin, 1994.
140. Adamus, G., Aptsiauri, N., Guy, J., *et al.*, *Clin. Immunol. Immunopath.* 78: 120–129, 1996.
141. Taviaux, S., Williams, M.E., Harpold, M.M., Nargeot, J., and Lory, P., Hum. Genet. 100: 151–154, 1997.

Charles E. Thirkill

Index

Interleukin-18 163, 167
Intra-arterial chemotherapy 141–143
Intraocular lymphoma 223–232
    AIDS related primary 230
    orbital involvement 225
Intraocular tumor 16, 73
Intratumoral cysts 8
Invadopodia 42, 43
Invasion 9, 35–46, 53–55, 59, 68, 103,
    142, 169, 177, 178, 180, 183, 188,
    197
Invasiveness 41, 42, 59, 183–185, 188,
    197
Iris cyst 2
Irradiation 24, 29

J8 45
Juvenile xanthogranuloma (JXG) 2,
    10–12

Kaposi's sarcoma 231
Keratinocyte growth factor 62
Keratinocytes 68, 180, 186–188, 191,
    243
Keratoakanthoma 7, 8
Ki67 171, 172, 177, 178, 212
Killer activatory receptors 101
Killer genes 132
Killer inhibitory receptor (KIR)
    114, 201, 202, 206, 207
Killer proteins 132
KIR see Killer inhibitory receptor
Kulchitsky cell 239

LAK see Lymphokine activated killer
LAR see Lymphoma-Associated
    Retinopathy
Lambert-Eaton Myasthenic syndrome
    (LEMS) 240
Laminin 36–39, 42, 44, 45, 55, 56,
    188
Laminin receptors 44
Langerhans cell-tumor cell-hybridoma-
    injections 180
Langerhans cells 102, 169, 170, 177, 187
Larynx carcinoma 103
LEMS see Lambert-Eaton Myasthenic
    syndrome
Leucocyte functional adhesion molecule
    (LFA)-1 39

Leukemia 230, 243
LFA-1 see Leucocyte functional
    adhesion molecule (LFA)-1
Light chain restriction 226, 232
Liver (Hepatic) metastases 74, 80,
    81, 104, 119, 120, 142, 143, 147,
    152
LMP2 94, 95
LMP7 94
Lomustine 144
Loss of allelic expression 108
Loss of cilia 8
Loss of heterozigocity 91
Loss of tolerance 237, 241, 242
Lymph node metastasis 44, 85, 87,
    164, 171
Lymph nodes 9, 16, 43, 124, 163, 164
Lymphatic drainage 16, 20, 74
Lymphocyte 17, 77, 79, 83, 84, 91, 94,
    102, 103, 118, 123, 148, 150, 152,
    169, 171, 174, 177, 186, 201–206,
    212, 213, 224, 226, 228, 229,
    231–233, 240
Lymphocyte activation 187
Lymphocyte homing 186
Lymphocyte priming 123
Lymphocytic leukemia 243
Lymphoepithelial lesions 212
Lymphokine 17, 201, 204–206, 208,
    207
Lymphokine activated killer (LAK)
    activity 201
Lymphoma 4, 10, 12, 79, 84, 164,
    201–205, 207, 208, 211, 212, 214,
    215, 217, 219, 223–233, 240, 247,
    243
    adnexal extranodal marginal zone
        B-cell 211
    AIDS-related lymphoma 230
    CNS 223
    histology 224
    immuno histochemistry 225
    intraocular 223–232
    cytokines 227
    molecular pathology 229
    orbital involvement 225
    pathogensis 232
    EBV associated 233
Lymphoma-Associated Retinopathy
    (LAR) 247

Viral oncogene 232
Viral retinitis 224
Virus-associated malignancies 84
Vitrectomy 224, 226, 227, 229
Vitreous 5, 18, 151, 223–229
Vitronectin 37, 38, 41, 43, 45, 56, 59
  spreading 38
Von Hippel-Lindau (VHL) gene product
  64

Von Hippel-Lindau (VHL) tumor
  suppressor genes 63
Vortex veins 44
VPF 151

Yo antigen 239, 240
Yo syndrome 240